THE NURSE
AS EXECUTIVE

SECOND EDITION

THE NURSE
AS EXECUTIVE

by
Barbara J. Stevens, R.N., Ph.D.

Director, Division of Health Services,
Sciences and Education
Chairman, Department of Nursing
Education
Teachers College, Columbia University
New York, New York

Nursing Resources, Inc.   Wakefield, Massachusetts

Library of Congress Catalog Card Number: 79-90379
International Standard Book Number: 0-913654-62-0

Typeset by A & B Typesetters, Inc., Concord, N.H.

Manufactured in the United States of America

For
my husband
Bill

Preface

The second edition of *The Nurse as Executive* differs from the first in several ways. First, it addresses management in the service setting only, reserving collegiate educational management for a separate book which will follow. The book's coverage is significantly expanded, with new topics such as political strategies, labor relations, and role theory. With these additions the book deals comprehensively with the domain of the nurse executive. This second edition also updates the book's treatment of nursing administration.

The new edition of *The Nurse as Executive* has been designed for a broad audience. The first edition was written for the practicing nurse executive who was inadequately prepared for her position. The second edition is designed to be used by professional students of nursing administration as well as by practicing nurse executives. In order to be useful to this larger audience, the second edition utilizes a central conceptual framework of nursing administration. It also presents advanced content of nursing administration. The book maintains, however, the practical, pragmatic approach which so many readers have appreciated.

This edition of *The Nurse as Executive* represents nursing management in a model with the following components: goals, structures, processes, resources, and controls. The *goals* are represented in the primary and instrumental ends of nursing care and management practice and in the philosophical and ideological values which determine those ends. The *structures* of nursing management are evident in those patterns by which the nurse executive organizes a nursing division and by which the division's goals are im-

plemented. These structures include the organization plan and the policies and the practices which direct the events of the division. Specifically they include the organization chart, divisional functions, staffing plans, assignment systems, structured communication systems, policies, procedures, and organized usage of time and space in the division. The *processes* of nursing management include such mechanisms as communications theory, strategies and politics, as well as use of role, problem solving, and decision theory. *Resources* include human and material resources. Restraints upon management (such as legal restrictions) are included in this consideration. *Controls* of nursing management include those regulatory processes which maintain and improve the nursing management of the division, in particular: quality control measures, performance appraisal, accreditation processes, education, supervision, and research.

In this model of nursing administration, management as a discipline is subordinated to achievement of the ends of nursing as the primary discipline. Hence nursing administration is a synthesis of knowledge of two disciplines: nursing and management.

Acknowledgement is given to the *Journal of Nursing Administration* for permission to reprint all or portions of several articles in chapters of this book: "Budget Generation and Control" is incorporated with other materials in Chapter 18; "Effecting Change" and "Management of Continuity and Change in Nursing" are incorporated in Chapter 13. Materials from "Use of Groups for Management" are included in Chapters 7 and 12. "The Problems in Nursing's Middle Management" is included in Chapter 15, and "The Head Nurse as Manager" appears in Chapter 16. Chapter 22 includes materials from "Systems of Measurement for Nursing Care," and Chapter 2 incorporates materials from an editorial, "Why Won't Nurses Write Nursing Care Plans?" Materials have been adapted from two additional *Journal of Nursing Administration* articles; "Performance Appraisal: What the Nurse Executive Expects from It" contributes to Chapter 23 and "Accountability of the Clinical Specialist: The Administrator's Viewpoint" is incorporated in Chapter 17. Acknowledgement also is given to Nursing Resources, Inc. for portions adapted from *First-line Patient Care Management*. Sections of the chapter, "What is a First-Line Manager?" from that book appear in Chapter 16 of this book.

Contents

x   Contents

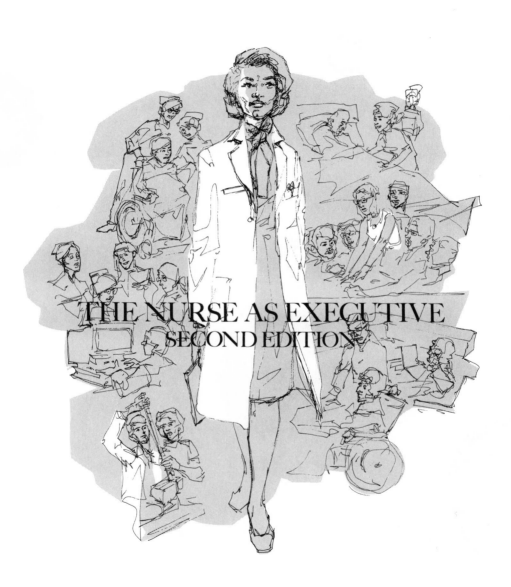

THE NURSE AS EXECUTIVE
SECOND EDITION

Introduction:

The Nursing Management Model

Components of the nursing management model used to organize this book are discussed sequentially, although they do not occur step-by-step in the real world. The components of this model represent not so much different elements as different perspectives on a single phenomenon; they include: goals, structures, processes, resources, and controls.

For those who prefer some imagery or analogy, the model may be compared to a chess game. As in chess, the *goal* is to win (checkmate). *Structures* are of two kinds. First, the design of the board itself constrains the moves, though one seldom is conscious of the board itself. Many structures constrain and design nursing management: the organization chart, the way in which certain kinds of patients are sent to certain units, the job descriptions used, and the staffing pattern. In chess the second kind of structure is the set of legitimate moves allowed for each playing piece. This is analogous to the rules for each employee according to the assignment system used, the particular tasks assigned in any given day, the policies and practices which control actions within the organization, and the schedules of the nursing division and each of its departments.

Processes are akin to the actual moves which a player makes, rather than the rules for movement. In our model, these processes involve communication, change, conflict, decision making, problem solving, political strategies, and other such techniques for dealing with varying and changing subject matter over time. *Resources* may be equated with the playing pieces of chess; in our model they become people, materials, equipment, supplies, and financial resources. To complete the analogy, the *controls* are those moves by the opponent which condition or dictate our response—the feedback which alters our next move.

GOALS

Management becomes uniquely *nursing* management when it is wedded to the ends, or goals, of nursing. It is the subordination of management as a discipline to the ends of another discipline, nursing, that establishes the new discipline, nursing management. Nursing management is not merely an application of management to the subject matter of nursing care. Rather, it is a synthesis different from the general disciplines of management and nursing from which it has emerged. Management goals and values are not lost in this synthesis, but they are radically altered in their subordination to the professional goals of nursing practice.

The chief end of most nursing service organizations is the delivery of nursing care to patients. Sometimes this primary goal is conceived of as a process of nursing acts (doing to or for the patient); sometimes it is equated with patient outcomes (end states of being or final learned performances). Many other conceptions are possible. The conceptualization of the care delivery goal varies depending on the nursing theories and philosophies accepted or enacted by the nursing division. For example, an institution implementing Orem's theory perceives nursing as a substitution for self-care[1]. Another institution using Levine's theory, in contrast, sees nursing as conservation of the patient's adaptive abilities[2]. Although nursing organizations share the goal of delivering nursing care to patients, closer examination reveals that this goal has different meanings in different organizations.

Where nursing goals are not elaborated in a specific nursing theory, they may be reflected to a lesser degree in the nursing division's statement of philosophy. Even where an elaborate theory of nursing is applied, the statement of philosophy adds to one's knowledge of a nursing division by indicating the division's other values and relationships. Nursing goals which are implicit in the nursing theory and/or divisional philosophy are typically further identified in statements of purpose and in identification of divisional objectives. In most cases such global, divisional statements are further elaborated in departmental or unit objectives. Some departments or units prefer to identify their own nursing theory or philosophy. For example, a rehabilitation unit might determine that a philosophy of nursing rehabilitation could be made without contradicting the divisional philosophy. Such a statement would help identify the specific framework of nursing within the special unit.

To date, most primary ends of nursing management deal with care of patients. It may be that as the discipline of nursing develops that may change. For example, there are now many institutions of medical care in which primary goals are those of research and medical education, with patient care being a secondary goal. Only time will tell whether nursing will follow a similar pattern or whether the nursing ethos will keep patient care predominant at all times, in all settings. Certainly education and research cannot become predominant nursing goals

until nursing acquires control over its own domain of practice.

Further goals arise from nursing's synthesis with management. Management values and indices, such as those reflecting economy and efficiency, are subsumed under nursing management. These goals do not become ends in themselves but are instrumental in the achievement of nursing goals. Whereas a business manager might seek to achieve a goal strictly for the sake of bottom-line profit, the opposite perspective is the case here. In nursing, managerial efficiency and economy will be striven for so as better to achieve nursing goals, either in quality or in quantity of services delivered. Although they are only instrumental, such management goals will be important in a society recognizing the limitation of its resources, and the nursing executive will be challenged to find ways to reach her nursing goals with more and more efficiency.

The nursing executive also will be challenged to weigh nursing goals against other societal goals and values. Every societal resource applied to health care, for example, removes resources available for other expenditures such as education, leisure, or cultural expression. The nurse executive must recognize that health (or nursing care) is only one societal value. It cannot be advanced as an absolute; it must be weighed proportionately against other values of the society. Given the society's growing sense of proportion about values, it is even more critical that managerial values be applied in the achievement of primary nursing goals.

It is not possible to talk about goals without discussing obstacles to their achievement. Indeed, most nursing management is a balance between activities directed toward goal achievement and those directed toward removing obstacles (problem solving). Excessive focus upon either of these managerial tasks can cause difficulties. If the nurse manager singlemindedly pursues goals while ignoring pressing problems, she will ultimately have difficulty improving her division. Similarly, if all her time is spent "putting out brush fires," the division she directs will never advance beyond its initial state. A balance between future-directed goal achievement and present-oriented problem solving is the key to any successful management.

STRUCTURES

Structures of nursing management may be perceived in diverse ways. Some organize *space*—for example, the architecture of a nursing unit, the layout of a classroom, the geographical units assigned to a given supervisor. Other structures organize *time*—for example, the step-by-step, sequential procedure or the cyclical procedure of allotment of days off to employees. Other structures may be seen as a critical integration of temporal and spatial elements, as in a disaster plan. Using an alternate construct one may envision structural elements as controlling *entities*, as does an organization chart, or *events*, as does an operating room schedule.

For purposes of this discussion, structures will be differentiated into those which are relatively *stable,* changing infrequently, and those whose content is subject to frequent *alteration.* For example, a staffing plan would change infrequently, but the schedule which implements that staffing plan might change weekly or monthly. Similarly, an organization chart might change slowly while the assignments of the incumbents in those organizational positions might change more rapidly.

In nursing management, the wise executive becomes aware of *all* the structures of her division, those that are evident, usually due to the frequency of revision, and those that are less obvious. For example, the designation of units by type of patient case is a major structure often overlooked by a nurse executive. Yet it makes little sense to have medicine control the distribution of patients over nursing care units. The physician spends less than twenty minutes per patient per day (a healthy estimate), whereas the nursing staff must plan 24-hour-a-day activities for care of those patients. Clearly, distribution of patients should be determined on the basis of nursing needs rather than medical needs.

Some nursing management structures receive constant attention in the nursing literature. For example, one always reads of new modes of assigning nurses, scheduling nurses, and centralizing or decentralizing nursing management. Other equally important structures, such as the distribution of patients, are seldom addressed. The structural interaction between nursing and unit management is another often-ignored subject. Similarly, procedure and policy books are frequently revised, entailing much review and attention, but job descriptions are seldom reviewed for analysis of assigned tasks per job. Nor are the job categories often considered as a whole in looking at the distribution of all tasks over the definitive jobs of the nursing division. Job description revision typically is seen as mere rearrangement in better format of preordained tasks. Here again the nurse executive may overlook a major structure in her organization—the task bundling, or combining of tasks to constitute a job. That is, she may not realize that the various jobs in the division are constellations of tasks, and the selection of those tasks presents a managerial option.

The nurse executive must become aware of all controlling structures and their interrelations. Simply assuming a structure exists but not questioning or reviewing it may mean the loss of a potential management tool. The effective nurse executive learns to recognize and use not only her divisional structures but the structures of the total organization of which it is part. The skillful nurse executive knows about and uses her knowledge of the structures of other organizations as well as of her own institution. Anywhere that her organization or division must interact with another, the nurse executive considers the compatibility of structural elements.

PROCESSES

In this nursing management model, the term *processes* is applied to mechanisms that are examined in their own right without specific reference to the subject matter to which they are applied. Hence, one may talk about change theory, or its managerial equivalent, management-by-objectives. Or one may talk about conflict theory, applying it to such diverse content as interpersonal relationships or formalized conflict such as occurs over the bargaining table. Communications theory and political theory are additional processes which may be discussed in their own right or applied in diverse content domains.

Process also includes the modes of thought used by the executive. Differences between concepts of problem solving and decision making, for example, dictate different approaches to the manager's role.

Processes are those components that are applied to and within the structural components of the nursing administration model. Processes direct changes within the managerial system; they are the moving forces in use of the management model.

RESOURCES

In the nursing management model, resources are those entities that comprise the organization environment, be they material, financial, or conceptual. In looking at the component, resources, it is easy to see the interplay of system components. Budget is discussed as a *resource* in this book because it represents a concrete entity, dollars, the resource with which things and services are purchased by the nursing division. Clearly, this placement of budget under "resources" is arbitrary. Budget could be perceived equally well as a *process* (budgeting) or as a *structure* for enactment of the division's objectives. Budget is also a *control* mechanism, as can be seen in its quarterly or monthly reports comparing allotted and used monies.

Most placement of a specific subject matter under a particular component of the nursing management model is somewhat arbitrary since, as can be seen with the subject of budget, a single subject may properly be addressed from the perspectives inherent in several components of the model.

Therefore I have selected what appears to me to be the predominant characteristic for each element discussed in this book, placing the given element in the model accordingly. The reader will recognize, however, that equally good arguments might be offered for alternate placements for most elements.

Discussion of legal elements of administration will be placed under discussion of resources because laws and their administrative acts will be treated as givens. This is not to indicate that the nurse executive should not be involved in the political process, of course. Nevertheless, at any given time, the laws of the moment represent constraints and opportunities which are givens in the environment.

Many of the major resources in the nursing division are intellectual. The nurse executive is a manager of knowledge workers since most employees of the health care organization are hired for what they know, not for repetitive mechanical acts. Not only is intellect a major resource of the nursing division, but the major expense for the division is payment for manpower. In a labor-intensive, not machine-dominated, industry, one that depends upon knowledge workers, the nature of management cannot be neatly separated from the content of the work to be done. This is why nursing management must be a synthesis of nursing and management if it is to be effective.

CONTROLS

Controls are the last component of the nursing management model. The term *control* is used here to represent several elements which are usually separate. The first sort of control is simple feedback: finding out results or effects of actions. For some parts of the nursing system, simple knowledge is the primary mode of control. For example, complaints from patients concerning noisy staff in the halls may be adequate control for correcting the problem.

Other mechanisms for control include direct action: supervising and assigning, as well as education. These actions are devised on the basis of feedback information along with goal direction. Where the appropriate action is not evident, control may take the form of research.

Control may be directed toward individual staff members through performance appraisal and coaching; toward patient group through various types of quality control, such as chart audit, observation, and interview; toward individual patients through nursing care plan evaluation; or toward the nursing organization itself through accreditation procedures.

Control in any portion of the nursing division usually requires an approach in which diverse measures are used simultaneously. For example, in the operating suite, one would simultaneously use ecological controls for the environment, quality control measures of patient care, performance appraisal of staff, and periodic evaluations of scheduling and logistic systems.

Controls, then, relate to the informational feedback system, to the correction and readjustment system, and to the reward and punishment system of the nursing division. Controls mediate among components of the nursing management model, adjusting a given management system by changing its goals, structures, processes, or resources. Further, there is a need for a superordinate control system—one that evaluates the quality and nature of the control mechanisms used in the system.

ORGANIZATION OF THIS BOOK

The chapters of this book are loosely organized according to the components of the nursing management model: goals, structures, processes, resources, and controls. Because these components are seen, not in sequence, but as existing simultaneously in the nursing management situation and because many elements of the nursing management situation may be perceived as involving several of these components, all aspects of the subject matter of an element will be discussed at the first presentation rather than presented repeatedly under each component. Thus when staffing is discussed, it will be viewed as to its goals, its structures, the staffing process, resources, and staffing control—all in a single chapter.

The book does not differentiate clinically related nursing aspects from aspects that are strictly managerial since it is my thesis that the very fusion of nursing and management is what makes nursing administration a unique and valid discipline in its own right.

REFERENCES

1. Orem, D. E. *Nursing: Concepts of Practice*. New York: McGraw-Hill, 1970.
2. Levine, M. E. The four conservation principles of nursing. *Nursing Forum,* 6(1):45–59, 1967.

BIBLIOGRAPHY

Arndt, C., and Huckabay, L. *Nursing Adminstration— Theory for Practice with a Systems Approach*. St. Louis: C.V. Mosby, 1975.

Claus, K. E., and Bailey, J. T. *Power and Influence in Health Care: A New Approach to Leadership*. St. Louis: C.V. Mosby, 1977.

Dietrich, B. J., and Miller, D. L. Nursing leadership— a theoretic framework. *Nursing Outlook,* 14(8):52–55, Aug. 1966.

Drucker, P. F. *Management: Tasks, Responsibilities, Practices*. New York: Harper & Row, 1974.

Hall, R. F. *Organizations: Structure and Process* (2nd ed.). Englewood Cliffs, N.J.: Prentice-Hall, 1977.

Kraegel, J. M. *Patient Care Systems*. Philadelphia: J.B. Lippincott, 1974.

Melcher, A. J. *Structure and Process of Organizations: A Systems Approach*. Englewood Cliffs, N.J.: Prentice-Hall, 1976.

Perrow, C. *Complex Organizations*. Glenview, Ill.: Scott Foresman, 1972.

Part I

Goals Of Nursing Management

Part I of this book examines the aspects of nursing management which relate to goal formulation. Chapter 1 examines nursing theory as a source of nursing goals. Chapter 2 looks at a nursing model based on the medical model. This model is presented because it still is the one most widely used in nursing service agencies; its presentation should not be taken as a recommendation for its adoption. Chapter 3 considers the relation of a statement of philosophy to goals. As does a nursing theory, a philosophy determines what goals are selected and in what ways they are approached.

Chapter 4 looks at the specification of divisional goals in statements of purpose and divisional objectives. It also looks at the mechanics of constructing objectives and purpose statements. Managerial and educational objectives are compared so as to il-lustrate differences which may be critical to the nurse executive.

Chapter 5 looks at the interrelation of nursing goals and managerial goals, completing the review of the goal component of the nursing management model.

Goal determination is a critical nursing management task, with clinical nursing goals as the ultimate focus of the nursing division. The nurse executive who wishes to lead the vanguard for the advancement of clinical nursing practice must show vision in her goals, but vision tempered by a realistic assessment of the resources and capabilities of her organization. The nurse executive must set goals toward which others may strive, and those goals must be realistic. By her selection of goals, the nurse executive bridges from the present to the future, from the status quo to the yet-to-be achieved.

Chapter 1   Analyzing Nursing Theories

Since the job of the nurse executive is to make nursing operational by delivering care to patients, it is essential that she understand the theory of nursing she is trying to implement. There has never been much agreement within the profession as to just what nursing is. That lack of consensus is probably a sign of professional health, for it enables nursing to retain the flexibility necessary for survival and growth. It enables the profession to develop various nursing models simultaneously, each with its own advantages and limitations.

TERMINOLOGY

Terms such as construct, model or paradigm, theory, and structure comprise the common language of theory development. Constructs are the basic elements of a theory. They identify the mechanisms that underlie the behaviors or events being studied. For example, the following constructs are used to explain certain nursing events: asepsis, tender loving care, reflective questioning, and rehabilitation. Constructs are abstract ideas; one cannot see a construct. One does see the behaviors that are attributed to the construct. One does not "see" asepsis; one only sees a nurse handling materials in a way that is quite different from what would be expected without such a concept.

A model (or paradigm) is simply a concrete representation of an underlying mechanism. Like a construct, it refers to an unobservable, explanatory, abstract idea. Some authors use the terms *construct* and *model* interchangeably. Others use the term model for representations that can be shown through replicas, reserving the term construct for representations that can be explained only in verbal terms. Tender loving care, for example, is a construct that would be difficult to model. On the other hand, one could easily depict a concept of communication, for example, as in Figure 1-1. Thus models or paradigms are simply analogies that serve to clarify thought about an abstract matter.

A theory unites and relates pertinent constructs that may be used to explain some complex phenomenon (in this case, nursing practice). It can be used to explain past behaviors or events and to predict future behaviors or events. A theory extracts from the behavior or event those principles that are supposed to be the controlling features. A theory is a kind of shorthand denoting the critical features from which a particular phenomenon is perceived to arise.

Because it is selective, a theory is necessarily a partial view; it selects only the most salient features by which to explain an event. Theories should not be thought of as true or false but as useful or not useful in dealing with the subject matter. Two different theories of nursing, for example, can be used to explain the same nursing incident. The question is not which theory is right and which wrong, but which theory can best ex-

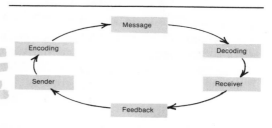

Figure 1-1. Communications Model

plain and make clear the events of the nursing incident. A theory is necessarily a simplified version of its subject matter, for it distills the features of the event that are seen as the ordering principles. If the theory is not simple, it will be of little help in understanding the nursing event; if it tries to explain every component of the event, it will be more like a television replay than like an explanation.

Constructs, models, and theories all are structures used to explain events or actions. They differ merely in form and complexity. In each case they lay bare an underlying structure that proposes to explain the subject matter.

COMPONENTS OF A NURSING THEORY

In order to look at differences in nursing theories, it is first necessary to establish some common subject matter. The following definition of nursing will serve to locate that common subject matter: Nursing is a derived activity applied to man in relation to health. As soon as one attempts to define nursing with more precision, conflicting interpretations appear. Nurses do not agree upon 1) how nursing activity is derived, 2) what nursing activity is, 3) how that activity applies to man, 4) what "man" is, 5) what "health" is, 6) how nursing activities relate to health, and 7) the relative importance to be given the component parts of the definition of nursing.

Let us examine briefly each of these variable components in an attempt to develop a basis for comparing various nursing theories. The first source of disagreement among nurse theorists is about how nursing activities are derived. The art-versus-science argument is perhaps the oldest theme concerning the derivation of nursing actions. Today nurse theorists increasingly opt for science as the primary source of nursing actions.

Even when nurse theorists claim to derive

nursing activities from science, however, there is no assurance that they mean the same thing by this assertion. Some theorists mean that nursing practice is derived and synthesized by a logical analysis of relevant facts (physiologic, pathological, psychosocial, and so forth). Others call their process scientific because they analyze patient outcomes rather than focusing on derivation of practice rules. Outcome-focused theorists are not particularly concerned about the original source of nursing action (tradition, logical derivation, trial and error, or pure accident), as long as the desired result is produced.

Other nursing theorists claim a scientific basis to their nursing on the grounds that they use a "scientific method." Various problem-solving nursing models can be identified in this category. Still other theorists claim that they are scientific because their model can be reduced to mathematical representations. Thus, how nursing activities are derived varies from one nursing theory to another, and nursing theories derived from quite different bases may call themselves scientific.

Not only does the derivation of nursing activity vary from theory to theory, but the perception of that activity itself varies. Some theories see nursing activity as primarily cognitive; others view nursing activity primarily in terms of its psychomotor output. In the latter category are those theories that tend to view nursing as a series of discrete tasks (bathing, feeding, changing dressings). This interpretation of nursing activity is presently promulgated by groups adapting systems analysis models to the practice of nursing. This discrete task concept also is utilized in computer-based or hand-calculated systems that attempt to quantify the nursing needs of groups of patients.

Where nursing is perceived primarily as a cognitive activity, theories may favor content components or process components. For example, one common process theory defines nursing as a definite sequential process of assessing, planning care, implementing care, evaluating and modifying care. A similar theory of nursing process is the one that follows the medical model, having components of nursing assessment, nursing diagnosis, nursing orders, and so forth. These theories view nursing from the basis of its thinking processes rather than from its action components. The acts such as bathing, feeding, and changing dressings have less significance in theories of this type; they merely represent end points in the total nursing process of determining care.

Many nursing theories stressing cognitive activity have content components rather than process components. Myra Levine's structure of nursing illustrates such use of cognitive components. Levine bases nursing on four conservation principles: conservation of energy and mass, conservation of structure, conservation of personal integrity, and conservation of social integrity. Instead of being given a process to follow, the nurse is given components to analyze.[1]

Other theories of nursing collapse the difference between derivation of nursing activities and the nursing activities per se. The theory that says nursing *is* problem solving is such an example. Here the derivation of the nursing (problem solving) is perceived to be the activity of nursing itself (problem solving).

How nursing activity applies to man also varies from one nursing theory to another. Some theories, such as that of Martha Rogers, see nursing as concerned with the "total man"[2]. In theories of this type, nursing care is perceived as concerning the gamut of human needs. Health needs are equated with human needs, and thus the total man becomes the field for nursing practice. Other theories tend to narrow this scope, perceiving of health as one human need among other needs.

Whether nursing theories relate nursing to the total man or to the partial man, most theories divide their components into manageable parts. Some theories divide *nursing* into components; others divide *man*

into component parts. For example, the nursing component may be divided into steps of a problem-solving process, or steps such as assessing, planning, implementing, evaluating, modifying. Some theories which divide man into components use the physiologic systems, following the medical school model. Other nursing theories compartmentalize man into a schema of potential needs that cover the scope of nursing care. Abdellah's 21 nursing problems is an example in which man is perceived as needs components[3]. Roy's four adaptive modes represent another such division of man into components[4].

The nursing theories discussed thus far perceive the nurse as an external force acting on man, the recipient. Many newer theories include interaction in which the nurse and patient act as partners in determining the content of nursing care. In such theories the patient and the nurse cooperate in determining some or all aspects of care. Goal setting is often a primary focus in the interaction between patient and nurse.

Two-way theories make the patient an active rather than a passive factor in the nursing model. These theories have difficulty in maintaining consistency, however, because many patients and their families may not be capable of fulfilling the conjoined role.

It is clear that there are many theoretical bases by which the nursing activity can be related to the recipient of that activity. This relating mechanism is an important part of any nursing theory.

Interpretations of man per se are seldom included in theories of nursing, but the particular compartmentalization of man, or the failure to compartmentalize man, gives some insight into the underlying philosophy of man in the theory. Some nursing theories are compatible with several different interpretations of man; others are not. Most philosophies of nursing profess the worth of man. Indeed, valuing man is essential to justify nursing actions. What is to be valued about man, however, varies from philosophy to philosophy. Many different philosophic descriptions of man exist; a few samples follow:

1. Man is made in the image of God, and this accounts for his value above all other creations. Indeed, the rest of the world was created for his use.
2. Man is just another animal; his "supremacy" is his anthropomorphic view of himself. He is differentiated by his advanced ability to use tools, but there is no reason why this trait is inherently "better" than the cat's ability to run faster or the fish's ability to withdraw oxygen from water.
3. Man is differentiated from other animals by his rationality; he is the only animal capable of abstract thought. Man is supreme by virtue of his mind.
4. Man is differentiated from other animals just because he asks the question, "What is man?" He is the only animal who questions his own existence and nature. Thus what makes him different is his ability for introspection, i.e., the reflexive nature of his thought.
5. Man, other creatures, and other objects do not exist in the usual sense of the world. What exists is what is perceived. therefore only mind has a real, separate existence; all other things such as animals, earth, and body of man exist only in so far as they are conceived to exist by the mind.
6. Man is simply a bundle of sense perceptions. He continually changes as his perceptions change. The sense of a single continuous "me" is an illusion; there is no durable, unchanging part of a man. Man is a flux of changing sense perceptions.
7. Man, like other animals, has a body and mind, but he is the only animal endowed with a soul. He is the animal who persists through time, i.e., his soul continues to exist when his earthly body and mind perish.
8. Man is a unity, a single substance. Perceived differences between body and mind are illusory. Mental and physical phenomena represent different expressions of the same substance. When this substance loses its vitality, there is no existence for man beyond his temporal being.
9. Man is an integral experience, a lived-body. He cannot be explained by reference to selected parts of his being, for parts cannot explain the whole. Nor can he be explained by psychic or physiologic states, because "states" indicate a staticness, a "standing still" that is not consistent with the continual change experienced by man. Man is a unified and ongoing lived experience.

For each of these philosophic definitions of man, it is possible to develop an argument justifying nursing activities; the same is true for most but not all other philosophies of man. As the perception of man differs, however, the object of nursing activities varies. Nursing philosophies, if not theoretical nursing models, need to take the philosophy of man into account in their explication.

Concepts of health also vary from one nursing theory to another. One consideration is the wellness-illness continuum of health. Traditional nursing theories focus on illness and health. Newer theories give equal weight to wellness. The National Commission for the Study of Nursing and Nursing Education, for example, proposes nursing specialties (distributive and episodic) based on a division between well care and ill care[5]. Health may be seen in perspectives other than the wellness-illness continuum. Health may be compartmentalized into divisions such as physical, psychological, and social. Some theories collapse differences between man and health by using a single-category system. Where this occurs, human needs and health needs have the same meaning.

Other nursing theories perceive health as homeostatic equilibrium. Theories also vary in whether health is perceived as a positive state or as a negative state (the absence of disease or deficiencies). Whatever the characterization of health, it is an essential part of any nursing theory.

How nursing relates to health is another integral part of any nursing theory. The comfort-care-cure arguments illustrate the relation between nursing and health. Some nursing theories subsume all these perspectives; others differentiate nursing and medicine by relegating cure to medicine and comfort-care to nursing. Orem's theory of nursing, for example, uses a perspective of this sort when it equates nursing with provision of missing aspects in self-care[6]. When health is perceived as homeostasis, nursing relates to health in the form of a vector force for correction of homeostatic imbalances. Johnson et al. espouse this theory of nursing[7]. Other theories relate nursing to health on the basis of desired health outcome; a common classification is that of preventive, sustenal, remedial, and restorative nursing care.

In analyzing a theory of nursing, it is important to determine what components of theory are most important for the author-theorist. As noted, some components may be collapsed together; others may be omitted entirely. Some theories have more adequate development than others, but no single theory is without its weaknesses when applied to the actual practice of nursing. Every theory is by nature incomplete, for it has selected certain aspects of experience (in this case, the nursing experience) to represent and explain a process that is more complex than the theory when viewed in its actual, phenomenal occurrence.

For this reason it is not essential or even desirable that the nurse executive give any single theory of nursing the status of a belief. The nurse executive who believes that her concept of nursing is right and all other concepts are wrong is limited in her approach to nursing problems. No single nursing theory represents an ideal way to view all nursing activities or problems.

The nurse executive should be eclectic and select from among numerous nursing theories the theory which is most effective in a particular situation. For example, the nursing theory that permits the best intensive care nursing may not be the theory that facilitates the best operation of a rehabilitation unit. The nursing theory that works best in exacting physiologic research may not be the theory that works best in a community health nursing practice.

REFERENCES

1. Levine, M.E. The four conservation principles of nursing. *Nursing Forum,* 6(1):45, 1967.
2. Rogers, M.E. *An Introduction to the Theoretical Basis of Nursing.* Philadelphia: F.A. Davis, 1970.
3. Abdellah, F.G. *Patient-Centered Approaches to Nursing.* New York: Macmillan, 1960.
4. Roy, S.C. The Roy Adaptation Model. In Riehl, J.P., and Roy, C. (Eds.) *Conceptual Models for Nursing Practice.* New York: Appleton-Century-Crofts, 1974, pp. 135–144.
5. National Commission for the Study of Nursing and Nursing Education. *An Abstract for Action.* New York: McGraw-Hill, 1970.
6. Orem, D.E. *Nursing: Concepts of Practice.* New York: McGraw-Hill, 1971.
7. Johnson, M., Davis, M.L., and Bilitch, M. *Problem-Solving in Nursing Practice.* Dubuque, Iowa: W.C. Brown, 1970.

BIBLIOGRAPHY

Andreoli, K.G., and Thompson, C.E. The nature of science in nursing. *Image,* 9(2):32–37, June 1977.

Cleland, V.S. The use of existing theories. *Nursing Research,* 16(2):118–121, Spring 1967.

Crawford, G. Evolving issues in theory development. *Nursing Outlook,* 27(5):346–351, May 1979.

Dickoff, J., and James, P. Theory of theories: a position paper. *Nursing Research,* 17(3):197–203, May–June 1968.

Dickoff, J., James, P., and Wiedenbach, E. Theory in a practice discipline. Part I: practice oriented theory. *Nursing Research,* 17(5):415–435, Sept.–Oct. 1968.

Donaldson, S.K., and Crowley, D.M. The discipline of nursing. *Nursing Outlook,* 26(2):113–120, Feb. 1978.

Ellis, R. Characteristics of significant theories. *Nursing Research,* 17(3):217–222, May–June 1968.

Ellis, R. The practitioner as theorist. *Am. J. Nursing,* 69(7):1434–1438, July 1969.

Hardy, M.E. Theories: components, development, evaluation. *Nursing Research,* 23(2):100–107, March–April 1974.

Hardy, M.E. (Ed.) *Theoretical Foundations for Nursing.* New York: MSS Information Corp., 1973.

Jacox, A. Theory construction in nursing: an overview. *Nursing Research,* 23(1):4–13, Jan.–Feb. 1974.

Johnson, D. Development of theory: a requisite for nursing as a primary health profession. *Nursing Research,* 23(5):372–377, Sept.–Oct. 1974.

McCarthy, R.T. A practice theory of nursing care. *Nursing Research,* 21(5):406–410, Sept.–Oct. 1972.

McKay, R. Theories, models, and systems for nursing. *Nursing Research,* 18(5):393–400, Sept.–Oct. 1969.

Newman, M.A. Nursing's theoretical evolution. *Nursing Outlook,* 20(7):449–453, July 1972.

Phillips, J.R. Nursing systems and nursing models. *Image,* 9(1):4–7, Feb. 1977.

Quint, J.C. The case for theories generated from empirical data. *Nursing Research,* 16(2):109–114, Spring 1967.

Smoyak, S.A. Toward understanding nursing situations: a transactional paradigm. *Nursing Research,* 18(5):405–411, Sept.–Oct. 1969.

Silva, M.C. Philosophy, science, theory: interrelationships and implications for nursing research. *Image,* 9(3):59–63, Oct. 1977.

Wiedenbach, E. The helping art of nursing. *Am. J. Nursing,* 63(11):54–57, Nov. 1963.

Chapter 2   A Model for Nursing Practice

MODEL COMPONENTS

Of the many nursing models, those most commonly used are the models that adopt the basic medical model; that is, they contain some form of the following steps: assessment, diagnosis, prognosis, prescription, therapy, and evaluation. Although nursing has adopted the basic categories of the medical model, it has developed its own terminology (Table 2-1).

The medical model would appear to be well suited to the needs of nursing if one were to judge by its extensive adoption. However, much of the advanced nursing literature stresses the need for nurses to follow one or more parts of the medical model more stringently, thus indicating some problems in its adaptation.

Problems in nursing's use of the medical model can be detected by looking at its implementing tools. Such tools tend to develop as aids to processes already underway. The first deficiency in adaptation of the medical model appears to be in the area of nursing diagnosis. If one looks carefully at the two categories, assessment and diagnosis, it becomes clear that nursing uses these in a way different from their use in medicine. The physician assesses the patient through examination and history taking. Using the information attained in assessment, he then makes a diagnosis. That diagnosis—diabetes, strangulated hernia, or myocardial infarction—is a different entity than those signs and symptoms that were observed in the assessment.

Nursing uses the terms assessment and diagnosis in an altered context. Seldom does the nurse combine all the discrete symptoms into some further entity called diagnosis. If,

for example, in her assessment of a patient, the nurse judges that the patient has a defect in visual perception and paresis of the left leg, she uses these assessments as diagnoses in her goal setting and care planning. Thus nursing seems to collapse the two categories of assessment and diagnosis. The nurse treats a patient assessment as if it were itself a nursing diagnosis. There are two possible explanations for this collapse of categories. One explanation is that nursing has failed to adequately define its own concept of nursing diagnosis, and that the deficiency should be handled by improving nursing theory and practice. To date, the work of groups trying to create nursing taxonomies has been inconsistent and generally unsatisfactory. Many different entities have been lumped together under the rubric of the nursing diagnosis.

A second possible explanation is that the medical model does not fit the nursing process. In this case, the solution is to identify the differences between the medical process and the nursing process and to evolve a unique model for practice which really reflects the nursing process.

Another problem in nursing's use of the medical model is the association between prognosis and prescription. The thinking in the medical model dictates the following sequence of events: 1) Prognosis establishes the realistic outcome to expect for this patient with this impairment. 2) To achieve that realistic outcome, or better, is the goal of therapy. The prognosis, in its form as the optimal realistic outcome of health, becomes the goal of therapy. 3) Prescriptions are then determined to reach that optimal goal. Such prescriptions may be partial measures at any particular stage in time (such as passive exercise now, with active exercise later), but they

Table 2-1.   Common Nursing Terminology and Related Nursing Tools

Category	Nursing Terms	Implementing Tools

Assessment	Patient assessment
	Identification of
	  patient needs/
	  problems
		Nursing interview
		Nursing history
		Physical examination

Diagnosis	Nursing diagnosis	Diagnostic tax- onomies
Prognosis	Goal setting	Nursing care plan
Prescription	Nursing order Nursing care plans	Nursing order sheet Nursing care plans

Therapy	Nursing
	  intervention
		Routine nursing
		  notes
		Nursing progress
		  notes

Evaluation	Quality assurance	Nursing quality control forms Nursing chart audit

all aim toward ultimate production of the goal.

In nursing, deficiencies in the prognosis and goal setting are common. Outcome goals are seldom defined, or else they are given in such broad terms as to be meaningless as a guide to prescription. The term *outcome goal* as used here means "the final nursing goal for the patient"; it represents the optimal realistic prognosis. Once again there are two possible explanations of the general failure of nurses to make adequate nursing prognoses as reflected in outcome goals. One explanation is that there is a deficiency in prognosis in nursing, and that nursing theory and practice should be improved in this area. The other possible explanation is that the outcome goal is not really essential to nursing prescription and practice. In this case, the problem is that the medical model does not fit the nursing process.

In considering which of these explanations is most adequate, it is valuable to look at the relation of outcome goals to immediate goals. Theoretically, immediate goals should

be interim steps toward the outcome goals. Indeed, they should be derivations from those long-term objectives. One should be able to justify any immediate goal as of value toward attainment of the outcome goal.

In practice, however, one often finds that nurses identify immediate goals but fail to relate them to outcome goals. This would seem to indicate that outcome goals are not necessarily seen as essential by nurses. It may be that open-ended prognosis is not a serious impairment for many nursing instances. For example, a nurse can base her immediate care of a patient with a recent cardiovascular accident on an assumption, true or false, of ultimate complete rehabilitation.

Other instances can be conceived, however, in which outcome goals would radically alter all immediate goals. A temporary versus a permanent sensory deprivation would be such an example for any patient in a post-critical phase of recovery.

Assuming that the medical model for the nursing process is one valid form for nursing practice, Table 2-2 is offered as a guide for the steps of that model.

PATIENT ASSESSMENT

Patient assessment usually combines in one form or another three techniques for assessment of present and prior health status: physical examination techniques, observation, and interview. Such techniques, singly or combined, appear in tools termed *nursing interviews, nursing histories,* and *nursing assessments.* The structure of these assessment tools represents ways of categorizing the important aspects of man or of nursing. Tools are used in assessment in order to make that process both systematic and complete. Schemes for categorization are manifold; the following are a few examples.

Group I

Scheme A

State of consciousness
Emotional status
Intellectual capacity
Sensory status
Motor abilities

Scheme B

Social status
Mental status
Emotional status
Sensory perception
Motor ability
Metabolic status
Respiratory function
Circulatory status
Nutritional status
Elimination status
Rest and comfort
Skin and appendages

Scheme C

Pain and discomfort
Body positioning
Mobility
Fluid and electrolyte balance
Oxygen supply
Learning needs

Psychosocial adjustment
Skin integrity

Scheme D

Structural integrity
Mass and energy conservation
Social integrity
Personal integrity

Scheme E

Physiological status
Psychological status
Sociological status

Group II

Scheme A

Disease-related needs
Therapy-related needs
Personal needs

Scheme B

Supportive needs
Therapeutic needs
Rehabilitative needs

Scheme C

Immediate, acute needs
Chronic maintenance needs
Rehabilitative needs
Well-health maintenance needs

Scheme D

Sustenal needs
Remedial needs
Restorative needs
Preventive needs

Scheme E

Preserving body defenses
Preventing complications
Providing comfort
Implementing prescribed therapies
Planning return to the community
Detecting changes in the body's
    regulatory system

The first group of schemes is based on categorizations of man, whereas the second group uses categories of nursing as its basis.

Table 2-2.   Components of the Nursing Process Based on the Medical Model

Steps in the Nursing Process	Objective	Criteria
Patient assessment	Develop a knowledge base on which to make nursing decisions	Normal health patterns and normal rehab-adapted patterns
Nursing diagnosis	Place a judgment upon assessment data	Implicit or explicit taxonomy of diagnoses (may or may not differ from medical diagnoses)
Goal setting	Use nursing diagnosis and patient assessment to set realistic health goals	Normal health outcomes for illnesses, patient's motivation, opportunity, capacities
Therapy planning	Identify care measures most likely to meet long-term and immediate goals of nursing and medical regimens	Documented relations between care activities and patient outcomes, logical prediction of care effects on outcome
Care implementation	Provide care measures needed to meet goals	Implicit or explicit standards of care
Care plan evaluation	Determine if plan is meeting goals	Implicit or explicit patient outcomes

Prerequisite Knowledge	Activities	Tools
Ability to identify needs and problems, knowledge of norms and ability to identify deviations	Assessment of physiological, psychological, social, and personal factors	Nursing interview Nursing history Physical exam and observation
What signs and symptoms constitute what nursing diagnoses	Place judgments upon assessment data	Nursing taxonomies of diagnoses
Knowledge of outcome norms, ability to modify outcome norms based on individual factors	Setting long-term and immediate goals	Nursing summaries Nursing care plan
Nursing theory relating nursing measures to desired outcomes	Identify nursing measures to be taken	Nursing orders Nursing care plan Nursing research studies
Ability to use nursing skills, manipulomotor and psychosocial	Provide needed care activities	Nursing progress notes Routine nurses charting
Patient assessment skills	Assess client progress and its relation to care given	Nursing quality control systems Nursing chart audit Case studies

Some agencies begin assessment with a categorization of man and then convert this information into a categorization based on nursing practice in an attempt to differentiate between them. Usual practice, however, is to use only one form or the other in a single assessment process. One's selection of a man-based or nursing-based criterion should be consistent with the philosophy and definition of nursing of one's particular institution.

It is important that the organization consider the suitability of the selected topics in each category. Errors of topic selection could include deficiencies or excesses in number of topics covered, selection of topics that are unwieldy for practical use, or selection of topics not consistent with the organizational philosophy and definition of nursing.

Several common sense rules can be applied to the evaluation of or construction of assessment tools:

1. The assessment tool should not duplicate investigations already available from other sources. There is no reason nurses cannot use information gained by others for nursing purposes. To submit the patient to unnecessary duplication in examination or interview is wasteful of nursing time and stressful to the patient.
2. Assessment processes should seek only information that will be used in the nursing planning. One often finds such inanities as a careful listing of each patient's food preferences in an organization that allows no variation in menus. There should not be interviewing for "interview's sake." No matter how weighty the subject may be in relation to the patient's life, unless it will actually enter nursing care planning, obtaining such information is an invasion of privacy.
3. The form should allow for discretion in collection of data. Compulsive form-filling is not an appropriate use of nursing time. One of the most valuable parts of an assessment may be the

nurses's decision that certain sections of the assessment tool are not pertinent for this patient and can be omitted without impairing the nursing care planning.
4. The assessment tool should be realistic in terms of the nursing actually practiced or practicable in the institution. Few institutions, for example, allot enough nursing hours per patient for ideal nursing care. The assessment tool should reflect the scope of nursing practice that is the realistic goal of the nursing division.

Patient assessment, then, is usually the first stage of the nursing process. Raw data are collected, but these data are selected through a preconceived screen of assessment tools based on the definition of nursing. In order to reduce assessment data to workable size, the method of exception is normally used. This means that only health patterns seen as abnormal or deficient are considered. To identify health abnormalities requires that two criteria be built into the assessment process: knowledge of usual health patterns and knowledge of usual rehabilitation-adapted patterns. The second criterion is just as important as the first. For example, the nurse must determine if the patient, who has been admitted for another health problem, has already adapted to his existing diabetes, blindness, amputation, or other impairment. She must take the patient's state of adaptation to standing deficiencies into account in her assessment.

NURSING DIAGNOSIS

In an attempt to apply the medical model in its entirety, nurses are now attempting to develop their own taxonomies of diagnosis. A nursing diagnosis usually is differentiated from a medical diagnosis as being a label for a condition identified by a nurse and amenable to treatment by nursing care. What is a diagnosis for one discipline, may be a symptom for another. For example, the medical diagnosis, cervical arthritis, might be derived, partly, from an extant "limitation in mobility" (a nursing diagnosis and a medical symptom). Although there is agreement that a nursing diagnosis is arrived at through assessment data, there is little agreement upon just what a nursing diagnosis is. The following entities have been called nursing diagnoses by various authors:

1. States of being experienced by the patient, e.g., anxiety, confusion
2. Physiologic deviations from the norm, e.g., irregular bowel function, impaired hearing
3. Patient behavioral deviations from the norm, e.g., obsessive compulsions, continual seeking for attention from nursing staff
4. Combinations of above classes with their underlying causes, e.g., pacing due to anxiety concerning upcoming surgery

Hence while many groups and individuals have produced lists and tomes of diagnoses, there is still no basic agreement upon the nature of a diagnosis and how it is derived from the assessment data.

Unlike its medical predecessor, the nursing diagnosis seldom is seen as a single entity. For example, numerous symptoms may lead the physician to a single diagnosis: myocardial infarction. Typically, this is not the case in nursing diagnosis. Hence the same patient might (depending upon the classification scheme selected) have several nursing diagnoses, e.g., pain, fear for life and future, resentment of dependent role. As with the medical diagnosis, these entities serve as conclusions based on assessments, and they lead to the next stage of goal setting. In other aspects they usually are dissimilar. It should be noted, however, that some authors deny the existence of nursing diagnoses separate from medical diagnoses. For these nurses, there is a single class of diagnoses, used by both professions.

GOAL SETTING

Goal setting in nursing can be loosely equated with prognosis from the medical model. Both are similar in that they represent anticipated patient outcomes. The nature of these outcomes is quite different, however. Medical prognosis is a practiced guess at the statistically likely health outcome for the patient. Where the term *nursing prognosis* is used, it usually has a similar meaning (statistically likely health outcome).

Goal setting differs from the statistical approach to outcome. Long-term nursing goals define the *desired* patient outcome, given the realities of the patient's impairment. While prognosis aims at the statistical average, long-term goals aim at the highest level of health outcome that can be realistically anticipated, given optimal health return. This realistic goal setting requires both knowledge of the usual health outcome for a given illness and ability to estimate the patient's motivation, opportunities, and capacities. Thus, statistical and uniquely individual factors are combined in setting long-term nursing goals.

In the medical model the prognosis is not further compartmentalized. The prognosis may change as the patient's condition alters, but the medical prognosis is always a unitary concept. Goal setting in nursing has a different nature. In the first place, goal setting (or nursing prognosis, where it is used separately) is seldom a unified entity. It would be more accurate to talk about goals setting or nursing prognoses. Since nursing diagnosis typically produces a series of discrete factors rather than a unified entity, it is not surprising that multiple factors appear in the goal setting and in nursing prognosis, too.

Not only does goal setting involve multiplicity in content, but each goal is further broken down into goal stages. A good care plan will indicate immediate goals and will show how each immediate goal is related to one or more long-term goals. For example, the following are immediate goals that might appear at one time or another on the way to the long-term goal of return to normal ambulation: 1) increase strength of arm and shoulder muscles for use of crutches, 2) ambulate safely on crutches without weight bearing on injured side, 3) ambulate safely on crutches with graded weight bearing.

In evaluating the adequacy of goal-setting activities, one should be aware of several sources for error in both long-term and immediate goal decisions: an inappropriate goal, omission of a needed goal, and setting an appropriate goal but for the wrong time.

THERAPY PLANNING

Conceptual Planning Problems

Goal setting is translated into action by conversion of immediate goals into nursing orders for therapies most effective in reaching those goals. Nursing orders are the ongoing plans for nursing care, and a nursing care plan represents the conformation of such orders on any one particular day. To make a judgment about nursing care on the basis of one day's nursing care plan is as limited a perspective as trying to judge the adequacy of a course of medical treatment by viewing the medical orders in effect on any one day of illness. Such a process totally ignores the need for longitudinal data that record permanently the nursing orders and the progression of changes in those orders. Nursing orders need to be kept as a permanent record in order to compare them with permanent records of patient progress. Only in this way will nursing be able to research and evaluate its own process and its effect on health outcome.

Therapy planning is more complex than its medical counterpart, prescription, because it must combine and coordinate nursing orders and physician orders. This summation usually takes the form of the nursing care plan. The effective care plan should be organized to show the relation between each immediate goal and its associated nursing and/or physician orders. It is important that the relation between goals and ordered-care activities be

documented, for this is another locus for needed nursing research. Many traditional nursing activities are assumed to be appropriate means for reaching certain goals on very little documented evidence.

Getting nurses to write care plans is still a problem in many institutions, even though most nursing administrators agree that written nursing care plans are necessary for quality care. Why is there such resistance to writing care plans? So many credible reasons can be given for use of the nursing care plan that the failure to write plans is sometimes puzzling. The following reasons for support of the care plan are the most common: 1) Nursing as a profession must be willing to identify its own content, above and beyond the carrying out of medical orders. 2) Consensus in nursing approach requires a written plan of care. 3) Continuity in nursing approach (over three shifts) requires a written plan of care. 4) Formulation of a written plan will help the nurse to clarify and solidify her nursing goals. 5) It is necessary to identify precisely components of nursing care in order to have a check against care omissions. 6) Nonprofessional personnel need to have clearly established and well-communicated nursing directives.

These and many additional reasons can be given for the use of written nursing care plans, yet the foot-dragging continues. Some administrators have resorted to compulsory care plan requirements. For example, a director may require that all care plans be written before the charge nurse leaves at the end of her shift. Such a plan, while useful as a training mechanism, does not guarantee the quality of those care plans; nor does it get at the underlying resistance to writing care plans.

Many explanations have been offered for this resistance. The staff nurse usually offers the excuse of time. "If I spent my time on writing care plans, I wouldn't have time to do the care!" Another, although weak, explanation is that the written care plan serves no purpose. "We do all the needed nursing whether or not we bother to write it."

Nurse administrators usually have a different set of explanations for the failure. Some claim that nurses lack the ability to identify the content of independent nursing functions. Others claim that nurses have difficulty in making nursing judgments. Still others state that the nurses lack the skills of patient assessment necessary to obtain the input on which the care plan is developed.

All these factors may be relevant in selected instances; however, they overlook some important issues in the care plan failure, conceptual as well as operational issues. One conceptual problem has its base in the nursing educational system. The nurse is frequently educated to think that there is a "right" answer for every nursing problem. During the years of her education, she is exposed to instructors who judge her class and clinical assertions as either right or wrong, good or bad. This same nurse is taught that she is a scientist and must plan her clinical care on scientific principles. Thus the nurse comes to expect that if she makes the "correct" decision, she can expect the "correct" outcome.

After graduation she soon discovers that clinical practice is not so simple. She plans a good teaching program for Mrs. A, but Mrs. A still fails to learn. She has a great plan for decreasing the anxiety level of Miss X, but Miss X remains as anxious as ever. Since her previous education has convinced the nurse that the correct decision produces the correct outcome, she soon comes to question her own planning ability. When she loses faith in her own planning ability, the last thing she wants to do is to commit her plans to paper, where everyone can see her ostensible shortcomings.

Thus the uncertainty of patient outcomes is one primary reason the nurse dislikes to commit her plans to any recorded system. The nurse tends to judge herself on patient outcomes rather than on the inherent worth of the proposed plan of care itself. This is not to assert that successful patient outcomes are not important, for indeed they are the aim of nursing. Indeed, when patterns in patient outcomes can be identified, the patterns help to delineate nursing care approaches that have high success or low success levels. (This interpretation concerns "probabilities" rather than rights and wrongs. It deals with empirical evidence rather than judging the inherent value and logic in a proposed nursing action.)

Too often the nurse is taught to ignore the distinctive character of practical activity, which is *uncertainty*. Individual situations are unique and never duplicated. No complete assurance of outcome is possible. No matter how prudent, the nursing plan is not the sole determinant of the patient outcome. Overt action cannot avoid risk, and nursing involves more overt action than most other health careers purely because the nurse interacts with the patient for longer time periods and concerning a broader scope of needs. Certainly it is the aim of nursing planning to decrease the number of variables that will negatively affect patient outcomes, but it is not possible to establish complete control over these variables.

Nursing, for example, involves more numerous acts of uncertain consequence than medicine. If the culture and sensitivity shows that an organism is sensitive to penicillin, the physician has little reason to doubt the outcome of this drug selection. If the nurse plans a strategy to encourage a disturbed new mother to accept her newborn, she has far less security in her selected strategy.

The more one has to deal with the behavioral and social sciences, the less predictable are the outcomes. A behavioral response can never be predicted in the same manner as can the result of a chemistry experiment. Even the nursing functions that rest on more secure bases, such as the physical and biological sciences, may go wrong in the area of practical activity. The nurse may know where the sciatic nerve "ought" to be, but that does not assure that it will be there for this particular patient. The nurse may put on a dressing with perfect sterile technique, but that does not assure that the patient will not "readjust" the dressing and contaminate it after the nurse leaves.

The solution to this problem obviously requires an altered concept of nursing intervention. The nurse must learn that patient outcomes are ultimately uncertain. She must accept that nursing input, even though it is extremely influential, is in fact only one variable in any individual patient outcome. She needs to accept that a good plan may fail, but that the failure is not the only criterion by which to evaluate the nursing judgments that made the plan. She needs to accept, without a sense of personal failure, the need to readjust a plan that is not working after a reasonable test period. Thus the first conceptual problem can be resolved by a general understanding that the rightness or wrongness of the nursing plan cannot be determined totally by the patient outcome.

A closely related conceptual problem is that represented by the view that there is only one *right* plan. Nurses need to realize that many different plans might be evolved to meet the same nursing needs, and that, indeed, one plan might be just as likely to lead to the desired patient outcome as another plan. The nurse must not be expected to find *the* plan to meet each patient need—many different methods can lead to the same patient outcome—she should be expected only to find *a* plan. She must not feel responsible for finding the one plan that suits her superiors; she is responsible only for determining a plan that seems to have a high probability of success. Obviously it is not only the staff nurse who must understand the multiplicity of potential methods. Until head nurses and supervisors recognize that different approaches to problems are possible, it is unlikely that any staff nurse will want to commit her ideas on care to paper.

One more conceptual factor causes nurses to be reluctant to make care plans. Care plans represent conclusions, but usually they fail to show the lines of reasoning behind those conclusions. In this case, care plans are just like physician's orders. When the physician orders that a leg be elevated, he does not include a long explanation of how he arrived at that decision. Care plans, too, are seldom constructed to show the reasoning behind

the nursing order. This practice also conflicts with the nurse's educational orientation. As a student, she had to detail her reasoning and give supportive principles for each nursing judgment.

Thus the nurse often wishes she had a written form by which to substantiate her written care plan. This desire is more than just habit, however; certain kinds of nursing orders (strategies) may actually work better and be better enforced if the care supplier understands the aim of the strategy. For example, the nurse may have a valid reason for requiring that a patient do a difficult dressing change himself, but if her strategy is not immediately obvious to the rest of the staff, they may hesitate to follow the plan.

Thus, in establishing a system for recording nursing orders, one needs to consider the nurse's need to explain her judgments and strategies. If such option is not available, the nurse may hesitate to write nursing orders that have complex derivations.

The Operational Problems

Operational problems also exist in instituting written care plans. If one analyzes the concept of the nursing care plan, it is apparent that the care plan is really a set of nursing orders. It will then be useful to contrast the treatment of nursing orders with the treatment of physician's orders. Many differences are immediately apparent. First, with the physician's orders, one physician has overriding responsibility and authority. Even when physicians work in teams, they have an established "pecking order." No intern sets out to countermand the attending physician's orders simply because he would like to see the case managed in a different way. Few nurses extend a similar professional courtesy to their colleagues.

Many head nurses work on a principle by which any nurse on duty can "contribute" to the nursing care plan by simply writing down her desired order or by deleting orders that do not seem suitable to her. This egalitarian plan leads to a simple management problem: if it is everyone's job to write care plans, it is really no one's job. Unless some particular person is held responsible for each care plan, there is no way to ensure that each care plan will be formulated. Thus the first operational problem is the need to center responsibility for each care plan in one individual.

Many head nurses have recognized the need to assign individual responsibility for nursing care plans. Too often, however, that principle is carried out by assigning the care plan as a daily function of the team leader or of the nurse caring for the patient. If either the bedside nurse or the team leader is responsible on a daily basis, as many as four or five nurses may be producing nursing orders for a single patient, on a single shift, in a single week. The crux of this problem is obvious: Many nursing plans involve a sustained effort over a period of time. Four or five different nursing approaches might all solve a particular patient need equally well. Daily alteration, however, from one approach to another, depending on the preference of the nurse on duty, is not at all as likely to solve the problem as a unified approach. How many times, for example, have two nurses frustrated each other over a decubitus because one nurse is trying to cure it by drying the decubitus with air and light, while the second nurse is trying to cure it on a different basis, by application of selected creams. This is perhaps an oversimplified example, but it makes the point that two approaches to a problem, both of which may be good in themselves, when combined, may be less effective than either one would be if used alone.

Suppose also that two nurses alternate care of Mr. C and that each nurse identifies the same nursing need, the need for increasing the patient's independence. Nurse A sets about meeting this need by a little calculated neglect, forcing Mr. C to feed himself by her absence. The next day, Miss B takes over, but she has a different plan. She intends to promote independence by first winning Mr. C's confidence. Her plan for establishing rapport is to meet his dependent needs for a

few days before beginning to move toward independence. Even though both nurses have the same goal in mind, Miss B's behavior will convince the patient that Miss A is cruel, and it will be more difficult for Miss A to help him in the future. Thus the care plan needs to be under the direction of one nurse over a sustained period of time if nursing strategies are to be consistent. A strategy that changes every day is no strategy at all. Certainly, lines of communication should be developed to permit recommendations from other staff members, and procedures should be established for instituting emergency changes as needed. The head nurse or other selected authority should be responsible for evaluating plans and guiding the assigned nurses in their care plan formulations.

Another practice, even more indiscriminate than that just discussed, is the practice of permitting any nursing staff member, including LPNs and nursing assistants, to write on the nursing care plan. While it is essential that such staff members have input system to the RN, where they have equal rights to add to or alter the care plan, it is difficult to substantiate the case for professional decision making.

While these conceptual and operational problems are not the only issues to arise in implementing a stable care plan system, they certainly are major factors to consider. The following principles may be helpful to the nurse leader in meeting these obstacles:

1. Evaluate each care plan on its inherent worth as well as on patient outcomes.
2. Be supportive of nursing care plans that are thoughtfully and logically developed by the responsible nurses, even if you would personally have selected other strategies. (Adherence to the approved care plan should be required of all staff; the care plan cannot be treated as an optional guide.)
3. Provide some means for the nurse to explain and communicate the reasoning behind her nursing care plans to other staff members.

4. Assign responsibility for a care plan to one particular nurse, over a sustained period of time.
5. Derive a system for staff input to the planning nurse.
6. Provide a system for review of care plans and of guidance to the planning nurses by a selected nurse expert.

If the staff nurse senses an attitude of acceptance for her planning, and if there is a clear system for the care planning tasks, then the nurse may be more receptive to the task of writing care plans.

CARE IMPLEMENTATION

Care implementation is the stage comparable to therapy in the medical model. Again, the nursing therapy has a complex structure because it involves implementing both nursing regimens and medical regimens. There are two tools for the care implementation stage. One consists in the routine nurses' charting, which is primarily a legal documentation system to validate the care given and includes recording of medications, treatments, diagnostic examinations, and noting baths and hygiene. These records primarily certify that selected care was given.

The record of primary importance in the care implementation phase is the nursing progress notes. Some institutions use one set of progress notes for both nurses and physicians; others use separate notes for each professional group. Either system is acceptable so long as it meets the objectives of the institution. It is important that nursing progress notes be just that, professional judgments of patient response to the related nursing and medical therapy. Nursing progress notes should be separated from the routine nurses' charting for two reasons. First, it should not be necessary to search through a vast amount of data to glean the few recordings that are pertinent to future nursing decisions. Second, until all nurses are capable of making professional judgments of patient progress, it is impor-

tant to separate this phase of nursing as a teaching mechanism.

CARE PLAN EVALUATION

Evaluation of the effectiveness of a care plan is an essential step in professional nursing. The two discrete parts to care plan evaluation concern the nursing process and patient outcome. The first part is the evaluation of those aspects under the control of nursing theory and practice. The second part is evaluation of changes that occur in the patient and are contiguous in time with the nursing process.

Evaluating the nursing process involves a step-by-step analysis of the decisions made for each phase in the nursing model. The model to be analyzed will be the model accepted by the particular institution. For the model used in this chapter, critical knowledge or criteria are identified in Table 2-2. Every criterion would need to be developed into a set of standards in order to create evaluation tools for each phase of the nursing process. In the case of this model, evaluation is needed of 1) the accuracy of the patient assessment, 2) the logic of the selected nursing diagnoses, 3) the fitness of the goals selected, 4) the adequacy of the therapy planning, and 5) the skill demonstrated in applying that therapy.

All these factors need to be evaluated, as they encompass the full span of health care. This evaluation requires two techniques: 1) cross-sectional sampling of multiple individuals who are in various phases of health care ranging from initial phases to rehabilitation phases and 2) longitudinal study of selected individual cases to evaluate complete courses of nursing therapy. Neither the cross-sectional nor the longitudinal approaches can be ignored in an adequate evaluation system.

Tools used in evaluating the nursing process are case studies, nursing chart audits, and nursing quality control systems. (Different types of quality control systems are discussed in Chapter 22.)

Analysis of patient outcomes is the second part of the care evaluation. Patient outcomes need to be evaluated at various stages of the recovery process. Some illnesses or conditions present clearly defined stages; others require arbitrary definition of stages for evaluation purposes. As was the case in evaluating nursing process, evaluation of patient outcomes requires the setting of standards. In this case, ideal outcomes will need to be established as criteria to which empirical patient outcomes can be compared. Once more, both cross-sectional and longitudinal studies should be carried out for adequate evaluation of patient outcomes. Outcome-based quality control systems and case studies can be useful in such research.

The relating of patient outcome to contiguous nursing process is the final step in care plan evaluation. This is the area in need of much nursing research and, clearly, it is the area that offers promise for establishment of new and validated nursing practices.

The medical model has been adapted by nursing with only slight variations. Generally the model appears to meet nursing's needs. Some of the problems of fit of the model have been pointed out in this chapter. It is interesting to compare nursing with social service in relation to the medical model. Both professions, because of their close association with medicine, began their practice by adopting this model. Social service, for example, began by doing a social assessment, establishing a social diagnosis, planning social therapy, and so forth. Over a period of time, nursing has taken the route of trying to expand its use of the model, whereas social service has adopted a series of other models upon which to build practice theory. The difference in response, with social service seeking other models, and nursing seeking to enforce better use of the medical model, has two possible interpretations. First, it may be that the medical model is a better "fit" for nursing than for social service, and this may account for the difference in response. A second possibility is that nursing should emulate social service in seeking models of its own that most adequately express the needs of its unique profession.

BIBLIOGRAPHY

Aspinall, M.J. Use of a decision tree to improve accuracy of diagnosis. *Nursing Research,* 28(3):182, May–June 1979.

Brodt, D.E. A synergistic theory of Nursing. *Am. J. Nursing,* 69(8):1674, 1969.

Dossey, B. Perfecting your skills for systematic patient assessments. *Nursing 79,* 9(2):42, Feb. 1979

Gebbie, K.M. Development of a Taxonomy of Nursing Diagnosis. In Walter, J.B., Pardee, G.P., and Molbo, D.M. (Eds.), *Dynamics of Problem Oriented Approaches: Patient Care and Documentation,* Philadelphia: J.B. Lippincott, 1975, p.65

Gebbie, K., and Lavin, M.A. Classifying nursing diagnoses. *Am. J. Nursing,* 74(2):250, 1974.

Kramer, M. Nursing care plans—power to the patient. *J.O.N.A.,* 2(5):29, 1972.

Lash, A.A. A reexamination of nursing diagnosis. *Nursing Forum,* 17(4):332, 1978.

Levine, M.E. *Introduction to Clinical Nursing.* Philadelphia: F.A. Davis, 1969.

McCain, R.F. Nursing by assessment–not intuition. *Am. J. Nursing,* 65(4):82, 1965.

Mauksch, I.G., and David, M.L. Prescription for survival, *Am. J. Nursing,* 72(12):2189, 1972.

Medical Programs Incorporated. Patient assessment: Taking a patient's history. *Am. J. Nursing,* 74(2):293, 1974.

Pardee, G., et al. Patient care evaluation is every nurse's job. *Am. J. Nursing,* 71(10):1958, 1971.

Roberts, R.W., and Nee, R.H. *Theories of Social Casework.* Chicago: University of Chicago Press, 1970.

Ryan, B.J. Nursing care plans: A systems approach to developing criteria for planning and evaluation. *J.O.N.A.,* 3(3):50, 1973.

Stevens, B.J. Why won't nurses write nursing care plans? *J.O.N.A.,* 2(6):6, 1972.

Woody, M., and Mallison, M. The problem-oriented system for patient-centered care. *Am. J. Nursing,* 73(7):1168, 1973.

Chapter 3   The Nursing Service Philosophy

The nursing service philosophy states the values and beliefs that influence the practice of nursing in a particular institution. The philosophy may be seen either as incorporating the theory of nursing or as a complementary document that relates the beliefs and values of the accepted theory of nursing to the larger domain in which nursing is practiced. In institutions that have not yet embraced a specific theory of nursing, the philosophy may be the only statement of values and beliefs. In such cases, the philosophy expresses some of the beliefs about nursing that would appear in a more formulated theory of nursing, were one to be accepted in the institution.

The discussion of philosophy to follow will assume that no specific theory of nursing has yet been chosen. Obviously, some elements included in this discussion of philosophy would be found in the theory documents were they simultaneously used.

The philosophy is considered here primarily as a *document* used to organize a nursing division. Additionally the dominant nursing ethos of an institution can be recognized in the *practices* of its members. This is "philosophy in action," but seldom will the "real" philosophy and the written document of philosophy correspond exactly. This is because the reality is in flux, while the document is only periodically revised. (This is a problem shared by *any* reality and its corresponding documentation.) The same problem occurs for documents stating purposes, objectives, functions, assignments, evaluations, or any other structures that organize a nursing service division.

The nurse executive will want to have her documents as current as possible in order that they reflect the current reality. But documents not only *reflect,* they *direct.* Hence the nurse executive will also want her documents (of philosophy and other structures) to lead to the future. Thus the document serves a dual purpose: 1) reflecting the present with some accuracy—otherwise it is misleading, and 2) indicating the immediate future toward which the organization is heading.

In writing a statement of philosophy, it may be that the greatest achievement is not the ultimate document, but the interaction among fellow managers which takes place when they thresh out the content of the document. Indeed, this interchange and examination of values is so critical that the philosophy must be discussed and examined again each time there is a major turnover in managerial nursing staff.

Another purpose served by the philosophy is orientation of new members. It also serves as a descriptive document to inform trustees, accrediting agencies, and others within the health care institution. Other operating documents share in these functions. For an operational document to fulfill these functions effectively, it must meet three criteria: 1) the document must be clear, precise, and meaningful in content, 2) the content must reflect the reality of the nursing practice, and 3) the document must give direction toward desired practice. Too often operational documents are seen merely as paper to have on file for needed occasions. Nurse leaders, for example, often meet *to write* but seldom *to think about* a philosophy that guides nursing practice. Operational documents need to be seen as minutes of operating decisions rather than as entities in themselves.

The problems that nurse executives have in writing an operational document occur when they assume that the document is the result of composition sessions rather than of idea sessions. A typical scene is one in which the nurse executive decides to review a certain operational document, the philosophy for example. She calls a meeting of her top management staff and gives each member a copy of the current document. Starting with the first sentence, the group then reviews the document, making both grammatical and content alterations as they progress until the entire document has been "revised." This process usually involves several meetings as sentence wording is a complex task. Finally a new document is produced for which there is either consensus or majority approval, and the task is complete for another five years.

What is wrong with this mode of operation? First, it is clearly a composition job, not a management operation. Second, the approach, starting with the "old" document, puts the management staff into a mind-set dictated by the old form. This mind-set is doubly reinforced if the approach to the task is one of line-by-line revision, a practice assuring that no attention will be given to the document as a whole or to its implications for practice.

What would be a better approach to producing a viable document? Suppose the nurse executive were to use the following procedure: She calls a meeting of her top management staff. She does *not* start by passing out the old philosophy; indeed, she requests that any copies of it be put aside. After appointing a recorder (ideally the person who will compose the final document) the nurse executive begins by asking for discussion of the philosophy reflected in the group's present nursing practice and the philosophy the group ought to have. The group then, instead of working with composition, works with ideas. The nurse executive tries to achieve consensus or majority approval on ideas, not on wording of sentences.

Once the ideas have been carefully discussed, sorted, approved, or rejected, the person assigned to draft the document can begin composition. This duty, of course, is assigned to an individual with writing ability. At a later meeting the document is reviewed by the group to see if it accurately reflects the meaning of their discussion. If not, the author revises it again. At no time does the group focus on composition; their job is to produce ideas that relate to managing the division. The same procedure pertains for any revision of operational documents. On a job description, for example, the group would discuss the job as reflected in present practice and the job as it ought to be.

In this way the documents ultimately produced convey the desired criteria: description and direction. By grounding the discussion of the operation in actual practice, one assures that the final document will not be some utopian vision, unattainable in the concrete work environment. By analyzing what the operation *ought* to do, one projects the needed future practice and assures that needless traditions will not be continued. Decisions produced in this way are realistic resolutions of the conflict between idealistic aims and the constraints of a concrete situation.

Unless there is an express theory of nursing, the philosophy is often the first operational document of a nursing division, a belief statement that characterizes the nursing practice in the institution. Too often the nursing philosophy is thought of as a general statement; on the contrary, it should be a specific statement representing a particular institution uniquely.

One does not need to be a philosopher to write a statement about nursing practice. The philosophy statement simply represents the central beliefs and values of the division relative to nursing and nursing practice. Philosophy statements are not right or wrong; they reflect accurately or inaccurately. Their content may vary from institution to institution, depending upon what values are perceived as central to nursing in a given setting. It is, however, difficult to write a nursing philosophy without talking about what nursing is perceived to be and how nursing relates to the patient and to the particular organization.

TYPICAL SUBJECT MATTER OF A PHILOSOPHY

The following content areas are found in most comprehensive nursing philosophies. If the division has no strong values concerning a given content area, the area may be omitted in the philosophy statement.

1. A specific nursing theory, which can either be referred to or incorporated in its entirety.
2. Nursing practice values, which may or may not include commitments to various practice modes and assignment systems.
3. Nursing education values, with respect either to staff education or to education of students, or both.
4. Nursing research values, with respect either to active research programs or to the application of research findings of others.
5. Relationship of nursing practice to nursing administration or institutional administration.
6. Relationship of nursing or the nursing division to the client (or patient).
7. Relationship of nursing to the extended client world, e.g., the community or the society.
8. Relationship of nursing to the rest of the organization, which may include reference to its modes of operation.
9. Relationship of nursing staff with other health professionals, or to other nurse professionals not among the nursing staff.
10. Relationship to the goals of other departments, e.g., to the research goals of medicine or the placement goals of social service.
11. Relationship to other value systems such as religious groups or societal groups.
12. Nursing management values (may include commitments to particular modes of management, e.g., participative management).
13. Relationship of the nursing division (or its members) to professional nursing— organizational or conceptual.
14. Relationships of nursing to other institutions of health care (coordinative and cooperative relationships).
15. Values related to patient rights and other beliefs about patients/people.
16. Values related to employee rights or concepts of professional or occupational growth and development.
17. Values related to promotions, retentions, and transfers within the organization.

It is important to note the *perspective* from which a given philosophy is written. It may be written from the perspective of the nursing administration: "We believe that each staff member should be provided with the inservice education needed to optimize his capabilities." While this statement does not identify its perspective as administrative, it clearly is the nursing administration which is responsible for the "providing" mentioned in the belief.

An alternate perspective for a philosophic statement is that of the staff: "We believe that it is our individual responsibility to maintain and update our knowledge of professional nursing." Here the "we" is the staff, not the administration. Other perspectives are possible: some philosophies are written from the perspective of the patient; others from the perspective of the total organization. If the document of philosophic statement is to have internal consistency and coherency, it is important that the perspective not fluctuate. One should be able to determine who—or what group or entity—is making the statement of philosophy.

A single statement of philosophy may be used by the entire nursing division, or, more commonly, each major nursing department may elect to create its own philosophy. Such a subordinate philosophy would have to be consistent with the divisional philosophy, but it might be better able to characterize the nursing care within the particular department. A brief sample subordinate philosophy for a psychiatric nursing department follows:

> We concur with the philosophy of the nursing division and support its beliefs and values.
>
> The specific philosophy of this department is based upon a belief that nursing can help patients improve in their ability to live more effectively with themselves and others.
>
> We believe in an interdisciplinary approach, working closely with physicians, social workers, and other health care professionals.
>
> We believe in an eclectic approach in psychiatric therapy. We believe the nurse should be skilled in various treatment modalities in order that she may support the therapy mode prescribed for each patient by his respective physician.
>
> We also believe that nursing is an independent profession, and that the psychiatric nurse makes her own professional judgments as to how to apply that treatment modality with individual patients.
>
> We are committed to the development of psychiatric nursing research by use of the longitudinal case study method. The nurse in this department believes that data must be kept to correlate nursing strategies with patient outcomes.

Although this philosophy may strike the reader as mundane, at least it differentiates between a divisional and a departmental statement of philosophy. Note that this philosophy did not repeat any generalities which might be found in the divisional philosophy. Instead it focused upon what was unique and different within the context of the department.

Philosophies may be more or less sophisticated, depending upon the capabilities and needs of a given nursing division or department. Even an unsophisticated document constructed by those who will use it is probably better than a sophisticated one imposed from above or created externally by an "expert."

PHILOSOPHIC IMPLICATIONS IN METHODS OF NURSING PRACTICE AND EDUCATION

Many nursing acts, events, or strategies (methods of one sort or another) have implications for philosophy, even if they are beyond the scope of the typical statement of philosophy used in most nursing divisions. The nurse executive should develop a sensitivity to these philosophic issues so that she will not employ methods which are inconsistent with her announced philosophy.

Many philosophic methodologies are applied in nursing practice. As demonstration models, two such philosophic structures, the logistic method and the problem-solving method, are discussed in this chapter. For purposes of contrast other philosophic methods are briefly described. The nurse executive does not have to become a philosopher in order to cope with philosophic issues in nursing. It is necessary, however, that she be analytical in her approach to nursing and nursing management. This means that she must recognize consistencies and inconsistencies, identify assumptions underlying ideas and actions, draw subtle distinctions between actions and ideas that are different in kind, and recognize categories that combine actions or ideas of the same kind.

The Logistic Method

The first example, the logistic method, is easy to understand and recognize in nursing practice. The logistic method might be viewed as the construction of a wall in which the worker is concerned with one brick at a time. He is interested in how each brick lines up with the last brick and how well it fits on the brick underneath; only at the end of the whole process does the composite wall receive his attention. In the logistic method each component (each brick) is handled as a separate entity. Then stress is placed upon the relationships among components such as cause and effect, time sequences, and logical sequences.

In nursing, the logistic method follows this pattern: The focus is on the parts and their relationships to each other rather than on some totality of nursing, of man, or of health. The logistic form is recognizable in traditional nursing education programs that divide into such separate parts as cardiovascular nursing, genitourinary nursing, and orthopedic nursing. Nursing is compartmentalized into discrete units, and when the student has completed all the compartments, she is ready to graduate. This curriculum form does not spend time defining the similarities in nursing needs of all ill persons, nor does it focus on a unifying concept of man. Universal concepts are not integral to the curriculum composition. Indeed, state board examinations themselves demonstrate the compartmentalized approach prior to 1981.

In the logistic form of curriculum, the compartmentalization takes place in three levels: systems within the body, diseases or conditions within each system, and defined components within each disease.

Relationships among parts are important considerations in the logistic mode. For example, the sequence for study of each disease from etiology through sequellae is guided by principles of cause and effect and of time sequence. Diseases are related to each other by their location in the same body system. Body systems are usually related by their place interactions. For example, the orthopedic injury is related to the accompanying neuromuscular injury. In this logistic system the "building bricks" of various diseases and body systems are discrete entities, capable of separation from each other. Since the logistic method focuses upon rela-

tionships of parts, it is first essential to differentiate those parts from each other.

The nature of logistic compartmentalization and relationship of parts can best be seen by comparing a logistic structure to a structure that represents a different philosophic method. For this purpose a cardiovascular course or a cardiovascular unit for patient care can be compared with a geriatric course or a geriatric unit for patient care. Whether in education or practice, the geriatric focus is a holistic view of man. The geriatric individual is viewed from the totality of his existence. The concept of geriatric life is not logistic for several reasons. First, it cannot be clearly differentiated from other components; there is no sharp division at which one passes from middle age to old age. Geriatric age is defined in global terms, with imprecise entry points and with variations in characteristics among its class members.

The nebulous borders of the concept of geriatric age can be contrasted with the precise divisions between logistic components. For example, there is a clear differentiation between a vascular injury and its related neuromuscular damage. These injuries may be closely related in understanding and in therapy, but no one has any difficulty defining where blood vessels end and neuromuscular tissue begins. It is not particularly useful to search for such relationships between middle age and geriatric age. Middle age does not cause geriatric age; it simply blends into it. Thus in the holistic philosophy inherent in the concept of geriatric age, there is no great need to concentrate on its relations to other components of its system (infancy, childhood, and so forth). The lack of interest in the "border" between middle and geriatric age can be contrasted with the careful attention given to the relations between the cardiovascular system and the renal system (logistic relations).

Another application of the logistic method is the use of systems analysis theory in nursing. The systems approach had its first impact in data collection and interpretation such as cardiac monitoring, computer-assisted histories, and computerized laboratory diagnostic processes. All these systems are logistic because of the nature and relationships of their parts. All have three common components: 1) some form of input, 2) central processing, and 3) output. These parts relate to each other in a precise order and in a specific, predictable way. In each case data are processed exactly as the system is programmed.

The apnea alarm mattress is a simple example of such a system. The input is the displacement of air in the mattress caused by respiratory movements of an infant. The central processing is a comparison of the rate of displacement with a preprogrammed minimum. (Many systems have both minimum and maximum criteria.) The output is the notifying alarm that sounds should the input fail to remain within the programmed limits of respiratory rate.

The systems models have also affected the concept of nursing itself. Nursing is logistic when it is described by a discrete structural model relating its identified parts. The following models show nursing from a systems and, therefore, logistic approach (Figures 3-1, 3-2, and 3-3).

All these models essentially define nursing or nursing education as a series of components put together in an invariable way. Each uses a critical-pathways approach in which arrows show the movements of the process and the lines of feedback. The important factor in these systems is the clear, prescribed relationship of parts to each other. These nursing models and their parts

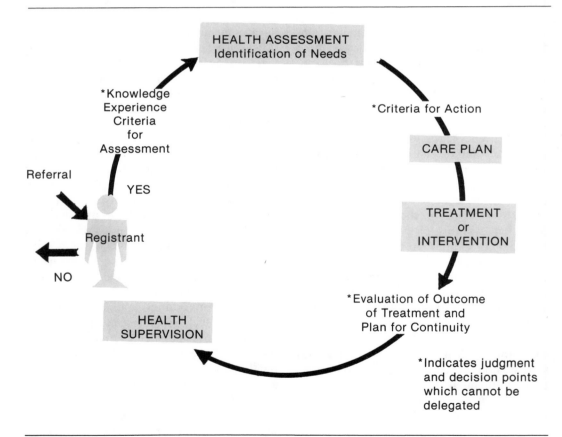

Figure 3-1.   Process of Providing Care (From Betty J. Hallstrom. Utilization of nursing personnel: A task-specific approach. *Nursing Outlook,* 19:665, 1971. By permission.)

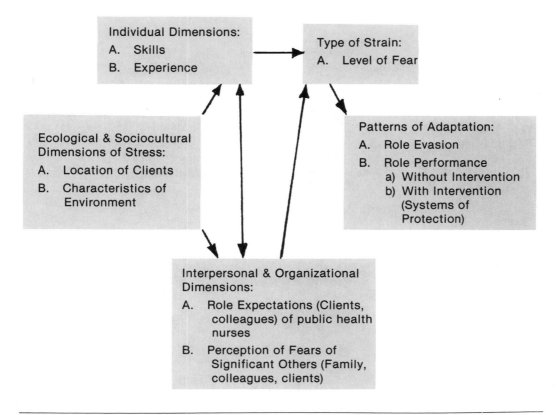

Figure 3-2.   Schematic Representation of the Interface between Ecological and Interpersonal Correlates of Stress in Public Health Nursing (From Mary M. Castles and Pat M. Keith. Correlates of environmental fear in the role of the public health nurse. *Nursing Research,* 20:248, 1971. By permission.)

remain stable, with unchanging relationships, regardless of the nursing situation in which the models are applied.

The logistic mode of philosophy fits the mechanization of present nursing processes and reflects new trends in education. Computer-assisted instruction is a good example of logistic teaching. If the student selects answer A, he is channeled into one path (continuation to a new concept); if he selects B, a wrong answer, he is channeled into a different path (one supplying corrective concepts). In either case, the student goes through the same program of basic concepts. All pathways feed back into the primary learning system. In a logistic system, not only do terms have univocal meanings, but meanings derived from combinations of terms are also unambiguous. The "correct" answer in computer-assisted instruction or in programmed learning (another logistic form) is the same for every individual who studies the content. One and only one response is accurate and acceptable. This contrasts, for example, with the problem-solving mode in which the learner is to identify alternate solutions. In a problem-solving mode, it is accepted that more than one alternative may be appropriate or that the right alternative for one person may be wrong for another.

What then are the advantages and disadvantages of a logistic interpretation of nursing today? The logistic structure has some definite disadvantages. The primary weakness is caused by the segregation of its

STUDENT'S LEARNING SYSTEM

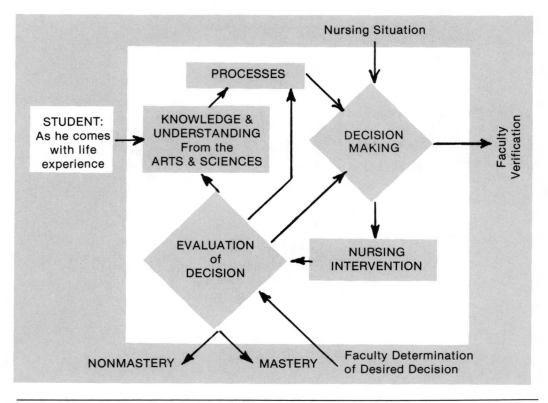

Figure 3-3.   Control Loop for Learning in Nursing Major. (From Alice Joyce Finch. For students only: A system for learning. *Nursing Outlook,* 19:333, 1971. By permission.)

units. Some learners fail to integrate the parts into a total concept of nursing. In other words, the learner may know and understand each "brick" without ever recognizing that he is building a "wall." The second weakness of the logistic system stems from the absolutist nature of its concepts. The nurse who adapts this structure may be rigid and resistant to change should future health care move in radically different directions.

The logistic structure, however, has definite advantages too: 1) it is compatible with specialty trends in patient care, 2) it is compatible with technologic developments in health care, and 3) it is compatible with trends in education. Thus it may help the nurse to develop a way of thinking about nursing that will enable her to make an op-

timal adjustment in common nursing practice settings.

The Problem-Solving Method

A problem-solving approach is another philosophic viewpoint that can be used in nursing. Since problem solving is often misapplied in nursing curriculum development, it will be discussed in relation to nursing education first. Problem solving in nursing education best succeeds when it is applied consistently throughout the whole program. If it is to be used, the problem-solving method should extend into all areas of the curriculum: classroom teaching, clinical teaching, and the learning tools used by the student. The faculty using a problem-solving method should ascertain that this method is evident in both joint and individual materials. The problem-solving approach should be immediately evident in the school's philosophy. The faculty members need to define nursing itself as a process of defining and resolving problems. The problems may change as the faculty develops or changes personnel, but the primary focus is on nursing defined as a learned method of problem resolution.

The conceptual difference between nursing viewed as a method and nursing viewed as content can be illustrated by two definitions of nursing: 1) Nursing is a science that meets the physical and psychosocial health needs of individuals. 2) Nursing is a planned process of identifying and meeting physical and psychosocial health needs of individuals. The second definition focuses on nursing as a *method* rather than as a specific *content*.

The concept of education in the faculty's philosophy should reflect the primary aim of education, teaching the student to think in a certain manner, to apply a problem-solving approach to nursing. The curriculum objectives follow the pattern by including objectives relevant to learning and applying the problem-solving process. Thus long before the faculty plans its individual activities, the necessary background for the problem-solving method is built into the system.

In the first nursing course the faculty provides the opportunity for the student to learn problem solving as a method. The methodology itself is given as actual content early in the student's learning experiences. While the steps of problem solving may be presented in different ways, with different terminology, generally the steps follow the sequence identified by John Dewey: 1) perplexity, in which one is involved in an incomplete situation, 2) conjectural anticipation, i.e., a tentative interpretation of the situation, 3) careful survey and exploration, 4) elaboration of a tentative hypothesis, and 5) taking a stand on a hypothesis as a plan of action for testing[1].

The guidesheet presented to the new student might identify some of the following items:

Steps Involved in Problem Solving

1. Recognizing that a problem exists
   a. Lacking the means to a desirable goal
   b. Difficulty in identifying the character of a situation
   c. Inability to explain unexpected events

2. Understanding the problem
   a. Delimiting
   b. Defining

3. Collecting data concerning the problem
   a. Evaluating possible sources of information
   b. Attaining adequate data for solution

4. Formulating one or more hypotheses
   a. Determining what, if anything, one might do about the problem
   b. Plan of action based upon one or more assumptions about the facts

5. Testing the hypothesis
   a. Choosing the most likely hypothesis for testing
   b. Deductive reasoning of the consequences of the selected hypothesis (... if H, then C)
   c. Determining a method which will test for evidence of whether the consequences do occur
   d. Evaluating testing results and modifying hypothesis accordingly

The usual approach in the problem-solving curriculum, after discussing the content of the problem-solving process itself, is to have the student learn the problem-solving method by application. The student is given practice problems in which she must identify each element of the problem-solving process.

From her first clinical experience and thereafter, the student is taught to approach the patient or the patient's situation as a riddle to be solved, a challenge in which she must identify the problem and find the solution. For the student's early experiences, the teacher may identify the problem for her so that the student may focus on the solving process. (This patient has difficulty breathing, . . . this patient is fearful of his coming surgery, etc.) On the other hand the instructor may choose to focus the student's attention on definition of problems. For example, she might assist the young student in utilizing interview techniques that elicit problem areas.

To use a problem-solving approach clinically places certain demands on the instructor. First, she must be flexible enough to accept the different solutions that different students may find to the same clinical problem. Problem solving recognizes that the problem solver (in this case, the student) is part of the situation she is trying to resolve. Since no two students are identical, it would be unrealistic to expect identical resolutions. Thus the teacher must rid herself of any axiomatic rules that place unsupported demands for uniformity on the students. For example, she must discard such rules as, "the sickest patient must be bathed first."

In the clinical application of problem solving, requirements are placed on the teacher acting as an individual; it is also necessary that the faculty as a whole consider the problem-solving methodology when they develop their clinical tools. Appropriate clinical tools can greatly reinforce the problem-solving process.

The nursing care plan, for example, can be structured to encourage the student in problem-solving thinking. The differences in the modes of thought required to fill out the sample care plans shown in Figures 3-4 and 3-5 are evident.

Figure 3-4 merely leads the student to "fill in the blanks"; Figure 3-5 forces the student to relate data and to specify how she relates problems to solutions.

The student clinical evaluation form can also encourage or discourage problem solving. The following forms illustrate this point. Figure 3-7 clearly reinforces problem-solving concepts. Just as the evaluation and

the care plan can support problem solving, so can every other clinical tool if appropriately structured.

Application of problem solving is not limited to the teaching of a method and utilization of it in clinical experiences and clinical tools. The curriculum itself should reflect the problem-solving methodology. The total curriculum can be seen as a problem to be solved; the courses provide specific problems, as do the class and clinical learning experiences.

One common content approach that is well adapted to the problem-solving process is orientation of the curriculum around the problem of homeostasis. The term *homeostasis* itself implies a problem, the maintaining of a balance, i.e., a principle of stability. The principle of homeostasis can be applied to psychological and sociological as well as to physical problems.

Each course in a curriculum of this design can focus around a specific problem in homeostasis. Examples of course foci might include maintaining nutritional homeostasis, fluid and electrolyte balance, problems in maintaining mobility, and so forth. In each case the course is seen as a problem to be solved, and in learning this course content, the student attains more knowledge toward solving the total problem of maintaining human homeostasis. To build a curriculum around the principle of homeostasis, however, is not a prerequisite for use of the problem-solving method. Any content that can be organized to present and solve major problems is adaptable to the method.

Just as the teacher can encourage student problem solving by use of the right clinical tools, so also can she encourage problem-solving behavior by appropriate classroom techniques. Lecture material, for example, can be presented in the problem-solving form, stating a problem and working through the steps to solution. This gives students a needed opportunity to observe someone else using the problem-solving process. Demonstrations also can be given, not as "steps of a procedure" but as the presentation of an objective and determination of various appropriate ways to reach that objective. Discussion groups can be led to conform with the problem-solving mode. Other teaching methods can be similarly modified to express a problem-solving method.

If a problem-solving approach is to be ef-

fective in a nursing curriculum, it must be applied in all the individual and jointly constructed faculty materials. It should be carried through from the broadest concepts to the philosophy and objectives and down to the most detailed and concrete structuring of each individual class presentation. Problem

PATIENT CARE PLAN

Name_____ Marital Status _____ Physician _____

Age _____ Diagnosis _____ Admission Date _____

Occupation _____ Surgical Date _____ Sex _____

Religion _____ Nationality _____

Brief History, Symptoms	Diagnostic Tests	Medicines and Treatments

Hygienic Care	Surgical Procedures	Diet

Figure 3-4.   Sample A: Nonproblematic Care Plan

PATIENT CARE PLAN

Name_____ Marital Status _____ Disabilities _____

Age _____ Diagnosis _____ Ethnic Factors _____

Occupation _____ Role in Family _____

Religion _____ Type of Dwelling _____

Physiologic Changes	Related M/S Intervention	Rationale for Intervention

Nursing Problem	Proposed Nursing Resolution	Rationale	Evaluation

Figure 3-5.   Sample B: Problematic Care Plan

NURSING PERFORMANCE RECORD

	A	B	C	D	E	F
Application of knowledge						
Application of principles of nursing care						
Organization and use of time						
Interpersonal relationships						

Figure 3-6.   Nonproblematic Performance Record

STUDENT CLINICAL EVALUATION

	Satisfactory	Unsatisfactory	Supportive anecdotes
Recognizes and identifies patient problems			
Formulates realistic nursing solution			
Identifies nursing activities which contribute to the solution			

Figure 3-7.   Problematic Performance Record

solving must infiltrate into every aspect of curriculum development; the student will learn to apply problem solving only if the faculty demonstrates the same consistent application.

The problem-solving methodology has recently become fashionable in nursing service and medicine due to adaptation of the problem-oriented medical record[2]. Here again is evidence of a clinical tool encouraging a certain form of thought pattern. This problem-oriented medical record system, when applied to nursing, requires that the nurse identify specific patient problems and relate each nursing action and observation to the appropriate problem in her charting.

Such enforced use of forms requiring the problem-solving process is far more effective in inculcating problem-solving modes of thought than is the use of any number of lectures on and about problem solving.

The nursing service executive who wishes to encourage problem solving can apply the same principle to other documents in addition to nurses' notes. Nursing care plans, for example, can be organized to solve problems. Even where the nursing service uses a simplified Kardex form in nursing care plans, the problem-solving principle can be applied. Many present care plan formats are structured so that patient goals are listed in isolation from the activities supposedly related to them. The nursing care plan shown in Figure 3-8 is a typical example.

Clearly the problem solving involved in making a nursing care plan is that of deciding what nursing activities will efficiently and effectively bring about the desired solution. The first form (Figure 3-8) gives no assurance that the nursing activities will be directed toward resolution. The second (Figure 3-9) in contrast, would require that the nurse planner do the required problem solving.

The same kind of problem solving can be encouraged in other documents. For example, a supervisor's bimonthly report to the director could take the form shown in Figure 3-10.

Thus a problem-solving philosophy can be instituted in nursing service by carefully designed routine forms. Education in the problem-solving process, of course, would assist staff members in using such materials, but even without special staff education the forms themselves promote problem-solving processes of thought.

NURSING CARE PLAN

Patient Name ————————————

Room Number ————————————

Nursing Goals:

| Date | Nursing Activities |

Figure 3-8.   Nonproblematic Nursing Care Plan

NURSING CARE PLAN

Patient Name —————————————————   Room Number —————

Nursing Problem 1. ————————————————————————
    Related Nursing Activities ————————————————————

————————————————————————————————

————————————————————————————————

Nursing Problem 2. ————————————————————————

    Related Nursing Activities ————————————————————

————————————————————————————————

————————————————————————————————

Figure 3-9.   Problematic Nursing Care Plan

SUPERVISOR'S REPORT			
Supervisor _____		Date _____	
Present Problems	Related Solutions	Present Status of Problem Resolution	Planned Strategies for Future Resolution

Figure 3-10. Problematic Supervisor's Report

Operational Philosophies in Nursing

In contrast to the logistic and problem-solving forms, an operational philosophy has a different effect on nursing behaviors. In this concept the focus is on the operations to be performed rather than on the recipient of those actions. Hospitals that classify patients into self-care, minimal care, intermediate care, and acute care units are following an operational mode. This type of division does not depend on anything about the patient per se (his physiologic systems, his problems); instead it is related to the kinds of activities to be performed for him. The criterion for division is the kind of work to be done. In one unit, for example, the nurses may specialize in actions maintaining life support systems; in another unit, the consistent "work" may be patient teaching.

Many health maintenance organizations make divisions on the basis of activities to be performed. Patients are separated into groups for well-care and health education, chronic maintenance care, and acute episodic ill-care. Again, the division is based on the work to be done, not on holistic concepts of the patient. The patient, over a period of time, is likely to move through several different sectors, each sector performing different functions for him.

Since health maintenance organizations have evolved partly in response to economic costs of health care delivery, it is not surprising that they have an operational form.

If nurses can successfully manage the operations involved in chronic maintenance care, however, there is no economic justification for having physicians do this activity. Clearly the focus is on how to facilitate things for optimal efficiency for the "operators." How these activity-directed systems affect the patient (the object of the actions) is of secondary consideration in such a philosophy.

In nursing education, operational programs of learning are becoming popular. In an operational curriculum the focus is on the learning operations of students. Such curricula frequently give the students a wide variety of learning experiences (operations) from which to choose in meeting each objective. In some of these programs students have the option of sequencing their own curriculum components. Often these programs rely heavily on audiovisual software to provide multiple learning activities. LEGS is a recent operational publication familiar to most teachers[3]. This compendium identifies wide varieties of learning experiences for most common content areas taught in nursing education.

Logistic, problem-solving, operational, and holistic philosophies are all evident in today's nursing. It is not important that the nurse administrator be able to apply some philosophic term to each nursing system she uses; it is important that she be able to support her choices with reasoned arguments. Put simply, it is important that her choices be appropriate for her nursing objectives. Philosophic methodologies do have important implications for nursing theory and for nursing action.

SUMMARY

The nurse executive will need to consider philosophy in two discrete ways. First, she will have to be concerned with the explicit values and beliefs which are expressed in the concrete statement of philosophy of the division. Next, she will have to be cognizant of some of the philosophic underpinnings of the methodologies and systems of care which she may elect to use in the division. Ideally, she will strive for conformity and complementarity among the explicit and implicit philosophic positions.

Although the philosophy of a nursing division (or of its director) is not in itself a goal, it clearly colors what goals will be selected and how those goals will be enacted. Philosophy interacts with the divisional purpose. It is useless to argue over which of these documents (or ideas) comes first, for philosophy impacts on purpose and purpose enacts a philosophy; they are interactive ideas.

REFERENCES

1. Dewey, J. *Democracy and Education.* New York: The Free Press, Macmillan, 1966, p. 150.

2. Hurst, J. W., and Walker, H. K. (Eds.). *The Problem-Oriented System.* New York: Med Com Press, 1962.

3. Roe, A., and Sherwood, M. *Learning Experience Guides for Nursing Students.* New York: Wiley, 1972.

BIBLIOGRAPHY

Abdellah, F.G. et al. *Patient-Centered Approaches to Nursing.* New York: Macmillan, 1960.

Arndt, C., and Huckabay, L. *Nursing Administration—Theory for Practice with a Systems Approach.* St. Louis: C.V. Mosby, 1975.

Coleman, L.J. *Development of an Administrative Protocol: The Relationship among Nursing Theory, Practice and Administrative Theory.* MSN thesis, University of Illinois, 1977.

Dietrich, B.J., and Miller, D.L. Nursing leadership—a theoretic framework. *Nursing Outlook,* 14(8):52, Aug. 1966.

Divencenti, M. *Administering Nursing Service.* (2nd ed.). Boston: Little, Brown, 1977.

Folta, J.R., and Deck, E. *A Sociologic Framework for Patient Care.* New York: Wiley, 1966.

Hadley, B.J. Evolution of a conception of nursing. *Nursing Research,* 18(5):401, Sept.–Oct. 1969.

Hegyvary, S.T., and Chanings, P.A. The hospital setting and patient care outcomes. *J.O.N.A.,* 5(3):29, March–April 1975.

Johnson, M., Davis, J.L., and Bilitch, M. *Problem-Solving in Nursing Practice.* Dubuque, Iowa: W.C. Brown, 1970.

Murphy, J.F. *Theoretical Issues in Professional Nursing.* New York: Appleton-Century-Crofts, 1971.

O'Connell, K.A., and Duffey, M. Research in nursing practice: its nature and direction. *Image,* 7(2):3, Feb. 1976.

Wolf, M.S. Group stages: one view of the development of the nursing profession. *Image,* 9(3):64, Oct. 1977.

Chapter 4

The Nursing Division's Purpose and Objectives

The divisional purpose and objectives are the major goal statements of a nursing division. Theoretically, other goal statements flow from these. Purpose and objectives will be reviewed separately, tracing their relation to each other.

DIVISIONAL PURPOSE

The statement of purpose gives the reason that a particular nursing division exists, the intent that it serves. Usually a statement of purpose is broad in nature, listing only major purposes of the nursing division. The purpose may be limited to one: the delivery of care to patients. Or the purpose may be multiple, possibly incorporating service and education. Few nursing service divisions yet display nursing research as a major purpose, but that is likely to change as the nursing discipline advances. In the purpose statement, these broad basic goals are usually qualified in some manner which attempts to characterize the individual nursing organization.

The purposes of a nursing division are usually constrained by several factors. First, the purpose of the division must be compatible with the purpose of the health care institution of which it is part. Indeed, the broad purpose of the nursing division is determined by that institution because it created the division in the first place. Usually, however, the nurse executive has the power to modify, add to, or determine the manner in which the purpose will be enacted. Furthermore, she is granted the professional right to qualify that purpose according to her knowledge of the nursing discipline. Therefore, though the nursing division's purpose must conform to the institution's purpose, there is usually considerable room for freedom in characterizing the purpose. Furthermore, many institutional purposes are so broad and generalized as to offer few, if any, constraints upon the nursing purpose.

A second potential constraint on the nursing division purpose is that of law. A division's purpose cannot deviate from the constrictions imposed by the nursing practice act of the state in which the institution is located. The major problem is one of scope of nursing practice; the nursing division may not assume a purpose beyond the bounds of legal nursing practice within the given state.

Further constraints on divisional purpose may be offered by credentialing and accrediting bodies. Although these may not hold the force of law, the desirability of accreditation or credentialing (for purposes of receiving financial, contractual, or status benefits) may act as effectively to control purpose as do laws.

The majority of purpose statements for nursing divisions are general, short (a paragraph or two), concise, and will usually deal with one or more of the following topics: delivery of patient care, provision or support of teaching programs, and provision or support of research efforts.

A statement of purpose may be worded from several different perspectives. First, it may state the purpose of the nursing division qua organization, i.e., the desired *structure* that provides for and controls nursing services. For example, "The purpose of this nursing division is to provide requisite nursing services for all patients admitted to the institution."

A second option is to word the purpose so as to describe the *process* of nursing desired.

In this case, the purpose envisions a particular concept of nursing as its goal: "The purpose of this nursing division is to provide problem-centered nursing care for each patient."

Other purpose statements are worded in terms of desired patient *outcomes:* "The purpose of this nursing division is to assure that each patient attains satisfactory health recovery and optimal health maintenance." Some statements of purpose choose to include all these perspectives: structure, process, and outcome.

Departmental Purposes

While the divisional statement of purpose gives the general goal of the nursing organization, it is not surprising to find that purpose broken down into subpurposes, usually by department. Several examples of statements of departmental purpose follow:

Operating Room Department:
The purpose of the Operating Room Department is to organize, direct, and deliver those specialized nursing services that effectively contribute to meeting consumer health needs during surgical intervention.

Intensive Care Department:
The purpose of the Department of Intensive Care is to provide continuous, comprehensive and emergency nursing care to the critically and seriously ill patient, to preserve life and maintain function during the critical episode.

Consumer Education Department:
The purpose of the Department of Consumer Education is to promote the optimum level of health for all clients by participating in the development of health counseling and education programs that best meet consumer health education needs.

Clearly, subordinate statements of purpose must conform to the purpose of the nursing division, but, as with departmental statements of philosophy, the clarification of departmental purpose may be a useful device for shaping goals.

NURSING DIVISIONAL OBJECTIVES

The nursing division purpose usually is elaborated into two specific kinds of objectives: permanent and temporary. Where subpurposes have been derived by department, they are complementary sources of objectives. Permanent objectives represent those ongoing goals which must be achieved continuously, over and over again. Thus they remain "objectives," even though they may be successfully achieved at any given time. A typical list of permanent objectives might contain statements like the following:

1. Advance the practice of clinical nursing within the division.
2. Implement useful new research findings in clinical nursing.
3. Provide adequate resources for implementation of nursing care at the determined level of excellence.
4. Provide nursing staff adequate in quality and quantity for implementation of nursing care at the determined level of excellence.
5. Foster an environment which encourages research, creativity, inquiry, and personal growth in staff members.
6. Retain a staff which is up to date in its knowledge, application, and conceptualization of nursing practice.
7. Maintain productive relationships with other divisions and departments of the institution.
8. Contribute productively to interdisciplinary research and education as well as to patient care.

Note that these objectives are permanent in that they demand continual achievement, continual monitoring, and ongoing effort. Although the nursing division will review its permanent objectives at frequent intervals, there tends to be a relative stability in the selected goals.

The temporary objective uses the principle of focus: certain objectives are selected for special attention, with the aim of improving the related nursing practices. Objectives to be emphasized usually are selected on a yearly basis, and the selection is based upon the present state of the nursing division. Usually these objectives are selected for the purpose of bolstering known weak spots. Some focus objectives also may be selected to improve on strengths or to develop special interests; some examples follow:

1. Improve quality control scores by 10 percent.
2. Decrease tardiness of staff by 20 percent in the next year.
3. Reorganize the nursing office for greater managerial efficiency.

Typically a focus objective will be supplanted by a new one after it has been achieved. Hence the focus is on the intermediate, one-time objective, rather than a permanent, ongoing goal.

Divisional objectives typically are distributed downward through the nursing organization. Hence some departments may be responsible for achieving some part of a given divisional objective, while others (or other levels of the organization) may be responsible for other components or subparts of the objective. This downward branching allows for objectives to be achieved at various levels (divisional, departmental, unit) in totality or in part (subobjectives). The nurse executive, then, may construct a schema of accountability for achievement of objectives throughout her division.

Often downward distribution of objectives is combined with an upward branching. In the upward branching, the lower managerial level constructs some objectives for itself—objectives which reflect goals specific to the managerial unit, goals which may not have been included in the conception of the divisional goals. For example, the

supervisor of the operating rooms may have certain ecological objectives which are unique to her area. She might impose these goals upon herself and her department. Often objectives of this sort are negotiated upward by presenting them to one's boss. Discussion and negotiation may then take place with the manager and the subordinate eventually agreeing upon a list of combined downward- and upward-oriented objectives.

The reader will recognize in this scheme the common managerial mechanism, management-by-objectives (MBO). In many instances descriptions of MBO are limited to downward-directed objectives. A few authors recommend only an upward flow of objectives, in which management (at least top management) becomes the recipient of ideas and decisions from below rather than the directing force for subordinate workers. In reality a combination of these two methodologies probably produces the best results.

Most nurse executives combine nursing and nursing managerial objectives in the same documents. Some few nurses prefer to differentiate out the management function, creating discrete and separate lists of nursing and management objectives.

Differentiating Educational and Managerial Objectives

Even though a division's objectives flow from the divisional purpose, the relationship usually is such that many different combinations of objectives could have been selected to enact the purpose(s). Hence objectives often are the first statements in which the individuality of the nursing division becomes apparent. Nursing service objectives often are mishandled as if they were educational objectives. In order to differentiate between managerial and educational objectives it is necessary to explore the purposes which such objectives serve.

Educational and management objectives are alike in that they define and set the goals of their respective nursing organizations.

They differ, however, in at least one important aspect. Attainment of educational objectives involves a change in behavior or, at least, a potential change in behavior on the part of the student. The successful acquisition of an educational objective increases the student's repertoire of possible responses in relevant situations. On the other hand, the management objective directs staff behavior by selecting among multiple, potentially available behavioral responses. Educational objectives provide the learner with new options; management objectives point out the preferred option for a given staff in a given institution.

Determination of both educational and management objectives involves value judgments. Selection of objectives in either an educational or a service program is a creative valuing process, essentially free from other constraints. Yet this creative process will structure the rest of the nursing program. Granted, the selected nursing objectives must be consistent with the philosophy and purpose of the organization, but they cannot be inferred from the philosophy and purpose of the organization. Selection of objectives is not a case of sorting out, in which objectives consistent with the stated philosophy are selected and those inconsistent with it are rejected. Instead, the process is one of selecting a reasonable number of attainable objectives from an infinite number of possible and philosophically consistent objectives. The constraint of philosophic and organizational consistency may be of some help in eliminating ill-fitting objectives, but it is of little guidance in selecting among the potential appropriate ones objectives from which the character of the whole program will flow.

In selecting objectives, many individuals or groups are unwilling to reject any worthy objective. This unwillingness leads to two problems: selection of more objectives than any one program can reasonably attain, and selection of objectives that are mutually incompatible. The program that tries to do everything it sees as good or desirable produces diffusion of effort and lack of direction and generally fails to create a unique program, one with which members can identify.

Both educational programs and management programs require a hierarchy of objectives. In management, the objectives follow the natural hierarchical work divisions: organization objectives, nursing division objectives, department objectives, unit objectives. In educational programs, the objectives follow the apportioning-out of work: school objectives, curriculum objectives, course objectives, unit objectives, class and clinical objectives. At each level there is some constraint and some freedom. The constraint is to carry out the higher level objectives that are applicable at this level, and the freedom is in the manner in which those higher level objectives are converted into lower level goals.

For successful translation of objectives into concrete actions, it is necessary to show how objectives at each level are distributed through objectives at the next lower level. Otherwise, it is easy to define objectives without ever putting them into effect. Most implementation of activities toward attainment of objectives actually occurs at the lowest level: curriculum objectives are translated into actions that occur in classes and in clinical experiences; most management objectives are translated into action on the patient units. If the nurse administrator cannot trace the extension of higher-level objectives down into lower-level programs, then she has no assurance that work is being done to attain them. To assure that an objective is implemented, it is necessary to trace its translation through objective hierarchies until it ends in one or more concrete activities.

Objectives serve several purposes: 1) they tell why a program has been created, 2) they justify the existence of a program by clarifying its purposes, and 3) they serve to direct the responsible individual in the selection of appropriate activities, be they learning experiences in nursing education or patient care activities in nursing service. The activities selected should be those most likely to lead to achievement of the objective.

Another function of an objective is to provide direction for the individual completing the selected activity, be it the student in a class or the staff nurse providing patient care. The objective tells the individual in what way, to what degree, and under what circumstances the activity is to be performed. The objective gives meaningful direction to the work; it also gives a criterion against which to measure and evaluate outcomes. Outcomes may be grades in a course or the patient's recuperation from a surgical procedure.

Foci for Objectives

There are three possible foci for objectives. They are the providing *structure,* the *process,* and the *outcome.* In education, the organization of the entire educational division constitutes the providing structure. This providing structure includes such things as how students are selected, how teachers are assigned, how classes are scheduled, how clinical facilities are contracted, and how the school program is administered. When an educational program identifies *structure objectives,* they are usually called school objectives, to differentiate them from curriculum objectives. Examples of educational structure objectives might be: To provide an educational program that will qualify the graduate to take state board examinations for licensure as a registered nurse or to establish academic counseling programs for all students. Most of the standards set by the National League for Nursing Accrediting Program for Schools of Nursing are structure objectives.

In nursing service, structure objectives relate to the management structures designed to deliver care. Examples might include: to ensure that each patient unit is under the management of a registered nurse at all times, to provide for ongoing evaluation and revision of nursing procedures and policies by committee review, or to establish and provide inservice education for all staff members. The Joint Commission on Accreditation of Hospitals has nursing service structure goals. The American Nurses' Association also publishes nursing service structure objectives.

In both education and service, structure objectives set goals for the organization providing the services. They describe a structure conducive to getting the job done.

Process objectives are goals for the work process itself. Thus, in nursing education, process goals concern the curriculum, the teaching, and the teacher; in nursing service, the process objectives concern nursing practice and the nurse. Some examples of process objectives follow:

1. Nursing education
   a. To teach the anatomy and physiology of the endocrine system
   b. To utilize a wide span of teaching methods and materials
   c. To participate in faculty governance

2. Nursing service
   a. To recognize abnormalities in electrocardiograph patterns
   b. To provide active and passive exercise for the patient with a cardiovascular accident
   c. To provide nursing care plans for one's patients

Process objectives focus upon what the "agent" should do: how the teacher should teach, how the nurse should nurse. In education such objectives are usually called teacher-centered objectives. Nurse-centered objectives can be found in many types of quality control forms. Most nursing service departmental objectives are formulated in the process model.

Outcome objectives define the desired goals for the client. Thus they are directed not to the teacher or the nurse but to the student and the patient, respectively. Some student-centered objectives follow:

a. To name and locate all the bones of the body
b. To explain the effects of hot wet dressings upon superficial and deep tissue circulation

Student-centered objectives are the type found most commonly as educational program objectives. Some patient-centered objectives follow:

a. To regain optimal health status
b. To learn how to calculate and administer insulin in self-care

Patient-centered objectives are commonly found in nursing care plan goals and in patients' bill of rights statements. Quality control forms also use this type of outcome objective.

It is important to notice the relations among the three types of objectives. For both education and service, it must be said that what ultimately counts is the outcome. If students learn well, pass boards, and have appropriate professional skills and attitudes, it really does not matter how the teacher taught or how the school was organized. Similarly, if the patient regains and maintains optimal health, it does not matter how the nurse nursed or how nursing service was organized. If outcome objectives are attained, success is assured.

If, however, the student fails boards or the patient fails to recuperate as anticipated, then one must ask why they failed (outcome). One can seek the defect in the student (she failed to study) or in the patient (he refused medications and ignored orders). If examining the client does not reveal the failure, one next asks how the teaching or the nursing was deficient, i.e., what went wrong in the *process*. If the providers seem to have proper skills, then one must ask how the organization failed to utilize those skills, i.e., what impediment occurred in the *structure*. Objectives thus form a logical series: outcome can be affected by process, and process can be affected by structure.

It is interesting to compare the focus of objectives as typically used in nursing service and nursing education. Nursing education programs usually focus on outcome objectives, and nursing service division objectives usually are stated as processes. There are several logical reasons for this difference. First, it is easy for nursing education to define outcome goals, for all students in the educational program have the same goal. Each student is expected to reach or exceed a set level of attainment of knowledge or skills for each course. For nursing service, it is not possible to set the same outcome goal for each patient. The only way such uniformity can be attained is to make objectives relevant to return to health, maintenance of health, and attainment of optimal rehabilitation. Outcome goals of this nature are too broad to direct nursing practice, so they are not especially valuable.

To attain useful outcome goals, the professional nurse must set individualized goals for or with each patient, considering his past health state, the nature of his present impairment, and his motivation, resources, and capacities. The educational program has similar outcome goals for each student; nursing service has a multiplicity of outcome goals since patients have different needs. Some inroads have been made in nursing service by setting unified goals for patients with the same impairment or health status: the obstetric patient, the amputee, and so forth. Still, the diversity among patients with similar impairments requires unique adjustments in the use of such group goals.

A second reason outcome goals are easier to evolve for nursing education than for nursing service is that students are active participants in the teaching-learning process, whereas patients may or may not have this status. There is a trend toward more active involvement of the patient in his own therapy and goal setting, and activation of the patient role appears to provide better outcomes. The model, however, does not fit all patients: some do not have the capacity for such participation. Even if the patient refuses an active role, therapy can still be done for him. The student, however, cannot take a passive role and still learn. Learning is an active process: teachers cannot "pour" learning into an empty receptacle.

Another problem with outcome objectives is that if they are not reached, they do not "tell" what went wrong. It takes an active investigation to find out what went wrong. If the patient has a bladder infection, one cannot immediately determine that it happened because Nurse X did process Y. An investigation must be made in order to determine the relationship of an outcome to ongoing processes. In education, since outcome objectives are the same for each student, the relation of outcome and process is less complex. If twenty students learn obstetrics in a satisfactory manner and one student learns nothing, it is usually fair to assert that the fault can be located in the student, not in the teacher. Similarly, if twenty students fail to learn, it is easy to infer that the teacher is the weak spot. Even here, however, the outcome failure does not say what was wrong in the teaching process.

The focus of objectives can be on structure, process or outcome. It would not be inconsistent to have objectives for all three foci, but most organizations do not adopt this procedure. Selection of a focus, be it on structure, process, or outcome, depends upon the nature of the content of the objectives or on the preferences of the nurse administrator. Often, accrediting boards may force such a decision on the nursing program.

(Unless the reader is particularly enthralled with the machinations of composition and structure of objectives, she will probably do better to skip this section. It may add confusion to what seemed clear in the preceding section. The expert will recognize that the preceding section made certain linkages for the sake of simplicity. Those linkages (structure to organization, process to nurse, and outcome to patient) should be adequate for the average user of objectives, but they are not absolutes, and one could consider structure, process, and outcome for each of the subject matters separately.

For example, the patient has structures—structures of body and structures of mind. Similarly he has processes—voluntary and involuntary body processes as well as learned performances. The organization, likewise, is more than structure; it has organizational processes and organizational outcomes. A similar case can be made for structure, process, and outcome for the nurse. Indeed any entity may be viewed simultaneously from these three perspectives where such detailed observation is useful. For most purposes, however, organizational structure, nursing process, and patient outcome will be adequate. (Organizational structure, process, and outcome will be addressed in a slightly different context in Chapter 5.) Furthermore, overelaboration of objectives may become a deterrent to action. Construction of objectives for all possible perspectives of organizational work becomes an overwhelming task, and implementation of such a plethora of objectives becomes impossible.)

Reference Sources for Objectives

It is impossible to talk about objectives without considering their degree of attainment and the way attainment is measured. Perhaps the most common reference against which objectives are measured is a *group norm*. A student's attainment of course objectives, for example, may be determined by her ranking among her classmates on a series of teacher-made examinations. In this case, the reference norm is that of her own class. If the teacher were to determine the student's attainment of course objectives by NLN examinations, the reference norm would be that of student nurses all over the nation. Thus, both teacher-made and standardized tests can be used to evaluate attainment of objectives by use of group norms. The teacher may also distribute grades (measures of attainment of course objectives) based on her concept of grade distribution. She may use a normal distribution or some other preconceived distribution curve of her own.

This is simply another way of creating norms for reference.

Nursing service also uses norms by which to evaluate objectives. Such norms are often unwritten, but they still exist. The nurse who determines that a new surgical patient is ready to ambulate has used a norm of readiness indicated by the patient's muscle strength, pulse status, and toleration of upright positioning. Similarly, the nurse has a norm which indicates when a dressing needs to be changed. She also has a norm that indicates when a postpartum patient is bleeding "too much." In nursing service, norms are learned primarily by experience. From multiple experiences with patients, the nurse derives norms by which to interpret and evaluate patient outcomes and care events.

A second reference source for objectives is the *behavioral statement of expected outcomes.* Nursing education often prefers this criterion-referenced system. In this case, norms are not used, but an absolute standard of performance is identified by which to measure attainment of the objective. With this concept, it would be possible for all students to receive A grades if they could attain the described behaviors. Mastery learning concepts are based on criterion-referenced objectives. This type of reference source is particularly useful in nursing for the following reasons: 1) Selection procedures in most schools of nursing usually result in a class population with academic talent well above normal. Thus it is not fair to submit these students to the normal curve distribution. 2) It makes more sense to have an absolute standard of professional competence than to let the attainment of objectives depend upon status within a particular class of students.

Quality control systems are the criterion-referenced sources in nursing service. When a determined criterion for the nursing unit is that no patients will develop decubitus ulcers, this criterion becomes the measure of the quality of nursing care. The nurse who remarks that it is "normal" for an obese,

paralyzed patient with poor circulation to have bedsores misses the point of the absolute standard. The criterion-referenced objective sets a goal which may or may not coincide with a norm.

A third reference source for objectives is that of individual growth. In nursing education, instead of being compared to other students or to some absolute standard, the student achievement in this system is compared to the student's own past record. He is evaluated on rate of change, amount of added knowledge, or on some established criterion which relates his present status to his own past status.

Nursing service often uses individual growth as a reference source. Evaluating the progress of a patient in a rehabilitation program typically takes this form. An objective for a stroke patient is set, not by what stroke patients "normally" do, nor by the ideal outcome for a stroke patient; instead the goal set is based on the patient's own progress to date.

Structure of Objectives

Bereiter identifies four different kinds of objectives: trait level, formal level, program level, and rule level[1]. Each type has a different internal structure and each serves a different purpose. It is important that the nurse adminstrator recognize each type of objective in order to judge its appropriateness when it appears in a given context.

Trait Level Objectives

The trait level objective describes, as its name indicates, aspects of the individual's makeup. Examples might include such items as emotional adjustment, flexibility, creativity, adequate self-concept. In nursing, objectives of this type often are found on student clinical evaluation forms and on employee appraisal forms. They include such categories as professional behavior, ability to organize, personal appearance, interpersonal relations.

Bereiter notes that objectives of this sort describe a state of being rather than an event. The aim of such an objective is not a particular behavior but production of a certain trait in the nurse. The presence or absence of this state of character is inferred from various sources of evidence. One problem with state of being objectives is that they are not generative of corrective measures for noted deficiencies. To tell a nurse, for example, that she lacks *initiative* in no way directs the nurse or the evaluator as to how to correct that deficiency.

Trait objectives have the further disadvantage of being taken as judgments of the character or personality of the nurse. The nurse is much more likely to be resentful and defensive if she is told, for example, that she is "disorganized" than if she is told that her sequencing of events is inefficient. In addition to these problems, the evaluator may have difficulty in reaching agreement with the nurse as to her status concerning trait level objectives. Since the asserted trait is an opinion of the rater, it is possible that the combination of observed events the evaluator groups as demonstrating a particular trait will not be accepted as evidence of that trait by the nurse or, indeed, by other evaluators. For example, the events that lead the rater to characterize the nurse as "inflexible" may be interpreted by the nurse as adherence to basic principles. Trait level objectives therefore are not particularly useful, whether the person being evaluated is a student or a nurse practitioner.

Formal Level Objectives

Bereiter's next type of objective, the formal level objective, defines a certain stage of development. Piaget's stages of concrete or abstract operations are examples[2]. An IQ of 120 is another example. A formal level is made up of numerous behaviors that are seen as "going together" to make up a particular plateau of attainment. This constellation of behaviors makes up the grouping structure.

In nursing education, NLN-required "level objectives" use the concept of the grouping structure. In nursing service, departments that differentiate levels of clinical performance (Clinical Nurse I, Clinical Nurse II, etc.) typically use grouping structures. In such formal level objectives, the acquired stage of development is inferred from behaviors in a number of tasks; these tasks are examined to ascertain if they reveal the grouping structure which is defined as a particular level. The question is: Does the behavior in aggregate conform to the criterion model?

Objectives of this sort have many of the same problems as do the trait level objectives. The formal level objective again describes a state of being, not an event. Thus, to say that a student nurse does not reach the "junior level" does not really say anything because it does not have a meaning without reference to the events that led to this interpretation. Thus, again, the objective is a composite opinion, removed from the actual nurse behaviors.

Formal level objectives have another drawback which is even more burdensome than that of the trait level. The trait level objective, at least, represents a single entity, whatever that trait may be. The stage of development in the formal level objective, however, represents a conglomerate of multiple behaviors. One then has great difficulty in judging if a nurse has reached a particular level. What if a nurse requesting promotion from Clinical Nurse I to Clinical Nurse II has reached several of the level components, excelled in a few, and failed to reach a few others? It is exceedingly difficult to describe this nurse in relation to a level she has partially met, partially not met, and partially exceeded. One then is forced into the weighting of categories and other sorts of gyrations to reach conclusions about attainment of such objectives.

In addition, formal level objectives, like trait objectives, are not generative of remedial programs. To tell a nurse that she has not reached the Clinical Nurse II level does not tell her how to get there. To be directive, one is forced to dig back into the materials on which the judgment was made.

Program Level Objectives

The third type of objective is the program level objective. A program level objective describes the desired performance on a task. Program objectives have the advantage of describing outcomes rather than traits. If the evaluator finds the individual deficient in an objective, the objective is generative of correction because it describes the outcome the individual failed to demonstrate. Program level objectives describe the desired goal for the nurse rather than telling what the nurse herself should be.

Process Approach. Program level objectives are not handled identically by all evaluators. Two different approaches can be identified. Some evaluators prefer a degree of precision whereby each objective spells out the exact task to be performed, with all the particular specifications. These process-approach objectives often are called behavioral objectives. Mager typifies this approach; his objectives are detailed so as to be self-teaching references[3]. Mager's rules for construction of objectives may be summarized as follows:

1. Identify the terminal behavior which is evidence of achieving the goal. (The writer of the objective describes the observable actual performance, what the nurse is doing when she demonstrates achievement of the objective.)
2. Describe the conditions under which the behavior is expected to occur. (Any qualifying conditions are identified and described.)
3. Give the criterion of minimal acceptable performance. (The writer tells to what extent, in what quantity, or how accurate the performance must be.)

An example of an objective meeting Mager's criteria might be: Given a drawing of the human skeleton, the nurse can correctly name 90 percent of the bones.

Gagne gives a similar set of rules for structuring behavioral objectives; they can be paraphrased as follows[4]:

1. Describe the stimulus situation.
2. Denote the observable behavior by action word or verb.
3. Give the term denoting the object acted upon.
4. Give the characteristics of performance that determine its correctness.

This form of program objective states in detail the actions of the individual in meeting the criterion; it states exactly what the person should do. Since these objectives describe the process through which the individual goes in meeting the objective, they can be termed *process objectives.*

The advantages of process objectives are clear. First, they provide a precise criterion for evaluation; second, they afford great assistance in selection of learning experiences; and third, they give the nurse an explicit description of the expectations.

There are, however, disadvantages as well as advantages. In order to specify objectives to the degrees suggested by Mager and Gagne, it is necessary to have objectives for small units. If, however, every curricular or nursing activity has its own objective, then part of the utility of objectives is lost. Objectives are usually seen as directing the learning efforts of students or the performance efforts of nurses to aspects of critical importance. If there are hundreds of objectives, this directivity is lost. Using the rules of Mager and Gagne, there is no way to group objectives into larger statements of goals.

Another problem with process objectives is that of the invariate behavioral response; only one discrete process is accepted as correct. Faced with stimulus X, the process objective expects each nurse to give identical response Y. Such invariate response is possible on lower levels of cognition or in psychomotor skills of a simple, repetitive nature. Such objectives do not allow for differences in behaviors as they occur in application, analysis, synthesis, or evaluation. Where different processes are equally capable of producing the same or equivalent results, the process objective cannot be used as a standard.

Product Approach. A less restrictive adaptation of the program level objective is used by many evaluators. In this mode, the behavioral outcome is defined without specifying the exact steps taken in reaching the goal. Samples of this form might include: "To describe the anatomic abnormalities present in spina bifida." "To meet the emergency nursing needs of the individual with massive internal hemorrhage." These objectives describe what the nurse does without placing restrictions upon how she does it. Thus they can be termed product objectives; they examine the product of the nurse's activity.

The difference between product and process objectives can be seen if one considers the related evaluating activity. For the process objective, any observer, including the nurse being assessed, clearly can see whether her behavior matches the objective's statement of behavior. For product objectives, correspondence of behavior to objective must be evaluated by the expert in the field. Take, for example, the educational objective, "To explain how arteriosclerosis affects blood pressure." Unlike process objectives, this objective does not direct the student's form of explanation, nor does it require that any two students go about meeting this objective in the same way. What is evaluated is the product of the student behavior; the quality and completeness of the student response is determined by the expert rather than being specified in the objective itself. A psychomotor task clearly illustrates the difference between process and product objectives. The process objective evaluates by detailing all the steps in the procedure; the product objective examines the finished product.

Product objectives have the advantage of being adaptable for different degrees of specificity. These statements allow one to combine many smaller objectives under one broad statement. Thus product objectives lend themselves to the creation of broad course and curriculum objectives or to development of hierarchical objectives for nursing service.

Construction and evaluation of the product objective follows a pattern different from that of the process objective. Construction of the product objective aims to describe the results of the nurse's activities as clearly as possible. The statement should be so phrased that it conveys the same meaning to all evaluators familiar with the content area. Evaluation of the product objective is more complex than that of the process objective. The process objective is constructed so as virtually to describe the test situation for evaluating the attainment of that objective. The product objective, however, does not indicate the means of testing its attainment. To rate a product objective, the evaluator must identify situations that will stimulate the nurse to create the product described in the objective. Not only must the test situation be capable of evoking the desired result, it must elicit that result from the nurse, if the result is within her repertoire.

Evaluation processes in nursing education regularly plan for such contrived testing situations. Nursing service, however, is more likely to evaluate the nurse behavior that occurs, given the present unit environment, rather than behavior intentionally elicited. This means that it is legitimate for a product objective on an employee appraisal form to be marked, "not observed," if the nursing environment was not such as to elicit that particular behavior. Even nursing service has some objectives that are not left to chance. For these objectives, employees are tested either at time of hiring or at periodic intervals following skill maintenance education.

Advantages of the product type of objectives are that they can be made for higher order mental activities requiring analysis, synthesis, or evaluation. Also, with the product type, objectives can be formulated for large units, such as entire courses (education) or entire nursing departments (service); this is not possible with the process type.

The disadvantage of the product objective is that there is greater possibility of disagreement between two judges as to the meaning of the product objective compared with the process objective. In addition, the product objective gives less guidance to the nurse in terms of estimating her level of attainment.

Rule Level Objectives

Bereiter proposes a fourth type of objective, which combines the advantages of both types of program objectives (process and product)[1]. His *rule level objective* describes specific behaviors like the process objective, yet has the advantage of allowing for multiple responses like the product objective. The rule objective is based on the structure underlying the assessed experience. Bereiter uses the example of language. When one understands a language, one can generate an infinite number of different, but grammatically correct, sentences. Rule objectives for language behavior seek out and identify the rules underlying language construction. For example, one rule objective would be, "every sentence must contain a subject and a predicate."

Rules for mathematic operations would be another example. To evaluate the attainment of any rule objective, sample behaviors are examined to see if they apply or fail to apply the rule. Clearly such rules can be identified for nursing behaviors.

Bereiter asserts that any important teaching is really the teaching of rules underlying some phenomenon. Use of rule objectives merely makes the evaluator responsible for making these rules explicit instead of implicit. In nursing, one can see application of rule objectives by examining behavioral modification programs in psychiatry. A rule such as, "If you don't socialize, you don't get tokens," applies the rule objective concept. Nursing education programs oriented around the presentation of nursing principles have adopted the rule objective concept.

In summary, several structures can be used in formulating objectives. To compare and contrast these structures, objectives with similar content (body mechanics) are given to illustrate each type.

1. Trait level. The nurse has grace and is well-coordinated in body movements.
2. Formal level (for student at "freshman level"). The student can state the basic principles of body mechanics. She applies these principles with assistance from her instructor.
3. Program level.
   a. Process type. Given a bulky object to lift, the nurse increases the distance between her feet by at least six inches.
   b. Product type. The nurse uses body mechanics in such a way as to protect herself from physiologic stress or strain.
4. Rule level. To lift a bulky object, one increases stability by widening the base of support.

OBJECTIVES AND PHILOSOPHY

Selection of objectives should be consistent with the organization's philosophy. In the following example, three different philosophies of education are examined to determine their effects on the statement of objectives. Essential points of each philosophy are given in Table 4-1. These philosophies have been selected to represent one middle and two end positions on a continuum relating man and his environment. In philosophy A, environment dominates as the important factor in learning, and in philosophy C, man predominates. B represents a middle position where man and environment interact on each other in a fairly equal ratio. These three points on the continuum should be adequate for purposes of illustration.

The relationship of man and environment has been selected as the pivotal criteria

Table 4-1 Philosophies

Questions Relevant to Teaching-Learning Process	A Association	B Interaction	C Process
What is primary in the relationship of man to environment?	Environment	Interaction between man and environment	Man
How does the primary element work?	Environment stimulates response (through senses)	Man and environment act on each other. Environment gives problems, man seeks ways to use the environment to solve them	Man is adaptive, uses *cognition*, is able to anticipate
What is man?	A programmed machine, programmed by others	An actor-reactor, a problem solver	An energy system in dynamic equilibrium
What determines behavior?	The environment	A mixture of environment and man	Man—his perceptions and drives, he is disposed to act in certain ways due to his goals
How does the individual affect the learning process?	Individual differences are secondary; environment is primary	Problems and solutions are unique for each learner	Dynamics of growth, are more important than status at any one time; individual differences are crucial; maturation is a basic concept
How does man learn?	By formation of a stimulus-response (s-r) bond, by association	By solving problems, selecting what stimuli appear as problems to be taken account of	By insight and cognition, reorganizing behavior to meet present demands
How does motivation work?	Learners seek to attain pleasure, to avoid pain; can use pleasure and pain stimuli to motivate students	The learner is motivated by realizing that a problem exists; what constitutes a meaningful problem depends on the environment and on the learner	Individual seeks an internal sense of adequacy; self-motivation is the rule
How do you teach?	Provide repetition for s-r conditioning, reinforcement by rewards and punishments	Situation set, help learner recognize problems, help him build methods of coping (problem solving)	Give him an opportunity to interact, and he'll learn patterns of adaptation
What is learning?	Association of desirable response with appropriate stimulus	Overcoming obstacles; learning to go about problem solving; adjusting the organism to the environment	Structuring a situation; establishing meaningful relationships
What about transfer of learning?	Transfer cannot be counted on—works only with "identical elements" in the training and transfer situations	Transfer takes place where appropriate generalizations have been learned; learner can use previous knowledge	All response is transfer, as all situations are new; transfer is learning; transfer is reorganization of previous response
What is the aim of learning?	Association of desirable response to appropriate stimulus, i.e., *the specific response*	Adjusting the man to his environment, *problem solving* is learning techniques of adjusting	Practicing *reorganization* in multiple situations

because of the nature of education. These philosophies are compared on issues relevant to the teaching-learning process.

How would philosophy A affect nursing objectives? It is clear that in this philosophy one stimulus yields one response (one specific behavior that is to be the same for all participants). Indeed, the aim of philosophy A is the creation of this specific product, i.e., the association of this response to this stimulus. Thus it would be logical to define an objective under this system as a specific behavioral response that is identical for all participants. Examples can be given of such objectives:

Basic education: The student, when given a list of 100 drugs, can correctly classify at least 80 among the categories of adrenergic, adrenergic blocking, cholinergic, or cholinergic blocking.

Continuing education: The nurse is able to place and attach 12 leads on the 12 appropriate body locations for the accurate recording of an electrocardiograph.

Nursing service: The diabetic patient, before discharge from the hospital, is able to accurately draw up in an insulin syringe any prescribed dose of insulin, using either U40 or U80 insulin.

These objectives correspond to philosophy A in several ways. First, they define the response expected from each participant. The objectives leave no room for variation; either the participant produces the right response or fails to produce the right response. The objectives describe the process by which the person responds. Clearly the program level, process type of objective is compatible with a stimulus-response theory of learning.

If one tries to apply process objectives to a type B philosophy, however, inconsistencies arise. The B philosophy admits that the participant has as much effect on the environment as the environment has effect on the participant. Therefore it would be illogical to expect any two participants to have exactly the same response, even if they were placed in identical environmental situations.

If one holds a philosophy of this orientation, it is not logical to state objectives so as to describe exactly how the participant will meet his goal. Instead, objectives should be stated in terms of identifying the problems that the participant must resolve. Examples follow:

Basic education: The student applies a sterile dressing to a wound without contamination.

Continuing education: The nurse is able to implement appropriate emergency measures for a patient with respiratory obstruction.

Nursing service: The patient with a leg amputation learns to walk safely with the use of crutches.

These objectives define the problem to be solved, without identifying the specific behavior which the participant will use in solving the problem. In the first example, two students might both successfully meet the criteria for applying a sterile dressing, one using sterile gloves and the other using sterile forceps. Thus, for this philosophy, fitting objectives would identify the problems to be resolved, leaving the participant free to utilize the environment in any way that will appropriately solve the problem. Focus is placed on clearly defining the problem situation; the aim is resolution of that situation, not some specific behavior. Whatever behavior resolves the problem successfully meets the criterion.

Philosophy B requires an event language because the resolution of problems is an interaction between man and his environment. Hence, to describe a trait or formal level for the individual would not give proper recognition to the part the environment plays in both defining and resolving the problem. Thus this philosophy clearly is compatible with product type program objectives. Rule level objectives would also meet the needs of this philosophy.

Philosophy C demands yet a different perspective on objectives. Here the focus is neither the participant's behavior nor the particular problem; the focus is the participant himself. Thus, consistent objectives would need to be stated in terms of growth and movement in the participant. The following examples are consistent with this philosophy:

Basic education: The student becomes efficient in organizing her work.

Continuing education: The nurse acquires needed skills for a Clinical II rating.

Nursing service: The patient progresses from dependence to independence in relation to self-care.

For this philosophy, with its focus on the learner, trait level and formal level objectives are fitting, for they tell something about the person rather than about events. The state of the individual is what counts in philosophy C, and that can be measured by two different methods: 1) comparing this individual to others (norms) or 2) comparing this individual to his own past status.

Clearly, selection of a format for objectives should be consistent with the organizational and divisional philosophy. The philosophy of education and the philosophy of nursing are likely to influence the reference source, the structure, the focus, and the content of both educational and management objectives.

SPECIAL CHARACTERISTICS OF MANAGERIAL OBJECTIVES

Much of the previous discussion of objectives has highlighted differences between educational and managerial objectives. A few more differences must be mentioned, especially since much literature on nursing management objectives draws so heavily from the works on objectives in education. There are several real differences which make the adaptation of educational literature less than ideal.

First, the educational literature assumes that the achiever of objectives is the single individual (the learner). In nursing administration, this is not always the case. While the staff nurse may be the achiever of some performance objectives, it is just as

likely that an objective will be achieved by some organizational entity (a unit, a department, or a whole division). The measure of achievement of objectives by complex, multiperson entities is more complex than the educational paradigm.

In addition the educational paradigm is one of voluntary activity involved with learning. Achievement of managerial objectives has as much to do with performing as with learning. Simply put, education is only one way to achieve managerial objectives—and not the major one. More actions are controlled by directive (supervision) than by education. Sometimes this educational paradigm gets in the way of good nursing management. When the nurse executive or subordinate manager assumes that everyone will do what they know (have learned), management may suffer from this naiveté. Ideally, this model should hold for professional behavior, but even here there is "slippage," requiring management and direction as much as education.

The educational model, moreover, deals exclusively with *acts,* whereas not all objectives in nursing administration deal with acts. One may deal with states of being, e.g., the fluid and electrolyte balance in a patient or the clarity of lines of relationship in an organizational chart. Again, not all nursing management—administratively or at the patient level—deals with voluntary acts. Furthermore, if one deals only with the educational paradigm, one becomes insensitive to the potential objectives concerning the structures in which nursing delivery acts occur.

Finally, educational objectives are concerned exclusively with outcomes. Earlier in this chapter, it was indicated that outcomes represent a final court of judgment as to achievement. Although this is true in one sense, it is false in another. For in addition to those outcome goals of a nursing division, there are secondary goals related to managerial efficiency. Hence, if a patient reaches the desired outcome goals following a cardiovascular accident, the judgment of success is contingent; first the nurse executive must ask if those desired objectives could have been reached equally well with fewer resources, fewer nursing hours of care. Effectiveness is only one measure in administration; efficiency is another which cannot be ignored, especially in a cost-conscious age.

SUMMARY

The purpose statement of a nursing division represents the first concrete document delineating goals. Typically the general purpose of the division is elaborated into a number of objectives, usually seven to ten, which are seen as being capable of achieving that purpose when taken together. These objectives usually are distributed through subobjectives over the entire nursing division. In this manner responsibility for achievement of objectives may be spread through the different organizational levels and structures according to a logical plan. Organizational levels and structures may contribute additional, usually more specific, objectives incurred locally by the special functions which these organizational entities perform. Taken together, the purpose statement and the elaborated divisional objectives represent the major goal statements of a nursing organization.

REFERENCES

1. Bereiter, C. Psychology and Early Education. In Brison, O.W., and Hill, J. (Eds.), *Psychology and Early Childhood Education*. Monograph Series No. 4. Toronto, Canada: Ontario Institute for Studies in Education, 1968, pp. 61–78.
2. Piaget, J. *The Psychology of Intelligence*. New York: Harcourt, Brace and World, 1950.
3. Mager, R.F. *Preparing Instructional Objectives*. Belmont, Calif.: Fearon, 1962.
4. Gagne, R.M. The Analysis of Instructional Objectives for the Design of Instruction. In Glaser, R. (Ed.), *Teaching Machines and Programmed Learning, Vol. 2. Data and Directions*. Washington, D.C.: National Education Association, 1965, pp. 21–65.

BIBLIOGRAPHY

Alexander, E.L. *Nursing Administration in the Hospital Health Care System* (2nd ed.). St. Louis: C.V. Mosby, 1978.

Bloom, B.S., Hastings, J.T., and Madaus, G.F. *Handbook on Formative and Summative Evaluation of Student Learnings*. New York: McGraw-Hill, 1971.

Brady, R.H. MBO goes to work in the public sector. *Harvard Business Rev.*, 51(2):65, 1973.

Cain, C., and Luchsinger, V. Management by objectives: applications to nursing. *J.O.N.A.*, 8(1):35, Jan. 1978.

Christman, L. Where are we going today? *J.O.N.A.*, 6(2):15, Feb. 1976.

Donovan, H.M. *Nursing Service Administration: Managing the Enterprise*. St. Louis: C.V. Mosby, 1975.

Drucker, P. *Management: Tasks, Responsibilities, Practices*. New York: Harper & Row, 1973.

Fiedler, R.E. A Contingency Model of Leadership Effectiveness. In Berkowitz, I. (Ed.) *Advances in Experimental Social Psychology*, vol. 1. New York: Academic Press, 1964, p. 150.

Lasagna. J.B. Make your MBO pragmatic. *Harvard Business Rev.*, 49(6):64, 1971.

Moore, M.C. Philosophy, purpose, and objectives: why do we have them? *J.O.N.A.*, 3(4):21, July–Aug. 1973.

Odiorne, G. *Management by Objectives*. New York: Pitman, 1965.

Palmer, J. Management by objectives. *J.O.N.A.*, 1(1):17, 1971.

Resnick, L. *Design of an Early Learning Curriculum*. Pittsburgh, Pa.: Learning and Development Center, University of Pittsburgh, 1967.

Skarupa, J.A. Management by objectives: a systematic way to manage change. *J.O.N.A.*, 1(2):52, 1971.

Stevens, W.F. *Management and Leadership in Nursing*. New York: McGraw-Hill, 1978.

Chapter 5   Nursing Goals and Management Goals

Nursing administration is a synthesis of two disciplines, nursing and management, in which both disciplines are altered because of their interplay. The nature of this interplay is especially important in relation to goals. The goals of nursing are primary—that is, they remain ends in themselves—whereas the goals of management are instrumental—that is, they have meaning insofar as their achievement advances the achievement of the primary goals. Management goals are not lost or ignored; they simply become instruments through which nursing goals are better achieved. (Nursing goals in this chapter refer to both the formalized and the informal objectives of the nurse executive for her division.) Clearly, to achieve an appropriate synthesis of nursing and management and of their respective goals, the nurse executive must have expert knowledge of both disciplines.

The effective nurse executive simultaneously fills two roles: nursing leader and organizational manager. By virtue of her managerial position, the nurse executive becomes the main spokesman for nursing within her institution. It is likely that the position gives her similar leadership opportunities in the professional nursing community and in the community at large. Hence it is critical that the executive use the authority and status of her position and her identity as leader for the advancement of professional nursing as well as for the advancement of nursing within her own institution.

The nursing goals, formal and informal, for a given institution, are derived from the interplay of several factors:

1. The nurse executive's vision of vanguard clinical practice, her idea of where nursing as a profession ideally is heading.
2. The situational context in the given nursing division, that is, the nature of the extant environment and the nature and level of nursing practice in the given institution at the present time.
3. The efficacy with which management goals, values, and techniques may be applied in moving the nursing division toward vanguard clinical practice.

PROFESSIONAL NURSING GOALS

It is important that the nurse executive be clear about her vision of nursing, where nursing is going, what future should be carved out for it. She must be able to identify and communicate her vision of nursing both within and outside of her institution. Her professional goals for nursing are important regardless of the "state of the art" in her own organization. The communication of this projective vision concerning professional nursing has a critical motivation potential. The nurse executive sets the tone of a nursing division, and part of that tone has to do with how she envisions and enacts professional nursing. Her perception of vanguard clinical practice is important, whether or not her division is yet ready to practice at that level.

Hopefully that vision of vanguard clinical practice will be one arising out of a personal philosophy and value system compatible with the nursing theory and nursing philosophy of the extant nursing division.

Ideally that vision will be one which conceives of nursing as a legitimate discipline, with its own domain for scientific inquiry. Obviously, since she is working in and through a health care organization, the executive will have a conception of vanguard clinical practice which is consistent with the notion of the organized delivery of nursing care. The nurse executive's vision of vanguard clinical practice serves to inspire others as well as to differentiate and define nursing practice. It serves as a banner and as a goal for those professionally oriented staff members who are interested in their personal professional development as well as in the advancement of nursing practice within their institution.

NURSING GOALS FOR THE DIVISION

Next, the nurse executive must determine her goals for nursing within *her* division. These goals may or may not coincide with her concept of vanguard practice, depending on the stage of development of the division. Since vanguard practice is on the frontier of nursing development, it is unrealistic to think that many institutions will be practicing this kind of nursing. Nevertheless, it is important for the executive to convey how her goals for the division link to that vision of ideal practice—how her divisional goals for nursing move the division in the right direction.

Even where executives agree upon the nature of vanguard clinical practice, the extant nursing practice in their respective settings may vary greatly. Different divisions may select different methods of reaching the same clinical goals, and different divisions may be at various levels of development toward those clinical practice goals. Nor can the nurse executive be judged by an absolute standard of nursing care produced. Obviously a director who takes a substandard division and elevates it to the level where it is providing good, safe nursing care, actually may be more effective than her counterpart who inherits a nursing division with a higher level of nursing care and does nothing to advance it. Professional nursing *vision* may not be limited by the developmental state of the organization, but it is clear that the specific nursing *goals* for a division are constrained by the situational context. A nurse executive in a small community hospital will oversee a different application of nursing than will the nurse executive in a major urban research- and education-oriented hospital complex.

Nevertheless, these two nurse leaders are likely to share certain professional values and objectives. They both will desire to implement the best possible nursing care, given the nature of their staff, their resources, and the patient populations served. Both will have a clear conception of what constitutes a safe level of nursing care in their setting, and neither will tolerate forces which seek to undermine safe practice. Further, both will be seeking to upgrade the level of nursing practice in their respective institutions, whatever the level of care already may be. Hence, because they share professional values and knowledge, nurse executives share in setting the boundaries for nursing practice: they determine the baseline beneath which practice may not fall, and they determine the level of practice toward which their nursing divisions should aspire.

Both vision and managerial instrumentality enter in determining the institutional nursing goals. The nurse executive uses her nursing vision and managerial skills to get the best possible nursing care given the contextual situation in which she finds herself. A director, for example, cannot create clinical specialists where few exist; she cannot hire many collegiate graduates if there are no college programs in the local community; she cannot improve the quality of the physicians' care as it affects nursing's domain. Nor can she wish for an ideal budget in an institution which is struggling to stay solvent in a hard economic year. These are situational constraints which must be taken into account (as must others like them) in determining nursing goals for a division.

Even in a difficult situation, an effective nurse executive can provide an environment where nurses are challenged to improve their practice and to respect professional nursing values. The nurse executive sets the tone; either she raises the vision, ambition, and insight of her staff or she fails to do so. Her vision of nursing—if it is respected and she is respected—will filter down through the nursing organization.

Thus, management goals and nursing vision combine to optimize on delivery of specific organizational nursing care goals. To be an effective leader in the achievement of nursing goals, the nurse executive must have both professional nursing vision and managerial effectiveness.

MANAGEMENT GOALS

Management goals, though instrumental, are important because if they are not achieved, nursing goals are not likely to be achieved either. The major management goals reviewed here are: control, effectiveness, economy, and efficiency. Note that these management goals are "process goals" in that they do not state *what* is to be controlled, effective, economic, or efficient. In other words, these goals could be applied to *any* content. In this case they are applied to nursing.

Even though these management goals are not content-specific, most of the management literature concerning these and other goals has been formulated by its authors with some underlying image of the context to which it applies. The management literature tends to explain goals in relation to some underlying ideology of the work world. Often this imagery bears little relation to the work world of nursing. Indeed, the managerial imagery often focuses on an industrial setting, usually that of the factory assembly line. For this reason, the management literature may seem inapplicable or may require significant adaptation for application to the nursing environment. Table 5-1 endeavors to contrast the typical work world ideologies of management and nursing. If the nurse executive is sensitive to these

differences, she may be better able to make appropriate applications (or modifications) of principles from the management discipline.

Given these ideological differences in setting and operations, it is not surprising that cure-alls suggested by managers unfamiliar with the hospital or other health care setting, frequently are inapplicable or, at best, inadequate. Where management programs fail to synthesize the management process and the nursing context (let alone the nursing goals), it is not surprising that inexperienced nurse executives cannot apply them. Experienced nurse executives must carefully consider contextual and ideological differences before they judge the application of a managerial principle or technique to be appropriate.

Control

Control is a major management principle; it specifies management's ability to monitor and adjust the work process. If one does not have control of the processes of production, one cannot be held accountable for—or effective in—achieving one's goals. Similarly, control is important for nursing as a discipline. No discipline can research and advance its practices unless it controls those practices and inquiry processes.

Control is likely to be problematic in the nursing context for several reasons. First, nursing takes place in complex organizations where it must negotiate with other power groups that traditionally have controlled or partially controlled nursing practice. Furthermore, the nursing division, as the hub of patient-related activity and as the custodian of the patient, is affected by more other individuals and managerial units than is any other health care unit of the organization. Indeed, functions of others such as the medical staff to a great degree dictate some specific work functions of nursing. At best, interdigitation with other individuals and units of the organization requires ongoing negotiation concerning who is responsible for what.

Table 5-1.   Comparison of Typical Management and Nursing Ideologies of Work

Subject	Management Ideology	Nursing Ideology
Raw materials (Entering client)	Uniform, with predictable reactions to processing	Diverse, not alike in all responses to processing
Process of production (Nursing)	Known, easily prescribed for each product	Some nursing acts known; many still being researched with relations to product unsure
Product (Exiting client)	Limited number of uniform products	Extensive number and classes of products, with each unit somewhat unique
Workers	Interchangeable; most do programmed tasks	Not interchangeable; many levels, few programmed tasks
Goals	Determined and directive of production	Under exploration, changing; negotiated between the ideal and the feasible
Time frame	Nine-to-five mentality; time to plan ahead as the norm	24-hour, continuous present; often crises with no advance planning time
Interaction with environment	Planned, controlled, based on production needs	Unplanned, uncontrolled, based on environmental needs (of patients and physicians), pressured
Decision making	Few key decisions yearly, usually made at the top	Critical and continuous decision making at all times, multilevel
Evaluation	Regulative, prescribed quality control procedures and systems	Problematic as evaluation techniques complex, often yet to be created; must evaluate complex phenomena

Finally, nursing has difficulty in asserting control of its own domain of practice because its client often is perceived of as "belonging" to the physician. Hence, if the physician objects to certain independent nursing functions or nursing research, he may demand that "his" patient be excluded from the given nursing process. Such intervention, if supported at higher levels, can do irreparable damage to nursing research attempts and can impair the consistent use of selected nursing strategies. Moreover, under present arrangements, it is not possible to ignore the economic power exercised by physicians in exerting their preferences. In present health care financing patterns, physicians have the power to withhold profit from an organization simply by taking "their" patients elsewhere. As nursing advances and differentiates its practices from that of medicine, patients should begin to select an institution on the basis of the nursing care rendered there. At present, however, it is still a fact that most patients are advised by their physicians as to which health care institution to enter.

Obviously, nursing as a profession must strive to make its aims, objectives, and services evident to potential clients. Individual nursing divisions need to establish mechanisms whereby the client can be informed concerning level and type of nursing care rendered.

Historically, nursing has made some errors in the exercise of the principle of control. For example, 20 years ago, the head nurse usually had total control of her unit. She gave orders to housekeepers, janitors, and secretaries as well as to nursing staff. In more recent history, nursing pulled away from the doing of "non-nursing" tasks by nurse practitioners. Unfortunately, this trend was accompanied by divesting nurse managers (head nurses) of the responsibility for managing non-nursing tasks. Nurse managers also were left "free" to "manage nursing." Today, for example, if the ward secretary is rude or simply incompetent, the head nurse may have to go through a separate management chain of non-nurse managers to seek a solution. Indeed, she may be unable to remedy the situation if these managers disagree with her interpretation of the secretary's behavior. Since separate organizational divisions and departments tend to develop their own unit-specific goals and measures of performance, there is even greater likelihood that such different interpretations may occur.

Today's head nurse is forced on all sides to use a negotiated order model of management in which she must reach agreement with other managers before action occurs. This is clearly a complex management

system and one without a great deal of inherent *control* in any one managerial position. Similar illustrations could be offered for all levels of nursing management in regard to loss of control (including the executive level). This trend toward complex, interdigitating, competitive control centers may be inevitable; yet one cannot help but wonder if nursing, in the name of "freeing nurses to do nursing," may have exchanged "control" for "freedom." Ironically, without control over its exercise, real freedom disappears.

Nursing management must strive to achieve the instrumental managerial goal of control if it is to advance its own discipline and its own practice. To do this the nurse executive must assess what control is necessary and sufficient for achievement of her nursing goals, and then she must set out, systematically, to acquire such control.

Effectiveness

Effectiveness, as a managerial goal, is the satisfactory achievement of one's objectives. In nursing there are several measures of effectiveness: 1) Quality control (quality assurance) tools and systems measure the statistical effectiveness of nursing care in reaching defined or selected patient care goals. 2) Performance appraisal tools and systems measure the effectiveness of performance of the individual worker. 3) The evaluation component of the nursing care plan determines the success or failure in the individual patient case. 4) External review standards, such as those of JCAH, and internally derived standards serve to supply criteria for evaluating nursing division operational effectiveness.

Some objectives of a nursing division represent absolutes, goals which are either achieved or not achieved—for example, the goal "to convert to planned program budgeting." Other objectives are such that they may be achieved, not achieved, or surpassed; an objective "to have an RN staff of whom 50 percent hold baccalaureate degrees" fits this category. Measures of effectiveness may be proportionate or absolute. For example, the following objective is proportionate: "that no more than 10 percent of clients receiving birth control education return with an unwanted pregnancy within three years." This would be absolute if stated as follows: "that no more than 30 clients receiving birth control education return with an unwanted pregnancy within three years."

Whatever form of objective is appropriate for a given measurement situation, it is the responsibility of the nurse executive to see that measures of effectiveness be determined for all major nursing goals. These measures give concrete data upon which to judge the overall effectiveness of the nursing division. They also provide the basis upon which one makes decisions concerning needs for alterations in the methods and resources used by the division. A measured failure in effectiveness indicates the need for a different delivery system for that particular element of the nursing system.

Effectiveness, then, is the management term which stands for the achievement of one's goals. Determinations of effectiveness are judged through the setting of standards relative to major objectives and the measurement of the achievement of those standards by various quality control systems. Nursing has had some long-standing quality control systems, such as performance appraisal. Other such systems, such as quality assurance of patient outcomes, are relatively new.

larger portion of its gross national product in health care. Nor is it logical for health care providers to demand that all health care needs be met before investments in other societal values (e.g., education, culture, leisure) be addressed. It is no longer feasible or reasonable to educate nurses to anticipate that they will be given the resources for "total patient care." Instead, they must be taught to set priorities, to differentiate essential care from provision of amenities, to relate care given to the cost of providing that care, and to make judgments which consider factors of cost versus benefit. Indeed, in an era of scarcity, one does not choose between the desirable and the undesirable but between the desirable and the more desirable. The attitude of careful choice for investment of resources begins with top management; the nurse executive must derive systems that monitor for economy, and she must impart a philosophy of economy to the nursing staff.

Economy is a management principle which usually is measured by financial indices. In nursing there is a tendency to connect economy with frugal use of supplies since their cost is evident. While frugal use of supplies is certainly important, the greatest expense in a nursing division is that of salaries. Hence careful use of employees' time is the greatest source for economy. For example, for a nurse executive to have many prolonged and unnecessary meetings attended by an excessive number of employees is the greatest waste of resources possible (even though it is not as obvious an economic loss as is the waste of supplies).

Economy

The management principle of economy dictates that the nurse executive get the most for her investment, that she be thrifty in the use of resources, be they financial, material, or human. In the present era with its focus on cost containment, economy of operations has even more significance than in the past. The nation's population has reached a point at which it is unwilling and unable to invest a

Efficiency

The managerial principle of efficiency will be defined here as a combination of effectiveness and economy, as meeting one's objectives with the least outlay of resources. Efficiency often is reflected in management ideologies as some index of units produced per time period. In nursing this idea applies in many cases: number of patients seen in a clinic per hour, the number of obstetrical deliveries per shift, the number of surgical cases per operating room per day, or the number of nursing hours per patient day. In nursing, however, such measures of unit/time mean little if, for example, the clinic patients processed did not receive appropriate nursing or if the nursing hours per patient day were inadequate for delivery of essential care. Hence the term, efficiency, as used here will reflect the quantitative element (units per time period, manpower per shift, equipment used per case), but that unit measurement will be deemed efficient only when it is both *economical* and *effective*—that is, when it reaches the objectives for the given activity.

Where measures of efficiency show deficits, several decisions are possible: 1) One may determine that the objective must be achieved in different (more economical) ways; this is cost effectiveness analysis. 2) One may determine that the objective should be dropped if it cannot be achieved at a reasonable cost; this is cost/benefit analysis. 3) One may reassess the appropriateness of the measurement standard which was applied for evaluation. Even where efficiency is achieved or where standards are surpassed it is still important to ask the questions that characterize these economic analyses: Could the objective be achieved even more economically? Is the achievement of the objective worth the cost? Are the standards too low?

SUMMARY

Nursing goals and management goals interdigitate in several ways at the nurse executive level. The nurse executive's vision of the professional goals for nursing, her knowledge of managerial instrumental goals, along with the context of her particular division and institution, all interplay in her setting of specific nursing goals for her division. Nowhere is it more evident that nursing management synthesizes nursing and management than in the selection of goals for a nursing division.

The nurse executive is responsible for building a system of evaluation and control so that she can know when her goals are and are not achieved. With this feedback she can alter the nursing system as needed to achieve—or better achieve—her goals. Much of nursing management has to do with the evaluation and subsequent modification of the nursing system so as to achieve predetermined goals. Instrumental management goals assist in both measurement and achievement of those nursing goals.

BIBLIOGRAPHY

Bracken, R.L., and Christman, L. An incentive program designed to develop and reward clinical competence. *J.O.N.A.*, 8(10):8, Oct. 1978.

Ethridge, P.E., and Packard, R.W. An innovative approach to measurement of quality through utilization of nursing care plans. *J.O.N.A.*, 6(1):25, Jan. 1976.

Felton, G., et al. Pathways to accountability: implementation of a quality assurance program. *J.O.N.A.*, 6(1):20, Jan. 1976.

Ganong, J., and Ganong, W. Strengthening the nursing service organization. *J.O.N.A.*, 7(7):14, Sept. 1977.

Hegyvary, S.T., and Haussmann, R.K.D. Monitoring nursing care quality. *J.O.N.A.*, 6(9):3, Nov. 1976.

Hegyvary, S.T., and Haussmann, R.K.D. Nursing professional review. *J.O.N.A.*, 6(9):12, Nov. 1976.

Hegyvary, S.T., and Haussmann, R.K.D. The relationship of nursing process and patient outcomes. *J.O.N.A.*, 6(9):18, Nov. 1976.

Hegedus, K.S. A patient outcome criterion measure. *Supervisor Nurse*, 10(1):40, Jan. 1979.

Malkiel, B.G. Productivity—the problem behind the headlines. *Harvard Business Rev.*, 57(3):81, May–June 1979.

Marriner, A. (Ed.) *Current Perspectives in Nursing Management*. St. Louis: C.V. Mosby, 1979.

McConnel, C.R. Why is U.S. productivity slowing down? *Harvard Business Rev.*, 57(2):36, March–April 1979.

Moloney, M.M. *Leadership in Nursing: Theory, Strategies, Action*. St. Louis: C.V. Mosby, 1979.

Weinstein, E.L. Developing a measure of the quality of nursing care. *J.O.N.A.*, 6(6):1, July–Aug. 1976.

Part II

Structures of Nursing Management

Part II of this book examines those aspects of nursing management which provide the structures through which the goals of nursing are realized, the structures that constrain and direct the events that occur within the nursing division. Chapter 6 explores the mechanisms by which purposes and objectives are converted into key functions and concrete activities for the division and its subunits. It also examines the cumulation of activities into constellations for role performance called jobs; standards used to evaluate functions and constellations of activity also are reviewed.

Chapter 7 examines the ways in which these functions and concrete activities are coordinated and grouped into large organizational units such as departments and committees. Principles and decisions for departmentalization are examined insofar as they relate to key divisional functions. Determinations of key functions and determinations for departmentalization interact, for departments are the managerial units which implement the functions of the division.

Chapter 8 looks at the quantitative estimates of activities resulting in assigning, staffing, and scheduling of personnel. Once again, these managerial activities are found to be highly interdependent, each system influencing decisions made in the other systems.

Chapter 9 explores how patients and staff are classified. Staff activities are examined as they relate to patient needs. Mechanisms here include various patient classification systems and clinical ladders for nursing staff. The chapter also considers how patients should be placed (on what units) within the health care organization.

Chapter 10 examines policies, procedures, and practices affecting the nursing systems. These rule systems specifically direct the events which occur in the division.

Structures of the nursing division take many forms. Some are relatively permanent: organization charts, assignment systems, job descriptions. Others are more fluid and changing: work schedules, assigned tasks, work policies. Together these permanent and changing structures organize the work of the division. Often these structures interact with each other. For example, the functions of the division partially determine what departmentalization scheme is selected. Conversely, where a departmentalization plan already is in effect, it may affect the selection of key functions for the division. Similarly, the staffing plan will interact with the assignment system; certain assignment plans require different staffing from others. The nurse executive cannot consider any structure in isolation; she must consider each organizing structure as it affects and is affected by other structures.

Chapter 6
Concretizing Goal Statements: Functions and Standards

To identify the purpose and objectives of a nursing organization is not the end of the administrative task. The executive must also determine how the goals set are to be achieved. Two mechanisms come into play: 1) determining what activities must be done to achieve the goals, that is, deriving functions and activity plans, and 2) setting expectations as to how well those activities must be done, that is, determining standards. This is the most critical stage of management because it is here that ideas are translated into action, where notions become—or fail to become—reality.

There are several types of so-called functions discussed in the nursing management literature. In this chapter we will look at three different sets: nursing divisional functions, job functions, and the functions of the nurse executive. These functions are derived primarily from the objectives for the division, the job, and the executive role respectively.

FUNCTIONS OF THE DIVISION

The functions of a nursing division represent the critical juncture where goals are translated into acts. The functions of a nursing division are the constellation of key activities perceived as necessary and sufficient for the achievement of the divisional goals (usually elaborated as a purpose and subsequent set of divisonal objectives). Objectives are assumed to achieve the divisional purpose if they themselves are achieved. It is important to recognize the obvious: that objectives are goal statements but that having goal statements does not assure that the goals will be achieved.

The next step in organizing is to ask what actions must be taken in order to achieve each objective. When a single objective is considered alone, the requisite actions designed for its accomplishment are identified in what is commonly called an activity plan. An activity plan is detailed; it tells who will do what, when, where, and how. This detail is possible because the activity plan addresses a limited subject matter (a single objective).

When a number of objectives are considered together, the actions required to achieve them jointly are usually called functions. Functions are the broad, key activities which, if taken together and successfully completed, assure attainment of the group of objectives.

The divisional functions which achieve the divisional objectives usually do not match objectives one for one. For example, a single function may accomplish three objectives. Conversely, a single objective may require a number of functions for its achievement. For example, the objective "to provide adequate and able nursing staff for competent care delivery" might be partially achieved by each of the following functions:

1. Develop and supply job descriptions for each level of personnel within the division.
2. Establish criteria and procedures for hiring, evaluating, and dismissing personnel.
3. Maintain an effective staffing plan which ensures adequate personnel placement.
4. Hire nursing division personnel as needed to fill the staffing plan.

One usually considers divisional objectives and functions as a constellation rather than individually, asking: Is this group of functions necessary and sufficient for the achievement of these objectives? Do these functions identify the key activities of the division?

Drucker notes that there are four kinds of functions: result-producing activities, support activities, hygiene and housekeeping activities, and activities of top management[1]. This observation is important because it identifies sources for functions other than goal statements.

Many organizations publish statements on functions of the nursing division. The American Hospital Association has such a statement specific to administration in the hospital setting[2]. Its brochure identifies functions related to: provision of nursing services; implementation of philosophy, objectives, policies, and standards; delineation of authority and duties; coordination within the institution; staffing; relations with patients and community; participation in personnel policy; record and report systems; continuing education; and relationships with formal education programs.

The American Nurses' Association has its own statement of functions, published in the form of standards[3]. Topics addressed include: philosophy and objectives; responsibility for quality of nursing practice; leader participation on policy-making bodies; integration of the nursing program into the organization; budgetary participation; departmentalization and organization; personnel policies; utilization of personnel; orientation and continuing education for staff; participation in student education; research activities; and evaluation of clinical and administrative practice. The National League for Nursing publishes a similar list of functions in a form termed "criteria"[4].

The American Nurses' Association also publishes standards (functions) for general nursing practice[5] and for specialized forms of practice[6]. These, however, address hands-on practice, and will not be dealt with here. In essence, most of these lists of standards represent some modified form of the so-called nursing process.

Objectives, Functions, Standards, and Criteria

It is important to note the difference among the three forms used by the American Hospital Association, the American Nurses' Association, and the National League for Nursing in their statements. Typically, a list of *functions* merely gives the topics to be included; such a list does not purport to give a mechanism by which to measure the performance of the included functions. The American Hospital Association chooses to use this terminology (functions) in its publication.

The term, *standard,* on the other hand, usually indicates a statement worded so as to enable one to judge its achievement. Standards are operationalized and allow the user to compare the actual performance or state with the written statement and to judge the degree to which a given function is achieved. The American Nurses' Association uses this terminology (standards) in its publication. Obviously, one may argue the merit of the selected terminology in any given case. Was the subject matter presented as topics or as evaluative statements? Was the appropriate terminology then applied?

The semantics is further complicated by introduction of an additional term, *criterion*. This term sometimes is used interchangeably with *standard*. Sometimes criteria are presented as those variables to which standards apply; in this interpretation, a criterion is a topic whose status is not evaluated until standards have been determined for it. While a *function* (whether or not it has been operationalized) indicates an action to be taken, a *criterion* (as commonly used) may give little indication of intent. For example a function might read, "provide an ongoing program of continuing education for staff." A corresponding criterion might be stated simply as "continuing education." Whether or not it is to be provided, avoided, or ignored would not be revealed until one read the subsequent criterion measures (sometime called standards). The National League for Nursing has chosen this terminology (criteria) for its publication.

The major message for the careful reader is to recognize that these common terms are not used consistently in the literature. Their meanings must be determined in the context of the document or article in which they appear. See Bloch for one useful interpretation of most of these terms[7]. For purposes of the rest of this chapter, the generic term *functions* will be used to refer to the key activities being described for the nursing division. It is important, however, that the reader become sensitive to the various forms used for statements of functions and to the purposes these forms purport to serve.

One also must differentiate between the entities discussed above—functions, standards, and criteria—and the entity termed the objective. Objectives are goals; functions are acts which achieve them; standards are the concretized acts which are taken as indices of the achievement of the underlying objectives. (As mentioned previously, the term, criterion, although used in diverse ways, still represents the measurement side of this issue.)

Where objectives are operationalized to a high degree, as recommended by Mager (see Chapter 4), it may be difficult to make such differentiations between objectives and standards. Usually, however, standards are seen as the measurements by which achievement of objectives is judged. Thus two or three concrete standards might be taken as evidence of the accomplishment of a single broad objective. Again, the reader is cautioned that use of the terms *objective* and *standard* may vary from author to author.

Some authors differentiate standards from objectives by reference to mini-max levels of achievement. In this conception, the term *objective* usually is used to refer to the higher level, the desired level of achievement, and *standard* is used to represent the lower level, i.e., baseline of acceptable performance. When achievement is weighed

between mini-max levels, another term, the *norm,* may enter consideration. Since the norm only speaks to the average condition, it may or may not coincide with a desired level. Often the norm is equated with the standard, but there is no reason why a standard might not be set higher than a present norm in reference to some given subject matter.

Distribution of Functions

Like divisional objectives, divisional functions represent an early phase of *differentiation* in the nursing organization. Indeed, divisional specialization begins when specific functions are assigned to different organizational units. It is equally important, however, to view and evaluate functions together as a whole. Only in this way can the *integration* of the nursing division be maintained. The organization of a nursing division is achieved with finer and finer discriminations, but always with a view from the whole. It is the function of top management to integrate and orchestrate that view from the whole. And each step of differentiation—selection of objectives, of functions, assignment of organizational units—must be viewed by the nurse executive as it affects the whole.

Divisional functions and their coordinated objectives are distributed downward through the organizing frameworks, the departments, units, and committees. As indicated in the introduction to Part II, the organizing frameworks themselves may be determined by the way in which functions are separated or combined. Thus one might create a staff education department if most staff education functions were kept together. If, on the other hand, staff education functions were dispersed, there might be no need for a single education department, and each nursing unit might be responsible for creating its own unique staff education program. In other instances, the nurse executive might treat her organizing framework of departments, units, and committees as givens, determining which functions she wishes to distribute in each of these "given" organizational entities.

Functions are distributed through several organizational structures. First, they are distributed by departments (main subclassifications of the nursing division) and by nursing units (subclassifications of the nursing department). Some functions, in contrast, are distributed within the committee structure of the division. Within those departments, units, and committees, functions are further delegated through various job descriptions and role expectations. Specific activities also are delegated through the assignment system.

The rules for derivation of divisional functions may be summarized as follows:

1. Identify the constellation of key activities necessary for achievement of divisional objectives.
2. Add functions required to *support* the activities identified as achieving the objectives. In a nursing division, such activities as continuing education and research might be considered supportive to a divisional objective of patient care.
3. Include essential hygiene and housekeeping activities required to maintain the division, for example, record keeping, employee health services, or secretarial services.
4. Add the key activities of nursing top management which have not been addressed under objective-achieving activities. These might include such activities as organizing the division or developing management staff.
5. Check to see if the selected functions are compatible with one another as a constellation of coordinated activities; revise as necessary.
6. Ensure that key functions are necessary and sufficient for achievement of divisional objectives.
7. Ensure that functions can be achieved within the division, given its departments, units, and committee structure; revise either structures or functions accordingly.

The rules which pertain for divisional functions also will serve for departmental and unit functions. All organization subunits also will need to specify their particular functions, those unique to the subunit and those in which they participate jointly with other subdivisons. Just as one objective might be distributed over several functions, so a single function may be distributed over several departments or units. Conversely, a given function might be assigned to a single department or unit if it requires specialization for its enactment.

JOB FUNCTIONS

Divisional functions (key activities) ultimately are differentiated into the specific tasks and responsibilities of which they are comprised. These discrete tasks and responsibilities are then sorted into relevant job constellations. Each constellation of functions should conjoin items of equivalent complexity, and the assortment of tasks and responsibilities in a single job should be of a compatible nature. Each job classification should represent a reasonable work pattern for a qualified individual. Obviously, the number of workers required for each job classification will depend on quantitative calculations: How many times do the job activities need to be repeated?

Considered as a whole, the job classifications of a nursing division should provide for completion of all tasks implied by the divisional functions. Job classifications are the final step of differentiation in organizing a nursing division and ultimately stem from the divisional functions. However, just as functions interplay with organizational departmentalization, so specific job tasks interplay with organizational policies. Policies may make the completion of tasks easier or more difficult. The nursing systems chosen to organize the work, such as the assignment system, also affect the nature of job descriptions. These interacting elements will be discussed in subsequent chapters of this book.

In a world without constraints or traditions, the nurse executive would determine her job classifications simply by logic and her sense of fit. Even today, the nurse executive is free to create many job classifications of her own choosing, but she is limited in the skilled professions by state licensing laws which restrict certain functions to certain classes of workers. Hence legislation, as well as tradition in nursing services, places some constraints on how job functions are bundled together. The nurse executive is likely to hire from established classes of workers such as RNs, LPNs, and various technicians. Nevertheless, even where established classes of workers are selected, their job functions may differ significantly from institution to institution.

The historical move to create institutional licensure was an attempt to do away with all constraints on job classification. As long as certain licensed groups of workers retain rights and privileges regarding performance of certain tasks, the nurse executive will have limitations on how she can bundle tasks and responsibilities. Nevertheless, most nurse executives accept this limitation as a small price to pay (in managerial flexibility) for the many benefits to be gained by maintaining discrete professional and occupational groups within nursing.

General principles in creating job classifications include the following:

1. The job classifications of a division should arise primarily from the necessary work to be done, not merely from the traditions and legal constraints.
2. Job classifications should clearly differentiate the expectations for different levels of workers, and the salary structure should reflect both required skills and job responsibilities. The nurse executive must be careful that the different levels in jobs are clear. For example, she should clearly demarcate staff nurse (RN) tasks and responsibilities from LPN tasks and responsibilities if she intends to justify having two separate job classifications.

3. Job classifications should be added, removed, or revised if the work of the division significantly changes. For example, advocates of all professional staffing claim a decline in unskilled or semiskilled tasks within the nursing division, necessitating removal of some lower-level job classifications.
4. In addition to considering each job classification singly, there may be a need for radical redistribution of all divisional tasks into new job classifications at some time in the history of a given institution. Some job enrichment programs focus on creating more meaningful collections of tasks within a given job. The differentiating out of certain tasks and responsibilities to secretary and unit manager classes of workers represented a major historical reshuffling of job classifications in nursing.
5. In some institutions job classifications are coordinated and classified institutionwide, according to level of difficulty and responsibility. In this case, the nurse executive must see that her job classifications are appropriately placed and coordinated with other institutional job classifications according to their required skills and responsibilities. Retrospective job analysis often is used in making such judgments or in revising job classifications which have become obsolete.

Job Descriptions

Constellations of job functions are documented in job descriptions. Job descriptions contain many other elements in addition to the tasks and responsibilities classified. An adequate job description contains at least the following elements:

1. A specific job title.
2. A job number or coding which indicates the level and classification of this job in relation to other jobs in the division or institution.

3. Reporting relationships (both to whom one holding the job is responsible and for whom one is accountable).
4. Summary description of the position, its key functions, and major responsibilities.
5. Substantive detailed list of responsibilities and/or tasks.
6. Real and potential hazards of the position: environmental, psychological, physiological, chemical, biological.
7. Qualifications for holding the position, usually educational and experiential. Some institutions also identify requisite personal characteristics if they can be clearly associated with success in the job.

Some cautions are in order regarding the writing of job descriptions. First, a job description should tell what is specific to a given position. One should not write a job description in which most functions are assistive in nature: "assists head nurse to . . . ," "assists head nurse in developing . . . ," "assists head nurse in managing . . . ." A job description of this sort does not give clear criteria for determining performance of the incumbent.

Second, as the position responsibility increases, the job description will be less programmed; as the responsibility decreases, the job description will be more programmed. For example, the job description for the nurse executive should describe many responsibilities but few specific tasks. This is because the nurse executive has the freedom to select those mechanisms by which to achieve the job responsibilities. The nurses' aide job description, in contrast, should list fewer responsibilities, and the ways in which those responsibilities are to be carried out should be specified as tasks: "takes TPRs as assigned" (a task) rather than "evaluates patient's physiological status" (a responsibility).

Even in contructing a job description for a position of limited responsibility, the nurse executive must be careful to allow leeway for unspecified tasks at the same level of skill and responsibility. To do so the list of tasks can be headed "characteristic tasks," so as to indicate the incompleteness of the list. Another device is the inclusion in the list of one general element which reads, "other tasks as assigned." It is important that a nurse executive not limit herself by trying to imagine and include all possible job eventualities in the job description. Consider one case, for example, where RNs carry blood samples to the laboratory while nurses' aides sit at the desk. The nurse executive in this situation was foolish enough to agree in a labor contract that nurses' aides would do *only* those tasks specified in their job description. Needless to say, she failed to think of every sort of appropriate task when composing that job description.

FUNCTIONS OF THE NURSE EXECUTIVE

The functions of the nurse executive in one sense blend the functions of the division and the functions of a given position. This is so because the nurse executive ultimately is responsible for all functions of the nursing division. Her job functions therefore necessarily reflect the divisional functions. Once again, the reader may find functions or standards for this position published by many nursing and related groups, namely, the American Nurses' Association[8], the National League for Nursing[9], and the American Hospital Association[10].

Rather than reiterate the divisional functions for which the nurse executive is accountable, this chapter will isolate the particular functions that the nurse executive performs either by herself or in conjunction with her top management team, the tasks which constitute the executive function. Whether performed with others or singly for simplicity the executive function will be discussed as if it were achieved by the nurse executive alone.

The Executive Function

The executive function includes those specific tasks and responsibilities which can be achieved only with a view of the whole, a view from the top. Thus only the nurse executive (or those few managers whom she allows to share her perspective of the totality) are capable of performing the executive function. The executive function includes several critical functions: providing vision, setting goals, solving problems, bridging, negating, and unifying. These are intellectual activities of the nurse executive, and her decisions in respect to these activities affect her entire division and the entire organization.

By providing vision, a twofold image of where nursing as a whole and her particular nursing organization are headed, the nurse executive brings about the envisioned future. She enacts in the present those conceptions of nursing which she wants to be real. Her conception of nursing, where it is going, and what that means for her nursing division comprise her vision. In providing vision, the nurse executive actively forms the future by her enactments in the present.

Her vision directly affects the major goal-setting activities of the division. Yet the vision itself is more than the specific goals selected; it is the ethos of nursing and nursing care which permeates the organization. Thus the nurse executive bears the burden of "setting the tone" of the division.

This is the ultimate, if subtle, meaning of leadership in nursing administration. The nurse executive who directs a division without vision, albeit with efficiency, ultimately fails in her greatest obligation and her greatest opportunity. Failure to see the significance of the vision into the future often is evident in those who argue that a non-nurse can function as a chief executive of a nursing division. While there are exceptions to any rule, it is rare that a non-nurse is so talented as to envision the future of nursing and to win the following of a division of professional nurses toward her vision for their profession.

Nor can this vision simply be equated with the goals set. Compare two nurse executives with a similar vision of nursing as a developing scientific, independent profession. One nurse executive might exemplify this vision by establishing an active nursing research department; the other, instead, might foster inquiry-based practice among her staff nurses. Thus the "vision" is broader than any specific goal exemplifying it, though it directs what goals will be set.

Similarly, the vision of the nurse executive will have an impact on executive problem solving. To a great extent, the executive's vision determines what problems are recognized, how they are cast, and what sorts of solutions are sought. Problem solving, here, refers to major problems whose resolution will affect the entire nursing division. Such problems typically are nonroutine, unique, nonrepetitive.

In addition to providing vision, goal setting, and problem solving, the nurse executive also plays a bridging role. Bridging takes at least three forms. In the first form, the executive bridges among the various departments and components of her division. This sort of bridging is represented in the well-known linkpin function; the director simply makes the organizational components fit together and function as a single machine.

The second form of bridging is between the conceptual and the actual. Here the executive bridges the gap from the world of idea, represented in her plans and planning documents, to the world of actual performance. In this bridging the ideas take on reality by being exemplified in nursing practice.

The third form of bridging is a temporal one from the present into the future. Present acts are created with future desired states in mind. Development of human resources for future organizational needs is a part of this bridging. Trend setting and working toward enactment of planned changes are part of the picture.

Another significant executive function, that of negating, is often overlooked. Yet it is critical that the dysfunctional, the impairing, be weeded out. Negating (or nest cleaning) is essential if the nursing division is not to be weighed down with unnecessary burdens of past policies and practices. Nest cleaning should be used like sunset laws (wherein an agency is not renewed unless it can substantiate its productivity and utility). In this case, the nurse executive needs to eliminate dysfunctional policies, practices, and procedures which have accumulated over time within the nursing division.

A final executive function is that of unifying the direction and purpose of all visionary, goal-setting, problem-solving, bridging, and negating activities. These functions must be coordinated and must complement each other. For example, the nature of the nest cleaning required may relate to concurrent problem solving; or goal setting may require special attention to various bridging activities. While attending to all these executive functions, the nurse executive simultaneously acts to stabilize and to unify the direction and purpose exemplifed in the executive functions.

The reader will recognize the foregoing executive functions as skills represented in Drucker's list of functions under the category top management. These functions affect the whole division and they must be achieved at the top. They represent the essence of leadership and direction for the division.

Organizing the Executive Function

Seldom is the executive function achieved solely by the nurse executive. Usually the director has a small cadre of top managers who share this responsibility. Sometimes the executive managers can be recognized by an organization chart; sometimes top management is an informal (nonofficial) group. For example, a nurse executive might have two supervisors (by whatever title) of surgical units. Both supervisors might excel in running their respective departments; but one might have extended communication networks throughout the organization, consult with other departments within the nursing division, and generally know the workings of the whole division. This supervisor might be part of the executive management, while her peer supervisor might not.

Top management often is an informal group for just this reason: managers gain entry to the group simply because of their ability to work from the view of the whole and to be effective in so doing. In addition to entry to top management by virtue of ability and manner of functioning, some positions are devised such that they necessarily give their incumbents top management status. An associate director's position, for example, probably carries responsibilities which place its incumbent in executive management. One almost always finds the director of staff education on the top management team. If this department is centralized, the communication network which is built by the successful incumbent ensures that she has the view from the whole which is the prerequisite for executive management.

The fortunate (or skillful) nurse executive will arrive at a complementary top management team. In this case there will be a natural division of labor based on preferences of the individual team members concerning those tasks which must be done at the top level. For example, if the director's own special skills are conceptual ones, she may want an energetic implementer (an action man) as one of top management. Similarly, if one member has excellent interpersonal skills on a one-to-one basis, there is probably a need for a top executive with a special talent for mass communication and public relations.

The nurse executive who tries to build her executive team out of members who are similar to herself is likely to have problems. Instead, she should strive for a balance of skills and preferred work activities. An ideal top management team exists when the division of tasks allows each member to do what she does best. This cannot occur where staff members share identical abilities and work preferences.

SUMMARY

The functions in the nursing division represent the enactment of purpose and objectives. Functions are the key activities that achieve the various goals of the division; divisional and job functions are two major types formalized in the operating documents of a nursing division. The functions of the nurse executive combine the divisional functions with the specific executive functions of top management; the latter may be the domain solely of the nurse executive or may be shared with an executive management team. It is important that the nurse executive and her staff seriously consider the functions whereby divisional objectives will be achieved. Objectives not incorporated into acts and functions are meaningless and unlikely to be accomplished. Ultimately, broad, generalized functions (key areas of activity) must be broken down into specific acts to be accomplished at specific times by specific persons. Some functions, like some objectives, are distributed downward through the chain of command to the extant patient care level; others are achieved at diverse levels of the hierarchical chain of command. Executive functions are achieved at the highest level of command.

REFERENCES

1. Drucker, P.F. *Management: Tasks, Responsibilities, Practices.* New York: Harper & Row, 1973, p. 532.
2. American Hospital Association. *Statement on Functions of a Hospital Department of Nursing Service.* Chicago: AHA, 1962.
3. American Nurses' Association. *Standards for Nursing Services.* Kansas City, Mo. ANA, 1973.
4. National League for Nursing. *Criteria for Appraisal of Departments of Nursing.* New York: NLN, 1978.
5. American Nurses' Association. *Standards—Nursing Practice.* Kansas City, Mo.: ANA, 1973.
6. See various other publications by the American Nurses' Association, such as those for practice in cardiovascular, emergency, and orthopedic nurs-

ing. Standards for specialty practice draw heavily upon the format determined in the generic standards for practice (noted in preceding reference).
7. Bloch, D. Criteria, standards, norms—crucial terms in quality assurance. *J.O.N.A., 7(7):20,* Sept. 1977.
8. American Nurses' Association. *Roles, Responsibilities, and Qualifications for Nurse Administrators.* Kansas City, Mo.: ANA, 1978.
9. National League for Nursing. *Role Expectations: Nurse Administrators, Governing Boards, Chief Executive Officers.* New York: NLN, 1977.
10. American Hospital Association. *Statement on the Position of the Administrator of the Department of Nursing Service in Hospitals.* Chicago, AHA, 1971.

BIBLIOGRAPHY

American Nurses' Association. A Plan for Implementation of the Standards of Nursing Practice. Kansas City, Mo.: ANA, 1975.

Finkelman, A.W. The standards of nursing practice and the supervisor. *Supervisor Nurse,* 7(5):31, May 1976.

Joint Commission on Accreditation for Hospitals. *Accreditation Manual for Hospitals.* Chicago: JCAH, 1971. Manual presently under revision. JCAH also publishes standards for other, specialized health services.

Moore, M.A. The Joint Commission on Accreditation of Hospitals: standards for nursing services. *J.O.N.A.,* 2(2):12, March–April 1972.

Nadler, G. *Work Systems Design: The Ideals Concept.* Homewood, Ill.: R. D. Irwin, 1967.

National League for Nursing. *The Role of the Director of Nursing Service.* New York: NLN, 1977.

National League for Nursing. *Nursing Administration: Present and Future.* New York: National League for Nursing, 1978.

Rotkovitch, R. The heartbeat of nursing services: Standard IV. *J.O.N.A.,* 6(4):32, May, 1976.

Stevens, B.J. ANA's Standards for Nursing Services: how do they measure up? *J.O.N.A.,* 6(4):29, May 1976.

United States Department of Labor. *Job Descriptions and Organizational Analysis for Hospitals and Related Health Services.* Washington, D.C.: U.S. Government Printing Office, 1970.

Chapter 7

Departmentalization and Committee Organization

Once the functions of an organization have been determined, the responsibility for them is distributed over organizational units such as departments and committees. As previously indicated, the nurse executive often determines both the divisional functions and organizational units simultaneously because of their interactions with each other. Just as in Chapter 6 functions were artificially differentiated out for close examination, in this chapter departmentalization and committee organization have been selected.

DEPARTMENTALIZATION

Departmentalization is the allocation of functions and responsibilities through a formalized arrangement of human and material resources in organizational units. Most health organizations are bureaucratic structures. This is true even for the nursing division which is highly decentralized. Even if the organization's head nurses were each to report directly to the organization's administrator, this would evidence some degree of bureaucratization, with control pyramiding up to a single responsible individual. Usually, even in the most decentralized institution, there are at least two levels of nursing management: head nurse (first-line) and director (nurse executive level).

Most nursing divisions, therefore, can be described by Weber's characteristics of a bureaucracy: 1) regular activities are assigned to fixed, official areas; 2) there are hierarchical layers and levels of authority such that higher levels control and supervise lower levels; 3) all important administrative directives are reduced to written statements; 4) people are selected and assigned to tasks on the basis of specialization; and 5) there is policy guidance for all activities of the organization[1].

Organization Charts

The organization chart is a graphic representation of the departmentalization process. Most organization charts are positional; that is, they are organized by title and rank, as in Figure 7-1.

Position and function, however, may or may not coincide. It is possible, therefore, to construct an organization chart based upon function rather than position, as in Figure 7-2. Unless function and position are closely tied, it usually is not possible to show both of these organizing principles in one chart.

Whether the organization chart is positional or functional, there are several common patterns for the distribution and relation of its components. The line pattern is strictly hierarchical, as shown in Figure 7-3. The line-staff pattern usually occurs where an organization is large and needs specialized functions (see Figure 7-4). In this example the two staff positions, or functions, are advisory extensions of the chief executive; they do not have responsibility down the line of command. Such staff positions are likely to be staff education, personnel work, accounting, or other functions that require special education or expertise. With the line-staff pattern, line people are relieved of a function that is better handled from a centralized position.

The third organizational pattern is typical of the institution that divides duties by function rather than by spatial congruence. This functional pattern is shown in Figure 7-5.

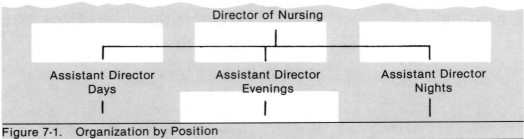

Figure 7-1.   Organization by Position

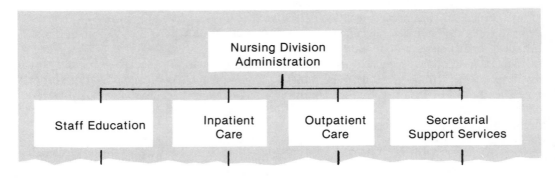

Figure 7-2.   Organization by Function

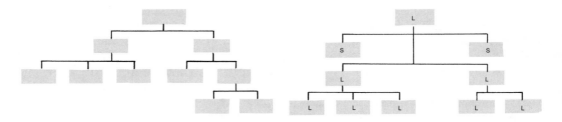

Figure 7-3.   Line Pattern

Figure 7-4.   Line-Staff Pattern

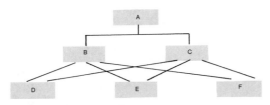

Figure 7-5.   Functional Pattern

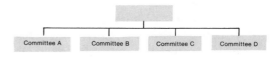

Figure 7-6.   Committee Pattern

Here, for example, C might be in charge of nursing care on units D, E, and F, while B might be in charge of general administration and materials management on those same units.

The fourth organization pattern is one in which committee structures are the vehicles for management (see Figure 7-6). This pattern of organization based on committee power is more common in nursing education than in nursing services. Its use as a mode of management in nursing service, however, is increasing as nursing services seek more and different ways to distribute nursing responsibilities.

Some few nursing divisions are organized by matrix rather than by hierarchy. This pattern is a complex construct in which an employee may be responsible to two or more bosses for different aspects of work. Figure 7-7 illustrates a matrix design.

In this illustration, a staff nurse is stationed on a given patient unit and is responsible to the head nurse of that unit. But if her patient care assignment includes an oncology patient, she also is accountable to Clinical Specialist I for the sort of care delivered to that patient.

Potential problems with the matrix type organization can easily be discerned. If, for example, the head nurse and the clinical specialist give conflicting orders to the staff nurse, her job may be untenable. Or the manipulative staff nurse may play her two bosses off against each other. Where a matrix organization is used, there must be clear decision rules. The employee must know which boss predominates when she receives conflicting orders or conflicting demands as to her work priorities.

Clear decision points will assist the employee but not necessarily the nurse manager. Suppose the staff nurse is to follow the head nurse's orders in case of conflict. Then the head nurse can make the clinical specialist's role very difficult if she so chooses; she can undermine her fellow manager by contriving to give countermanding orders until the specialist has lost all credibility with staff nurses as a manager.

Nevertheless, a matrix organization can be productive where clear rules are established and where good will predominates among peer managers. A sense of give and take and the ability to cope with a negotiated-order management model will enable the manager in this organization to develop a viable and productive role. The matrix model has solved problems of organization in many complex health settings.

Departmentalization in nursing is further complicated by the fact of 24-hour-a-day operation. Often there is a different organization chart for each shift. (The organization may need to be different because the functions of each shift may vary.) This situation is further confounded if certain units work 8-, 10-, or 12-hour shifts, respectively. When different organization patterns pertain during different hours, the authority and responsibility of these different organizational units and their interrelationships with each other must be clarified. Some organizations attempt to

	Head Nurse A	Head Nurse B	Head Nurse C
Clinical Specialist I in charge of oncological nursing practice	X	X	X
Clinical Specialist II in charge of cardiovascular nursing practice	X	X	X
Clinical Specialist III in charge of neurological nursing practice	X	X	X
X = Staff nurses			

Figure 7-7. Matrix Organization

simplify this organization problem by having a single organization plan, with 24-hour responsibility inherent in the positions of the officers of each department and/or unit. Whether 24-hour responsibility is realistic is a question to be answered in each extant case.

Besides considering departmentalization within the nursing division, it also is important to consider the departmentalization of the nursing division itself in relation to the rest of its parent organization. Even today, some nurse executives find that they fail to control all nursing practice in the organization. It is still not unusual to find that nurses in an emergency room, an operating room, or some other specialized unit may report to some manager other than the nurse executive. Where this pattern exists, it should be the nurse executive's highest priority to gain control of all nursing practice within her institution.

The nurse executive also will be concerned that the linkage of her department to the rest of the institution take place at an appropriate level so that she is reporting to the proper institutional officer. Given the size and significance of the nursing division, the nurse executive usually should report to the chief officer of the institution.

Criteria for Partitioning of Divisional Units

There are many criteria for determining organizational units. A nursing division usually combines several of the following criteria.

1. *Function.* The nursing division itself is an example of an organizational unit based on a function (nursing care). Within the nursing division, departments organized around function might include an inservice department, a quality assurance department, and an emergency room. In some instances, the functions which determine the organizational units are managerial, e.g., a nursing office or an accounting department. In other instances, the functions are based on nursing rather than managerial processes, e.g., an operating room suite or a coronary care unit.

2. *Customer.* An outpatient department might, for example, provide many different functions for a defined body of customers (nonhospitalized persons). Similarly an obstetric department might be seen as serving a specific clientele. In this case, one could argue the presence of two criteria, both customer and function, since similar processes occur for all customers of a like kind.

3. *Objectives.* Even where functions and customers differ in many respects, the criterion of desired outcome or objective may determine organizational units. For example, patients on a rehabilitation unit may exhibit all sorts of different impairments requiring diverse nursing therapies. Nevertheless, these patients may be gathered on a single unit since the staff shares a single objective for them all—optimal return to independent living.

4. *Geography.* Often a nursing department is created out of physically adjoining nursing units. Hence a supervisor may acquire 3 West, 3 East, and 3 North as her department, not because of similarities in patients, functions, or objectives, but because of their physical proximity. Geography almost always is a criterion for a head nurse's unit of responsibility. Even here, there may be exceptions. For example, a given head nurse may be responsible for all patients entering her geographic unit, whether or not they remain there. A discharge planning program, for example, may assign postdischarge care to the manager of the unit to which the patient originally was assigned. (In these cases, the criterion of customer takes precedence over the criterion of geography.)

5. *Logistics.* With this criterion, patients or subordinate units are joined under a single department if heavy interaction among units (or patients) is anticipated. Hence, postpartum mothers and newborn infants will be found in the same department even though they require different functions and are different customers. Similarly, preoperative, operative, and postoperative

units often are grouped under a single managerial department since they are linked by the sequential passage of patients through all three units.

In nursing management, it is important to examine the control question concerning departmentalization. Who makes the departmentalization decisions? Often nursing is expected to form its units according to criteria which better suit medicine than nursing. Where medical groupings consist of persons who need similar nursing care, e.g., a genitourinary unit, this may not present a problem. On the other hand, a medically determined neuropsychiatric unit may present the nursing department with diverse clients having diverse nursing needs. Nursing, since it provides a 24-hour ongoing service, ought to have control over its own departmentalization decisions rather than having that control in the hands of medicine, a service that only provides intermittent services.

Other Factors Impacting on Departmentalization

Several factors affect decisions about departmentalization, namely, span of control, number of hierarchical levels, centralization versus decentralization, and unity of command. These will be briefly reviewed.

1. *Span of control.* No nurse executive can manage effectively if too many persons report directly to her. An ideal (if abstract) span of control might consist of eight reporting persons. The nurse executive who has 20 head nurses reporting directly to her with no intervening management layer probably has exceeded a practical span of control. (This span might be acceptable only if the head nurses already were expert managers on their own, needing little day-to-day supervision or guidance.)

In contrast, an individual with fewer than four persons reporting to her may not really be needed. For example, an organization that has 10 head nurses reporting to five supervisors probably should reduce its supervisors to two or three in number. Professional organizations, however, tend to use smaller spans of control where the consultative process is frequent and necessary between superior and subordinate.

2. *Hierarchical levels.* The organization that has more than five, or at the most seven, levels of workers from the top person to the lowest-level employee is probably top-heavy with managers. The organization should aim for the lowest number of levels that can exist given the appropriate spans of control. The fewer the levels, the less distortion between management goals and the actual work done. Obviously, the larger the organization, the more hierarchical levels it tends to have.

Of necessity there is an important interplay between span of control and number of hierarchical levels. Where one increases, the other decreases. For example, if the nurse executive decides to eliminate the supervisory layer (a decrease in the number of hierarchical levels), then, instead of having four supervisors reporting directly to her, she will have 20 head nurses reporting directly to her (an increase in span of control).

3. *Centralization versus decentralization.* A division is highly centralized if major decision-making power and responsibility for key functions are concentrated in the top levels of that division. A division is highly decentralized if decision making and responsibility for key functions are delegated to the lowest possible managerial level in the division. Thus a centralized nursing division might have major decisions made by a council of the director and the associate directors. Such a division also would be likely to have many major functions, such as budgeting, staff education, quality assurance, and nursing research, in separate departments reporting directly to the nurse executive or her associates.

In contrast, a radically decentralized division might place most decision making at the head nurse level, with each head nurse running her unit independent of the decisions of her peer head nurses. Unlike a head nurse in a centralized division, the head nurse in a decentralized division would provide for budgeting, staff education, quality assurance, nursing research, and staffing of her unit from her own personal and unit resources.

Nursing organizations vary greatly in degree of centralization. The degree may differ for different tasks and responsibilities. There are general advantages and limitations to each mode of departmentalization. A highly centralized division, for example, usually commands considerable power, achieves economies of scale, and develops expertise in the specialized functions which are served by discrete departments. A limitation of a highly centralized operation is that it may not attract ambitious first-line and middle managers, those who are looking for authority and control over their own units. A highly decentralized division has the advantage of placing the decision making near the action; it also allows for diverse responses from managerial unit to managerial unit. Limitations of the decentralized form are that it loses economies of scale and that it sometimes shifts responsibility and authority to managers unprepared for them. For example, the supervisor who is responsible for providing inservice education to her own staff may not have the educational expertise required for the job.

4. *Unity of command.* According to this principle, each employee should report to one and only one boss. It is not fair to hold a person responsible to more than one boss, for to do so may expose him to conflicting demands. The reader will recall that this principle is broken by the mode of departmentalization in which different bosses are responsible for different functions. Hence a head nurse might be responsible to her supervisor for the quality of care on her unit and, at the same time, be responsible to another supervisor for staffing and scheduling. In this mode of organization, the possibility of conflict is supposedly removed because of the clear differentiation of tasks. The head nurse would always be accountable to Supervisor A for task A and to Supervisor B for task B.

A matrix organization further confounds the principle of unity of command. Here the employee might be responsible to two bosses for the same task. For example, the staff nurse might be responsible to the head nurse for the care of all her patients; at the same time she might be responsible to the clinical specialist for the care of those particular patients who fell within that specialist's practice domain.

COMMITTEE ORGANIZATION

The nurse executive's committee structure offers her another mechanism for distributing functions in addition to her departmentalization plan. The committee structure may be used for those functions which necessarily cross department lines. The nurse executive must be aware of a major difference between departments and committees, however. Departments have mechanisms for distributing functions downward to *both* groups and individuals. Committees, on the other hand, usually function by group activity. Since group activity is more costly, it should be used only where individual action is inappropriate.

It is important that the nurse executive understand the different bases of group formation so that she can select those options most useful for her own situation. The following kinds of groups or committees will be considered: 1) standing committees, 2) design groups (or task forces), 3) groups based on organizational position and job function, and 4) interdivisional committees that involve nursing with non-nursing divisions.

Standing Committees

The nurse executive reveals her operational definition of nursing in the selection of *standing committees,* for these committees represent the focal point of action in providing nursing services or nursing education. The following demonstration model compares the standing committees of two hypothetical directors of nursing services to illustrate how standing committees reflect the concept of nursing. Analysis is limited to the three primary standing committees for each director. (See Table 7-1).

A comparison of the committee structures of the two hypothetical directors will show some clear differences in their concepts of nursing. Director A is making a division of operations into products (things), procedures (actions), and patients (people). This is certainly a valid approach and tends to be rather comprehensive. In this approach to nursing, each sector is treated as a separate entity. In each case the committee has a specific output that clearly "belongs" to its particular sector (for example, a new product, a new procedure, a new care plan). There is little if any confusion about committee tasks; the job of each group is clearly delineated. This is probably one of the greatest strengths of a division into things, actions, and people. Under this committee structure, a change in any one committee can produce the necessity for a change in another committee. A new product, for example, might require a new procedure, but each committee is still very clear as to its own particular function. The committee structure gives a view of nursing as being composed of a series of separate parts which, when added together, comprise the totality of nursing.

Director B has a different concept of nursing. She tends to view nursing as a process rather than as consisting of parts. Her committees seem to flow from each other; work of the Care Evaluation Committee naturally leads to the work of the Care Improvement Committee. Similarly, improving patient care will call for changes in nursing systems. All three of these committees may involve things, actions, and people. All three focus on processes rather than on discrete entities. Some of the items that were *ends* for Director A (products and procedures) here become *means* to the goals of Director B.

For Director A, two out of three of her primary committees (new products and procedures) focus primarily on tasks. Her concept of nursing is that of a series of activities

to be done. For Director B, on the other hand, two out of three primary committees focus on the patient. Her concept of nursing reflects a needs-oriented approach. Director B starts with patient needs, while Director A starts with nursing tasks.

This difference can be illustrated by comparing the approach to a new product that each director might take. For Director A, a product is considered simply because it exists and had come to someone's attention; that is enough reason to evaluate it. Director B, on the other hand, does not approach products this way. When a particular patient need is identified, she then has a criterion for a products search, if a product is required to meet the need. In one system, the movement is from the product to the patient; in the other, it is reversed, from the patient to the product.

No one division of standing committees is right or wrong. There can be as many possible organizations of standing committees as there are different executives to think of them. The real question is whether the selected committee structure accurately mirrors the definition and philosophy of nursing of the organization. If an executive tries to indoctrinate her staff in a nursing philosophy which is not facilitated by the committee structure, she will have great difficulty. For example, an administrator who desires to implement a needs-oriented philosophy of nursing will have difficulty accomplishing this through a task-oriented committee system. Internal consistency among nursing concepts, divisional goals, and committee structure will simplify the work of the division.

Design Groups

A new trend which has put vitality into many nursing organizations is the increased use of design groups. The *design group,* sometimes called the task force, is a temporary committee, brought into existence to investigate and to propose solutions for a specific problem. The design group is a problem-solving, problem-oriented unit which ceases to exist

Table 7-1.   Comparison of Committee Structures

Director A	Director B
I. Procedure Committee 　A. Evaluates ongoing nursing practices 　B. Reviews and updates the procedure manual 　C. Composes new procedures as needed to accommodate new equipment, new supplies, or advances in nursing II. New Products Committee 　A. Assumes responsibility for keeping up to date on advances in equipment and supplies. 　B. Arranges for demonstration of interesting new products 　C. Evaluates utility and cost of each new product and recommends acceptance or rejection 　D. Implements purchase of selected new products and introduces the products to appropriate staff members III. Patient Care Committee 　A. Evaluates ongoing patient care 　B. Recommends changes in nursing care practices 　C. Evaluates and promotes patient safety 　　1. Reviews accident/error reports 　　2. Promotes safe working practices 　　3. Promotes a biologically and physically safe environment 　D. Recommends needed educational programs 　E. Develops new tools for use in patient care 　　1. Patient data forms 　　2. Nursing care processing forms	I. Patient Care Evaluation Committee 　A. Establishes criteria for evaluation of patient care 　B. Conducts quality control checks of patient care 　C. Conducts periodic nursing chart audits 　D. Provides for feedback to the nursing units and to nursing administration II. Patient Care Improvement Committee 　A. Uses feedback from Patient Care Evaluation Committee, accident reports, and other available data as a basis for instituting changes in patient care 　B. Identifies recurrent problems in patient care and seeks means of solving these problems 　　1. Identifies the care problem 　　2. Decides the appropriate avenues for solution 　　3. Institutes change 　C. Serves as an advisory group to the nursing staff education section III. Nursing Systems Improvement Committee 　A. Identifies problems in nursing delivery systems (examples: means of giving patient reports, means of assigning staff, means of distributing drugs) 　B. Proposes solutions to delivery problems by modifying old systems or creating new ones 　C. Plans and coordinates changes in nursing systems within the institution

once its problem is satisfactorily solved. Design groups tackle many different kinds of problems: administrative, procedural, interdepartmental, patient-oriented, or student-oriented. Indeed, they may be used for any problem which best can be solved by a select, informed group.

The composition of the design group is dictated by the problem itself. Those persons who have the most knowledge and experience to bring to bear on the subject are appointed to the committee. For example, a staff nurse with broad experience in primary nursing care might be chairman of a committee investigating the primary care system, and head nurses and supervisors might be among the committee members. The goal of the design group is to utilize the organization's best talents for a particular problem. Thus no two task forces are likely to have a similar composition. Some design groups also draw upon resource people outside the nursing division itself.

Groups Based on Organizational Position and Job Function

Groups based on organizational position and function exist in most nursing divisions. A *head nurse group* or a *steering committee* of nurse managers are examples. In determining whether such groups should be formally designated, the nurse executive needs to evaluate the desirability of providing a vehicle for group cohesion and power. For example, a nursing service director might want her supervisors to meet regularly in order to promote problem solving and acceptance of responsibility by the group. On the other hand, she might not want a committee of nursing assistants if she suspects that it would provide a nucleus for unionization. Even if the power of a group is limited, its existence as a formal body can serve as a nucleus for demands and actions.

It is the prerogative of the nurse executive to decide what groups will exist and what amount of authority will be granted to them. A group becomes formally recognized when on-duty time is granted to its meetings and its proceedings are recorded.

Most nurse executives find it useful to create an administrative council to provide a source of communication and participative management. There are a few factors, however, that should be considered in selecting the membership for this council:

1. Any group much larger than 10 or 12 in number seldom works as a single unit. Larger groups tend to break down into factions.
2. A group can comfortably combine persons with different functions if they share similar objectives.
3. The advantages of representation from nonmanagement groups against the efficacy of administrative privilege must be weighed if the council is to be a group that will make administrative decisions and recommendations.

As with committee structures, it is important that groups based on organizational position exist only if they serve a useful purpose. For example, that an organization "has always had a head nurse committee" is not a good enough reason for maintaining the committee. Its goals, however, may be different from the goals of other committees, being broad-based rather than limited to a select number of projects.

The functions of groups based on organizational position differ from the functions of regular committees. These ongoing groups typically monitor and respond to the changing work environment. They tend to be responsive to immediate administrative problems of diverse kinds, and function to grease the wheels of day-to-day operations. The content with which they deal varies greatly over time.

One function of groups whose members hold comparable jobs is the support, education, and role training of individual members. Thus the output of such groups may be measured in the improved performance of individual members as well as of the group in relation to specific projects.

Evaluation of the group must take into account the assistance which it offers to individual members. Functions of information sharing, mutual support, and member education are seldom evidenced in minutes of such groups. The nurse executive must therefore evaluate benefits for individual members in other ways. The best method of evaluation is that of attending meetings and listening attentively. The nurse executive will soon know if such gatherings are merely social, or work productive, or productive though social. Effectiveness of the group can also be measured by the use of questionnaires, asking group members to identify the significance of the meetings from their own perspective.

Interdivisional Committees

Another kind of committee is that which crosses divisional lines. Usually interdivisional committees result where the following conditions arise: 1) coordination of goals and activities is necessary, such as between service and education or among members of a health team working toward a common goal, and 2) recurrent problems occur because of conflicting goals or systems, as may occur between nursing and dietary or laundry departments. Situational problems between two divisions can best be ironed out in interdivisional committees of members who have firsthand experience with the problems that occur when the divisions interact. A head nurse can offer a much more accurate evaluation of a proposed plan for altering tray service than can a nurse executive, for example.

In addition to the assigning of appropriate level personnel to interdivisional committees, the total number of such committees may need to be limited. The demand for interdivisional committees is usually higher than the nursing structure can logically support. Thus priorities and limitations should be assigned. Standing interdivisional committees should not be allowed to evolve unless they serve a valuable and sustained purpose. Alternative routes to problem solving can be used in many instances.

One common problem in interdivisional committees is failure of leadership. Often, in attempting to give equal consideration to each group, a dual leadership is created with one member from each division serving as a cochairman. As in any other situation, a committee that is the responsibility of more than one person is really the responsibility of no one. It is better to alternate chairmen than to split the chairmanship. In establishing interdivisional committees, it is also important that the executive consider the structure and power of the committee. Seldom will she want to bind herself to the decisions of such committees without qualification. Committee power to recommend is usually a safer policy.

SUMMARY

Departmentalization and committee organization represent two of the mechanisms by which the nurse executive distributes the functions of her department. The organization of these units (departments and committees) affects the selection of functions; and the selection of functions affect the selection of units. Some constraints exist on the selection of departments and committees in most organizations. These constraints may consist of patient groupings desired by medical staff, constraints of space and geography, or past practices of the nursing division. Other constraints may be present in the form of resources. For example, if the nurse executive lacked experienced supervisors, she would be foolish to decentralize her division to this unprepared level of managers.

There is no single "right way" to organize a nursing department. Each nurse executive must determine the right functions and departments for her division, given the unique characteristics of her setting and her institution.

REFERENCES

1. Weber, M. Bureaucracy. In Mills, C.W. (Ed.) *Images of Man*. New York: George Braziller, 1960, pp. 149–191.

BIBLIOGRAPHY

Anders, R.L. Matrix organizations: an alternative for clinical specialists. *J.O.N.A.,* 5(5):11, June 1975.

Blau, P.M., and Scott, W.R. *Formal Organizations: A Comparative Approach*. San Francisco: Chandler, 1962.

Etzioni, A. *Modern Organizations*. Englewood Cliffs, N.J.: Prentice-Hall, 1964.

Gaynor, A.K., and Berry, R.K. Observations of a staff nurse: an organizational analysis. *J.O.N.A.,* 3(3):43, 1973.

Johnson, N.D. The professional-bureaucratic conflict. *J.O.N.A.,* 1(3):31, 1971.

Levey, S., and Loomba, N.P. *Health Care Administration—A Managerial Perspective*. Philadelphia: J.B. Lippincott, 1973.

Marciniszyn, C. Decentralization of nursing service. *J.O.N.A.,* 1(4):17, 1971.

Moore, F.I., and Singleton, E.K. A "temporary systems" approach to nursing education in a health care organization. *J.O.N.A.,* 8(7):7, July 1978.

Newhauser, D. The hospital as a matrix organization. *Hospital Admin.,* 17(4):8, Fall 1972.

O'Donovan, R.R. The department head and health care delivery. *J.O.N.A.,* 6(1):32, Jan. 1976.

Prouty, M.P. Making an organization chart. *J.O.N.A.,* 4(1):32, Jan.–Feb. 1974.

Schaefer, M.J. Managing complexity. *J.O.N.A.,* 5(9):13, Nov.–Dec. 1975.

Schaefer, M.J. How should we organize? *J.O.N.A.,* 6(2):12, Feb. 1976.

Smith, D. Organizational theory and the hospital. *J.O.N.A.,* 2(3):19, 1972.

Chapter 8   Assigning, Staffing, and Scheduling

The conversion of objectives into functions represents the first translation of goals into actions. The subsequent distribution of functions through departments, units, committees, and job descriptions is the next step in organization of those actions. A further distribution and differentiation of actions is done through assigning, staffing, and scheduling of personnel. Here the quantification of divisional actions occurs. In the prior decisions concerning departmentalization, committee structure, and job descriptions, work was distributed by type; but in assigning, staffing, and scheduling, work is allocated by specific tasks (or responsibilities) and concrete amounts of work to be done by concrete numbers of workers. This chapter will look at assigning, staffing, and scheduling as they pertain in the patient care unit.

Assigning, as used in this chapter, refers to the manner in which the total work of the nursing unit is divided up among personnel. *Staffing* refers to the plan for how many nursing personnel, of what classifications, will be needed for each unit on each shift. *Scheduling* is the ongoing filling (or approximating) of that staffing pattern by the designation of individual personnel to work specific hours and days on specified units. Scheduling, therefore, represents the enactment of the staffing plan.

Each of these areas—assigning, staffing, scheduling—presents problems and issues of concern for the nurse executive. Assigning and staffing present major areas for decision making. Scheduling presents a subordinate class of problems, logistic and mathematical.

Assigning and staffing decisions interact in the same manner as do decisions about functions and departmentalization. The reader will recall that departmentalization could be designed to optimize delivery of a specific group of functions. Similarly, a group of functions could be selected so as to be compatible with already extant departments. Usually, however, decisions concerning functions and departmentalization are derived by considering both aspects simultaneously. A similar situation occurs with assigning and staffing.

The planned or actual number and mix of personnel will place constraints upon the selection of an assignment system. For example, a staff with minimal personnel of whatever mix may be drawn toward a compensatory functional assignment system. In the opposite case, when an assignment system is selected before the staffing pattern is planned, then the staffing pattern will be based on the nature of the assignment system. For example, if a primary nursing assignment system is selected, the staffing will be planned to allow for an adequate number of primary nurses.

Ideally, an assignment system should be selected first. This selection would be based upon a decision concerning what system could best serve the patient care goals of the division. Next a staffing pattern would be devised to fit the demands of that assignment system, and finally, a schedule would be devised to suit the staffing plan. Seldom, however, does the ideal situation pertain. For example, if the community is short of professional nurses, the staffing may require a modification of the assignment. Similarly, if the institution has limited financial resources for salaries, staffing may affect assignment decisions. Typically, the staffing pattern and the assignment system are mutually determined.

ASSIGNMENT SYSTEMS

Assignment systems have an interesting evolution in nursing. Each new system is greeted as if it were the answer to all the problems of nursing care delivery. Indeed, each new assignment system can be seen to "cure" the major deficiency of the preceding system. Each system, in its turn, brings forth its own set of problems and deficiencies.

Nursing in this country began with the one-to-one, *case method* (private duty) model, where one nurse accepted and stayed with a case until her services were no longer needed. The first major deviation from this method was the so-called *functional assignment*. The functional assignment system is based on a division of labor, as on a factory assembly line. Hence in this method, one nurse distributes medications, another gives baths, and yet a third provides treatments. This method, which was required by a wartime shortage of nurses, "cured" the major problem of case method: the inefficiency of needing one nurse for each patient. The functional method allows fewer nurses to care for more patients than does any other assignment system.

Team nursing assignment, the next major system, in its turn cured the major defect of functional nursing. That defect was the focus upon tasks instead of on patients. The team method assigned a group of patients to a small group of workers under the direction of a team leader. Ideally, a patient was assigned to a team member capable of meeting most or all of that patient's needs. Team leaders often compensated for deviations in the scheme themselves, for example, by giving medications to patients assigned for care by aides.

In theory, the team method assigned patients, not tasks, and it allowed the workers the satisfaction of seeing a "total finished product": a patient who recuperated and was discharged (or who died a peaceful death). Even though team nursing is concerned primarily with the patient, the team leader still has to concentrate on tasks, for she still has to see that "everything is done."

Primary nursing assignment, in its turn, cured the major defect of team nursing: lack of professional accountability. The team method was a loose control system, for when a team (everyone) is responsible, no one really is responsible. Primary nursing made the individual nurse accountable. (In primary nursing, each patient is assigned to a primary nurse who has ultimate responsibility for planning his care—and delivering or monitoring that care when on duty. Often she assumes 24-hour responsibility for decision making related to the patient's care. Primary nurses carry case loads which may vary from three to ten patients, determined, usually, by a difficulty factor.)

Some people claim that primary nursing is a dialectical return under a different name to the original case method. That is not quite true. The private duty nurse of yore was virtually the sole care giver, usually on a 24-hour basis, often sleeping near the patient and waking if he required nursing services. The present primary nurse is *not* responsible for 24-hour care giving. Indeed, she is present only 40 out of 168 hours in a week—less on a week with a holiday, a conference meeting, or any other intervening event. Hence her ongoing responsibility is not primarily for care *giving* but for care *planning*.

It is interesting to speculate on what are the deficiencies of primary nursing—and what assignment system might ultimately replace it. One major problem with primary nursing is that it is only as good as the individual primary nurse. Were all nurses equally capable, this might not be a problem.

It is useful to examine each major assignment system still in use in nursing organizations, reviewing the strengths and weaknesses of each. Three staff assignment systems are in common use: functional, team, and primary nursing. Multiple variations of these systems are practiced. Let us use four criteria for evaluating each assignment method: 1) administrative efficiency, 2) patient needs satisfaction (effectiveness), 3) staff needs satisfaction (happiness quotient), and 4) economy.

The Functional Assignment

In theory functional assignment is the most administratively efficient of the assignment methods because of its division of labor according to specific tasks. Each employee has a clearly defined set of tasks, different from the assignments of others. There is little likelihood of confusion over who will do what. Minimal time is spent coordinating activities among staff members. Further, each member can become highly skilled if he does the same task repetitively.

One should not overlook the tendency of most nursing units to fall back on a functional system during periods of critical staffing shortage. Obviously nurses find the functional method most efficient during pressing shortages. (Note that no system of assignment should be judged out of the context in which it is normally applied; systems are more or less satisfactory, depending on the circumstances in which they are used. Hence comments here about systems give general patterns which may or may not be correct for any given context.)

The functional system, while high on efficiency, is judged low on the criterion of patient needs satisfaction because of the regimentation it involves. Patient needs can be overlooked if those needs fail to fit the "compartments" or task categories of the functional system. For example, the patient who has a need to limit human contacts will not have this need met in the functional assignment system. Nor will the patient's need for relief from anxiety necessarily be met—there is a "medication nurse," but not an "anxiety nurse." Aspects of need which fall outside of the task categories may be missed.

This criticism of the functional method should not be accepted without question, however. Although it is certainly true that regimentation of duties into rigid, discrete compartments is likely to result in failure to attend to issues that do not fit the classification system, mature professional judgment on the part of the nursing staff may help compensate for this potential deficiency. In some instances the functional system may even have considerable merit in satisfying patient needs. In an environment where patients have similar needs, like a newborn nursery or a recovery room, regimentation may have its advantages. If the anticipated, routinized patient needs are built into the task assignment system, it may be that these needs are met with more consistency than in other assignment systems.

Experts also give the functional system a low rating on staff satisfaction. The system of division of labor gives each worker repetitious and therefore potentially boring tasks. In addition, the worker does not have the satisfaction of seeing a "complete piece of work"—a patient who gets well because of the worker's singular efforts. Such judgments are based on an abstract analysis of the work design and an assumption about what people like. Although there are many cases of staff dissatisfaction under functional assignment, it is also a fact that many staff members are best satisfied by this task-oriented system, for many workers feel more secure in repetitive, task-oriented jobs. This may be especially true for the nonprofessional staff, who may need such structure to make sense of their complex environment.

Since functional nursing can be done with the smallest possible staff, it is the most economical of all methods. This economy is calculated on a basis of task per salary paid. Functional assignment also is the method best designed to take advantage of different levels of skill. Hence economy may also be realized here by always assigning tasks to the lowest possible level of personnel who may legally do the function.

The Team Assignment

The team method of assignment evolved as an attempt to increase patient and staff satisfaction even at the cost of administrative efficiency. There are several sources for the potential loss of efficiency. Use of each staff member is curtailed to care of a limited group of patients. When the mobility of staff is decreased, there is loss in overall unit efficiency. Another source of inefficiency in the team assignment is the increased time spent in coordinating delegated work. Since individual assignments are less regularized than under the functional method, more time is spent in conferences and in checking up on workers.

Further, the delegation of work is done by a team leader with less managerial experience and education than that of the head nurse who used to perform this function. Indeed, one often finds insecure team leaders doing work which should have been assigned to others, simply because they are uncomfortable with the task of delegation. This managerial deficit clearly decreases efficiency. Logistics also may impair team function; suppose, for example, that ten nurses must crowd around a medicine cabinet in an old hospital which was designed to support functional nursing with one, or at most two medication nurses.

Not all experts agree that the team system is less efficient than the functional method. Many believe that the closer interaction among the staff members provides an esprit de corps which compensates for time expended in conferences and work coordination. Most advocates of the team system, however, rest their support on the increased satisfaction of patient and staff needs.

In team nursing it is recognized that if a nurse has responsibility for one-half or one-third of a unit of patients, she can know more about each patient than if her responsibility is to all patients on the unit. With a smaller number of staff and patients, the nurse can better match staff abilities and patient needs in care assignments. In addition she can provide more direction for each worker on the team. Effectiveness in care is the anticipated outcome. Theoretically, the patient's needs are better met by the team system because he is cared for by a limited

number of personnel who know him better. Needs that could be missed on the functional system are carefully identified in the team method.

Increased effectiveness in care, so it is reasoned, results not only from identification and resolution of patient needs but from the opportunity for more therapeutic, closer patient-nurse relationships. These gains in effectiveness, however, may be somewhat offset by the increased likelihood of errors. The worker doing multiple, different tasks is much more likely to make a mistake than is the worker who is repeating the same task over and over. In almost all cases, the team assignment system is associated with patient-based rather than task-based division of work. Each staff member is likely to be doing many different tasks for a limited number of patients rather than a single task for a large number of patients as occurs under functional methods. Since this system increases the likelihood of errors, much more time must be devoted to monitoring for such mistakes.

Theoretically each staff member should feel greater satisfaction in team than in functional assignments due to increased guidance and better matching of assignments to skills. In addition, by working with fewer patients the team member has a clear sense of his own contribution to patient outcomes.

Economically, team assignment is probably the most expensive mode of delivering patient care. The employee time spent in conference and coordination is costly. The limited use of staff to one team requires more staffing. Even where staff are supposed to cover for other teams, one often hears, "It's not my team," as an excuse for not attending to overt patient needs—such as a lighted call signal. Where team members and leaders are frequently changed, then even the original economy (of expert knowledge of a few patients) is lost.

Modular nursing is "more of a good thing." If giving the nurse a team is more effective than giving her a whole unit, then giving her a smaller module of patients should be even better than giving her a team. Most arguments for or against team nursing can be applied to modular method. Again, a little more efficiency is lost because of staff mobility being reduced even more than in the team method. The smaller number of patients, however, permits closer monitoring of care than is the case in team nursing, probably decreasing the percentage of care errors and increasing the chances that patient needs will be identified.

Often modular nursing is dictated by the architectural layout of the patient unit. Many new designs break patient areas into small pods, modules, or subunits. In these cases, it is logical to reverse the old architectural principle and let function follow structure. (With luck the design of the unit will have been selected by the nursing division so as to best carry out a form of nursing already determined.)

Modular nursing is not addressed here as a major assignment system for two reasons: 1) Its application has been limited; many institutions converted from team nursing directly to primary, with no modular system even tried. 2) The principles of modular nursing are identical to those of team nursing; the difference is primarily one of size.

The Primary Nursing Assignment

The premise for primary nursing care is different from that of team and modular methods. In primary care each patient is assigned to one nurse for his total hospitalization. She is responsible for planning and organizing his care. Some institutions allow LPNs to function as primary nurses; most do not. The danger here is the assumption that a "simple" patient will stay "simple," and that an LPN will recognize if and when his needs exceed her abilities.

The focus in primary care is on who *plans* the care more than on who *does* the care. The RN may be assisted in the care of her patients by other staff members assigned through various systems. Often a modular assignment is used, but not always. Interestingly, this is the first assignment system

that can subsume other assignment systems within it. This is because of the predominance of planning over doing; it is a system which gives predominance to the cognitive acts of nursing.

In this system each professional nurse has a certain number of patients, and she is responsible for all nursing care planning for these patients. Usually this care planning is seen as a 24-hour responsibility, and the primary nurse may be called at irregular hours for important changes in her patient's nursing needs.

Administrative efficiency is lost by limiting each nurse's knowledge and mobility to the care of only a few patients. The system may permit, however, mobile use of other staff members. In addition, the detailed written care plans may help increase the efficiency of these other personnel. On the other hand, it is likely that the primary nurse will generate more nursing orders than would appear in any other assignment system. Any efficiency gained through clarity of orders and mobility of lower-level personnel is likely to be lost through the increased work requirements. Clearly, efficiency is traded for increased care effectiveness in this system. It should be noted, however, that in this work-generating system, the primary nurse may be easily frustrated if she does not have enough time (or staff support) to carry out the generated work. She will be acutely frustrated by having determined subtle needs which are not addressed in the care given.

One source of gain in efficiency in primary nursing care is the elimination of many positions in the chain of communication. The physician and other health workers are encouraged to deal directly with the primary nurse; less time need be spent in passing on orders. It also may improve effectiveness by decreasing the number of care errors that occur with multiple relaying of orders.

Effectiveness apparently is improved by this primary care mode. The system claims a high score on the criterion of patient needs satisfaction because each patient has his "private nurse planner." The method assures that at least one staff member has a vested interest in his case, and his problems are more likely to be identified and resolved under this system. Another source of effectiveness, the probable decrease in care errors, has already been described.

Primary care is an attempt to increase the professionalism of nursing by establishing accountability for individually designed and administered nursing care. Theoretically, primary care should increase the RN's satisfaction with her career because now she has "products": patient outcomes that are the direct result of her own work and decisions. This form of assignment allows the nurse to operate at the peak of her professional capacity. The system is not overly concerned with the satisfaction of staff members other than the primary nurse, though they may benefit from her clear nursing orders and guidance. Where not all RNs are primary nurses, there may develop a status system which is not conducive to satisfaction of all nurse members.

In real situations staff and patient needs satisfaction is greatly dependent on the preparation of the nurse for a primary care role. A nurse who does not feel secure in nursing care planning will feel threatened by primary care assignments. In addition, the patient whose primary nurse is not capable is much worse off than the patient under team or functional nursing who is exposed to many nurses, any one of whom might plan for his needs. In primary nursing, the success or failure of the system rests heavily on the selection of nurses for the primary role. It should be noted that preparation of today's students for primary roles inevitably will increase their sense of professional accountability. It may well be that the greatest gain from this assignment system will be the attitudinal and educative changes produced in tomorrow's practitioner.

Economically, there is little agreement as to the cost of primary nursing versus team or functional. Conflicting positions have been offered in both the popular literature and in several nursing studies. Primary nursing has been touted as more expensive, equal in cost,

and less expensive by different sources. Unfortunately, many of these studies combined two changes in the cost calculations: a change to primary nursing along with a change to professional staffing. (*Professional staffing* has been used to mean at least two different things: 1) all RN staffing and 2) all RN and LPN staffing.) In either case, when two changes have been made simultaneously, it is not possible to attribute cost changes to either one with accuracy. In most of the reported cases, professional staffing was accomplished by reducing aide positions, usually by attrition, and replacing them with higher-level staff. Two separate replacement mechanisms have been cited: 1) one-to-one staff replacement (keeping the same number of staff, but with a new mix) and 2) replacement of staff on a basis of financial parity, by hiring one professional each time enough monies for a professional salary were made available by the attrition of lower-level personnel. In the latter plan, the total number of staff is decreased.

Logically it appears likely that much of the reported cost saving probably is due to the professional staffing element rather than to the primary nursing assignment system, where the two elements are both present. This can be accounted for in several ways. First, many urban hospitals were negotiated into poor contracts with nurses' aide groups, contracts in which aides received high salaries for greatly restricted work assignments. Indeed, in some locations where aides were unionized and nurses were not, the difference in salary scales was so slight as to be ridiculous. Where this pattern pertained, aides often priced themselves out of the market, particularly in an environment where more and more patients were admitted with more serious illnesses, needing ever more highly technological nursing care. In such an environment, it makes sense that smaller staff—but professional staff with a work orientation—could deliver more care for the same or smaller cost. (Conversely, one also can see why professional staff would be more expensive in a different context, one where aides' salaries were not disproportionate and where patients seldom needed highly professional care. Here may be one of the explanations for contradictory findings in cost studies.)

Another reason many cost studies may have been favorable is that they were done while the primary assignment and professional staffing systems were still in the honeymoon period in addition to experiencing the Hawthorne effect of being studied. In such a period, the energies of a committed professional staff often run high, and effort will be sustained beyond the norm. (In some of these settings, primary nurses reported to the author of spending 10-hour days as the norm.) Certainly, this is cost effective when one "buys" 10 hours of work for eight hours of pay.

Unfortunately, these professionals often suffered "burnout." On returning to two such settings where primary care and professional staffing had been instituted three years before, for example, I found a drift away from primary nursing, back to team nursing. I believe that this was not a reflection on primary nursing per se, but a reflection on the unrealistic expectations established for the staff. Indeed, the staff reported that they had suffered acute frustration in devising excellent care plans and not having the manpower to carry them out.

This reaction seems to be a logical response to a work-generating system when it lacks appropriate resources. Hence, it would seem logical to expect that primary nursing, when divorced from the professional staffing issue, should be more costly specifically because it does generate more work for each person. It is illogical to think that "more and better" can be had for less cost, over a sustained period of time.

Comparison of Systems

The role of the staff nurse differs greatly from assignment system to assignment system. In functional care the nurse mainly organizes and sequences a number of given tasks. Her job in the functional system is to complete these tasks on time. A large part of her job involves organization and management.

Team nursing makes analysis of patient needs and problem solving a bigger part of the job of the staff nurse; it increases her sense of responsibility for patient outcomes. Team nursing does not decrease the staff nurse's need for organization and management, however. Since her tasks are now more variable, her role complexity increases. Whether she is a team leader or a team member, she has more kinds of tasks to organize than she did under the functional system. Not only does she have more of her own work to organize, but she must coordinate her assignment with that of other team members.

Modular nursing, by cutting down the size of the functional unit, cuts down on organizational tasks and increases focus on patient care. Primary care further decreases organizational tasks for the staff nurse and increases individual accountability for specific nursing care regimens.

The role of the head nurse also varies within the three major assignment systems. In functional care the head nurse is a manager in the strict sense; only she has the overall view of the whole unit. Only she is responsible for seeing that all the "pieces" of work are delegated, completed, and coordinated. Since many different nurses are likely to see each patient under the functional system, the head nurse is fairly sure that any gross defects or omissions in care will come to someone's attention. Therefore her evaluation activities are usually limited to a process of nursing rounds once or twice a day.

Under the team system the head nurse delegates many of her day-to-day management duties to team leaders. This should allow her more time for long-term planning for patient care and staff education needs. From the head nurse's perspective, the team system should be ideal; she has optimal distribution of management tasks and a minimal number of persons requiring close assistance and evaluation (two or three team leaders). This ideal is seldom realized, however, for the head nurse soon discovers a whole new set of duties that devolve upon her.

The head nurse's assistance to and evaluation of team leaders turns out to be more complex than her relations to staff under a functional system. The head nurse must observe and evaluate team leader skills of organization, coordination, and technical skills of nursing as well as interpersonal relationships. The team leader typically is a nurse who has little preparation for the management role. Thus the head nurse is required to teach both management skills and nursing skills in the team system. Team leaders must be taught skills such as how to make appropriate assignments, how to assess staff capabilities, and how to assume the authority of their positions.

A factor that increases the complexity of teaching management to team leaders is the inherent difficulty in managing patient-based care as opposed to task-based care. The team leader's job in patient-based care is more complex than the job of the head nurse in task-based care; it calls for far more coordination and cooperation with others; it involves more problem solving; and it requires greater involvement with both staff members and patients.

Under the team system the head nurse cannot evaluate the effectiveness of the care on her unit simply by seeing that all tasks are completed. The amount of time the head nurse spends observing, teaching, and evaluating is greatly increased under the team system. The head nurse can no longer assume that someone will make up for care deficiencies. Now only one-half or one-third of her professional staff are likely to see any given patient. The head nurse's evaluation activities must increase to assure safety and adequacy of care. Daily rounds are no longer adequate as the single assessment device.

These same points hold for modular and primary care systems. As the care systems limit the patient's contacts to fewer professional nurses, the head nurse more and more must assume the role of clinical care

evaluator. In the extreme of primary nursing care, it is vital that the head nurse evaluate the care planning of each nurse. In this system the nurse's mistake or error of judgment is not likely to be corrected unless the head nurse finds it.

In the evolution from functional, through team and modular, to primary nursing systems of assignment, the head nurse role evolves from that of an organizer and manager of tasks to an evaluator of clinical care and a teacher of nurses. These role variations demand distinctly different abilities. Hence an excellent head nurse under one assignment system may be a poor head nurse under another.

Trends and Issues

It is important to note that the primary nursing system in one sense attempts to mimic the one-to-one, professional-to-client relationship common to medical practice. The movement into independent practice in which the nurse has her own case load of patients outside the organizational setting, similarly is patterned after this one-to-one mode of relating to clients. It is difficult to interject such an assignment pattern into nursing simply because most patients need round-the-clock nursing (whereas they need only intermittent care by physician). The need of patients for continuous care necessarily makes nursing an organizational role, dependent on groups of nurses to share the ongoing, continuous care needs. This makes for a more complex work pattern than is necessary in a discipline where each practitioner can be relatively independent of others in his discipline.

Primary nursing, when it is seen as a care planning system rather than as a care giving system, offers an interesting compromise between placing accountability *individually* and *sharing* care giving functions. Ultimately, when viewed only as a care *planning* model, primary nursing is no longer an assignment system. Indeed, as a planning model, it is compatible with any care delivery system.

Indeed, most of the problems in applying primary nursing stem from viewing it as a care delivery system. Then one must make all kinds of elaborate plans for who may do what when the primary nurse is absent. Such major issues include: 1) Must every nurse be a primary nurse? 2) Should a primary nurse be responsible for another nurse's case load in her absence, and, if so, how does this affect her own case load? 3) How are lower-level personnel to be "shared" among primary nurses?

It is interesting to note the popularity of mentorship and "buddy" systems just at the time when primary nursing is taking hold. Indeed, these movements may be attempts to compensate for the relative isolation in which each nurse works in primary nursing. Indeed, it may be that the lack of casual apprenticeship opportunities will be the greatest deficiency of primary nursing. If each nurse works primarily alone, with her own patients, her learning and advancement in the craft of nursing may suffer from lack of role modeling. One may argue that increased use of consultants fills some of this need, but it still does not replace the day-to-day observation of an excellent, experienced nurse at work.

STAFFING

It has already been noted that staffing and the assignment system interact to deliver on the goals and functions of the nursing division. When any of these elements are changed, the impact on the others must be reviewed. Throughout the history of nursing, many controversies have arisen concerning the relation of staffing and assignment systems. For example, the functional assignment system has been promulgated as the method that enables fewer staff members to achieve more work by adopting industrial style division of labor. At present one hears contradictory arguments concerning the relation of staffing and primary nursing assignment systems. One finds arguments that primary nursing calls for increased, identical, and decreased staffing from past practices.

When fuller study is done on the relation of staffing patterns and assignment systems, it may be found that some assignment systems tend to use more or less staff than others; it also is likely that other variables in the environment will be found to affect the relationship between staffing and assigning. For example, the assignment system which is efficient in use of manpower in a large, complex medical center using high technology for seriously ill patients, may be inefficient in a small, community hospital with few critically ill patients and a lower level of technology. These subtle relations between staffing, assigning system, and contextual setting have yet to be studied systematically.

Although the following section will review staffing as if it were a separate entity, the reader is cautioned to remember its interaction with the other components of the total nursing system.

Staffing has two major components: 1) a *staffing pattern* indicating how many persons of what job classification should be on duty per each unit, per shift, per day, and 2) the *staffing plan,* a scheme mathematically derived to indicate how many people of what job classifications must be hired in order to deliver on the staffing plan. These two components each present a different set of problems for the nurse executive.

The Staffing Pattern

A staffing pattern for a single patient care unit is given in Figure 8-1. A final staffing pattern is the cumulative design; it incor-

3 WEST

	DAYS	EVENINGS	NIGHTS
	1 HN		
	4 RN	2 RN	1 RN
	2 LPN	1 LPN	
	2 NA	2 NA	2 NA
	9	5	3

Figure 8-1. A Staffing Pattern for a Single Patient Care Unit

porates counts for all units of the nursing division.

A staffing pattern is a relatively permanent document, built on several assumptions:

1. That each given unit will continue to admit the same type of patients in the same numbers, for the total period in which the staffing pattern is in effect
2. That patient needs can be "averaged out" per unit on a daily basis and can be converted into the number of required nursing hours (as reflected in the determined staffing)
3. That the converted number of nursing hours will remain relatively constant from day to day

If these assumptions fail to hold up, then the *constancy* of the staffing pattern is called into question. Obviously, these assumptions (and the efficacy of the staffing pattern) can be overturned by any change that causes a deviation in the estimated nursing hours per patient day, for example alterations in:

1. Patient acuity levels
2. Actual patient days
3. Nursing or medical technologies (where those changes cause a difference in nursing time required)
4. Assignment systems
5. Nursing care goals
6. Interface with other departments and divisions (where those altered interfaces cause more or less "work" for the nursing unit)
7. Physical plant or equipment
8. Nursing delivery or management systems

Where trends in these variables can be forecast, then staffing patterns can be adjusted accordingly. The staffing pattern of a nursing division usually is reviewed at least yearly for modifications required by changes in patient numbers, care trends, or contextual variables.

Determining the Staffing Pattern

The staffing pattern is a quantitative statement of patient care delivery. It reveals how many hours per day per shift per unit will be worked by each level of personnel. This critical conversion to a finite number of hours of work as compared to patient needs presently is done in two distinct ways. 1) Patient acuity/classification systems focus on patient needs: patients are sorted according to various descriptive categories, and each category is associated (usually through past experience) with a number of nursing hours required per patient in that category per shift. 2) Task-quantifying systems focus on nursing acts: common nursing tasks are related directly or indirectly (through various patient care units, PCUs,) to a time-per-task measure. This measure also may be arrived at through past experience, possibly through time studies and task analysis methodologies.

These conversion systems may be primitive or complex, accurate or inaccurate, correctly or incorrectly applied. The more sophisticated systems of both sorts break down final hours to be worked according to level of nursing personnel required to give the care. Some sophisticated systems combine a patient classification mechanism with a task quantification system. All these systems will be discussed in detail in Chapter 9.

One system of determining the staffing pattern will be presented here, though it oversimplifies a complex process.

1. Develop a system of identifying and codifying individual patient needs. (This usually involves use of a patient acuity/classification system.)
   a. Sum all patient needs per unit per shift for a per-day tally.
   b. Also differentiate needs as to complexity and summarize by complexity level.
   c. Cumulate need tallies for a long enough period to derive a needs norm per unit per shift per day.

2. Develop a system of relating patient need norms to quantitative care delivery norms. This requires that one:
   a. Determine the quality and quantity of nursing care that will be given in response to patient needs, and
   b. Apply a nursing task quantification system.
   c. Include relating complexity of needs to level of personnel.
3. Develop a mechanism for relating care delivery data to job descriptions of care deliverers. (Either job descriptions may be constructed to fit care delivery data *or* care delivery data may be compared to extant job categories in order to determine number of employees of each job category necessary to deliver the required quantitative sum of care hours.)
   a. Remember to include indirect nursing time if the quantification system used did not do so.
   b. Remember to correct norms if there is a goal of improving quality of care delivered. (It is true that nurses can "work smarter" in the same amount of time, but most upgrading also involves increased expenditure of nursing time. It is not reasonable to expect "more and more" for no increased cost in time involvement.)

Staffing which takes into account patient needs and/or specific nursing tasks to be done, is an advancement over old systems based on 1) number of beds per unit or, slightly improved 2) average census per unit. These old norms ignored the fact that even if census were stable, one group of 30 patients might need far more care than another group of 30 patients. Indeed, this fluctuation of amount of care needed (even among equal numbers of patients) was long reflected in a common quantitative measure of nursing care, the nursing-hours-per-patient-day (NHPD) unit. This measure is calculated by adding together all nursing personnel on a unit for 24 hours, multiplying them (singly or together) by the number of hours worked, and dividing this figure by the number of pa-

tients on that unit for the day (the census data). Thus one might calculate:

May 5, 1979:

$$\frac{20 \text{ personnel over} \times 8 \text{ hours each} }{3 \text{ shifts} \qquad \text{of worked time}}{40 \text{ patients}}$$

equals: 4.0 NHPD

One of the first alterations in staffing patterns based on the NHPD was the intensive care unit staffing. Here it was possible to group all patients requiring "excessive" hours of nursing care, determine the NHPD norms of this unit as compared to "average" nursing care units, and charge patient fees accordingly.

The NHPD is a norm which may be useful to the nurse executive. For example, she may compare typical NHPD figures for like units among different hospitals. Such data reach most nurse executives whose organizations participate in nationwide data collection through the American Hospital Association. Past data from her own organization also will be useful in providing normative values.

The use of the NHPD unit in reaching staffing decisions is limited, however. First, it is normative rather than prescriptive, i.e., it tells how many hours of care (roughly) *are* being delivered, not how many hours *ought to be* delivered in relation to either patient needs or in relation to any given level of care. Further, those hours incorporate all nursing staff hours, both those used in giving care and those used in administrative and other activities. Finally, the NHPD index combines three shifts without any mechanism for differentiation, in spite of the fact that the work loads may differ significantly on those shifts.

Indeed, there was a time when most staffing patterns were based on the NHPD (or census, or number of patient beds). Once a staffing number was determined for a whole day, then the nurse executive distributed that number on three shifts based on either her intuitive or her investigated notion of the proportion of care that was needed on each shift. Again, another set of norms arose—those of percentages of staff per shift. One common pattern was that of: days, 45 percent of the staff; evenings, 35 percent; and nights, 20 percent. Alternate patterns also were given and supported. Obviously, such a norm was interesting but useless in any given case because the tasks assigned per shift varied from institution to institution as did patient needs per shift.

Present staffing systems, relying on data concerning patient needs during a shift or nursing tasks during a shift make the shift, not the day, the unit for consideration in staffing decisions. In this way one avoids unnecessary extrapolation concerning how the shifts compare in work load.

It is important to consider the NHPD index and its impact historically on nursing administration. First, it has the advantage of being a figure which is easily calculated and which allows for comparison among institutions. Indeed, many unsophisticated nurse executives found themselves prisoners of this index. (Many hospital administrators who fail to understand professional nursing did—and some still do—see the NHPD as a norm applicable to any institution. The administrator of such limited understanding was not above using this figure as a measure for the achievement of the nurse executive in administering her division.)

Obviously, this norm became a burden in situations where contextual or patient variables significantly increased the nursing care tasks. Further, the calculation of this norm became more problematic. As numbers of workers on a nursing unit increased in types, calculations were made differently by different nurse executives. For example, one would include secretarial personnel if those employees were considered personnel of the nursing division. Another nurse executive might not count secretarial personnel if they reported to another division. It is not surprising that some nurse executives manipulated the NHPD counts to their statistical advantage. Indeed, at the present different mechanisms for calculating the NHPD are being proposed and followed for various purposes. What is important is that the nurse executive recognize the limited purpose which this calculation serves, and that she be able to understand and explain her NHPD data in light of the nature of that calculation.

Both the patient classification system and the task quantification system are attempts to create indices which overcome the poverty of the NHPD index. Both of these systems ultimately aim to relate patient needs (or nurse tasks) to staffing. NHPD only relates time-put-in to staffing, reflecting neither patient needs nor nursing tasks.

Variables Affecting Staffing Pattern Determinations

As indicated throughout this discussion, there are many variables that may affect staffing determinations. These include:

1. Nursing organization factors
   a. Patient care objectives
   b. Determined "levels of patient care"
   c. Nursing division/department/unit functions
   d. Assignment systems
   e. Services to staff, e.g., inservice hours allowed
2. Patient factors
   a. Variety of patient conditions
   b. Acuity
   c. Length of stay
   d. Patient numbers
   e. Age groups
   f. General health status and health goals
   g. Care expectations
   h. Fluctuations in numbers, acuity, variety, etc.
3. Staff factors
   a. Job descriptions of the division/organization
   b. Educational level of staff
   c. Experiential level of staff
   d. Work ethic of groups of staff members
   e. Expectations of staff from the organization

4. Health care organization factors
   a. Financial resources available
   b. Personnel policies, especially regarding work time
   c. Support services within the organization
   d. Number and nature of interfaces within the total institution
   e. Number of beds per unit or module
   f. Architecture and functional space layouts
5. Extraorganizational factors
   a. Staff mix available in the community
   b. Staff number available
   c. Coordinating patterns with community health agencies

Obviously, there are too many variables to allow one to derive a single, simple formula for staffing. Staffing judgments often are a mixture of scientific (or logical) derivations plus pragmatic knowledge of what works in a given situation.

Problems Related to Staffing Patterns

There are several problems which make staffing decisions difficult. Several will be briefly reviewed here: 1) staffing mix, 2) use of supplementary staffing patterns, 3) peaks and valleys in the work load, and 4) planned alterations in levels of care.

Staffing Mix. The nurse executive must decide how many RNs, LPNs, nursing assistants, or other workers are to man each nursing unit. Staffing decisions also include determining how many RNs of what categories are to be used (when a nursing ladder or other plan differentiates among RNs). Differentiations among levels of RN practice will be discussed in Chapter 9. The remaining discussion here will focus upon differences in professional and occupational work groups.

Decisions concerning mix will be dictated partially by the supply of skilled personnel available in the community (or who can be attracted to the community). Additionally, the types of patients to be cared for will influence such decisions. More seriously ill patients and patients requiring highly technical care will require higher levels of professional staffing. Efficiency in utilization of personnel plus quality in care are the basic criteria for determining mix.

Often mix is determined by an assessment of a task quantification system. Here each "task" is assigned to a given level of worker, and by a cumulative count of tasks per level, one can establish a ratio of staff mix. This method may be deceptive if it is applied without thought. First, many systems which time tasks only time activities done in direct contact with a patient. Hence they may allow no time for professional planning and just plain thinking. Such a system tends to recommend a staff mix at a lower level than actually required. Further, such a system may overlook the fact that a "low-level task" in any given instance may need to be done by a higher-level worker than normal because of other intervening patient-related factors. Thus just because "taking temperatures" is assigned to an aide level, one cannot assume that every temperature should be taken by an aide. Nevertheless, in a cost-conscious society, it is certainly reasonable to aim for a situation in which most employees are working (at most times) at their highest level of capability.

Some nurse executives believe that the use of tasks to estimate levels of staff personnel is not the way to attain maximum efficiency. Nurse executives favoring professional staffing give the following argument: When staff is heavy with lower-level personnel, there is an increased need for supervising, directing, and followup. This need for management alters the role of the professionals, their time is used in management, not in patient care. By staffing with higher-level personnel, whose role concepts and education prepare them for self-direction, one produces more and higher-quality patient care with a smaller total number of personnel. Elimination of the heavy amount of supervising, directing, and followup enables fewer personnel to deliver more advanced nursing care. Decrease in the number of staff is compensated for in quality of care provided.

Two other factors support the move toward professional staffing. One is the increasing complexity of the nursing technology, decreasing the need for employees with little education and few skills. The second factor is the increasingly high salaries for nursing assistants (often under unionized conditions); these salaries often allow for replacement by more highly skilled workers with little extra investment in salaries.

In addition to mixes of personnel for patient care, mixes of nursing and non-nursing personnel on the unit must be considered. Use of unit managers or secretaries is common to most health institutions; these workers take over various unit activities, freeing the professionals for actual nursing care. This division of nursing and non-nursing functions on the unit probably has solved more problems than it has created, but the division has brought with it a set of difficulties in coordination. Such difficulties can be forestalled by accurate understanding of and preparation against potential conflict situations.

Two sorts of problems are likely to occur with unit management systems: 1) logistic problems and 2) power struggles. Logistic difficulties occur when the unit management staff gives less than peak performance. Services of unit management can be compared to the supply lines that serve an army. The soldier on the battlefield gives little thought to such supportive service until the ammunition fails to arrive; then suddenly the supply services have a direct and critical effect on his ability to fight.

The nurse is in a similar position. Stocking of sterile supplies, for example, is not really important to her until she cannot obtain materials to do a dressing. When this occurs, one no longer can say that stocking of supplies is not a critical function in nursing care.

When unit management services are perceived clearly as *means* to the *ends* of nursing care, the division of functions is effective and everyone works toward the same goals. A problem arises, however, when a unit manager develops a sense of his job as an end-in-itself. This can happen easily, and the person who takes extreme pride in his work may be more susceptible to this fault than is the less conscientious worker.

Compared to the world of the nurse, the world of the unit manager is orderly, routinized, and relative stable. He deals with inanimate objects that stay where he puts them (except for interference by nurses); he has supplies that are used up at regular rates (except when nurses unpredictably use "too much" of an item at one time); he has supply charges that can be processed through clearly defined standard operating procedures (except when the nurse forgets to write down which patient used the supply); and he has temperatures that can be transferred routinely to patient charts (except when the nurse is slow to record them on the temperature board).

Clearly, from the perspective of the unit manager or secretary, the biggest obstacle to his work is the professional nurse. This obstacle is particularly frustrating if the manager sees his job as an end in itself. The unit manager has a job with a high degree of task routinization and a low level of technology; the nurse, on the other hand, has a job with great variation in tasks and a high level of technology. The nurse cannot develop routinized behavior where patient needs, priorities, and surrounding events cannot be predicted with certainty.

Where the unit manager sees his job as one of helping the nurse to cope with this irregular environment, the relationship between nurse and manager can be effective; such a manager can take pride in his ability to assist professional staff in meeting exigencies. Unit managers are most likely to develop this attitude when they are responsible to the head nurse.

Where a unit manager is a coequal with the head nurse, then means (support systems) have been equated in value with ends (nursing care). A manager in such a system may try to substantiate the equality of his position by adapting the environment to the needs of his own job of low technology and routinized tasks. This presents the problem of two bosses demanding that the same environment conform to the needs of diverse work perspectives. The problem with such an arrangement is not a confusion of tasks but a confusion of means with ends.

The power conflict is further exacerbated when an institution hires the brightest of young men as unit managers. These men, not unexpectedly, fail to find their routinized tasks challenging; their duties fail to live up to their conceptions of what a manager does, and they readily turn their attention to power plays for control of the unit.

A relatively simple solution to these potential problems is to make the unit manager directly responsible to the head nurse. In this way better nursing care will remain the objective of the support systems.

Appropriate staffing decisions concerning the numbers of secretaries or unit managers to be hired can be made by assessment of the kind and number of non-nursing tasks completed on each nursing unit.

The unit manager issue also illustrates an instance where nursing staffing may be constrained by the organization of personnel in other divisions. For example, if other divisions house unit managers, transporters, or other service personnel of some sort, it is likely that these positions historically originated in nursing. Now, however, when a staffing mix which is ideal might call for more professional staff and fewer support personnel, the nurse executive may find herself in a position of trying to divest other institutional power sources of positions in order to expand positions in her own division. While such a move may realistically be called for on the basis of current patient care needs, it inevitably will be perceived as a move on the part of the nurse executive to extend her domain and her power. Thus the negotiation across divisional lines where other positions interface with and affect nursing positions is a delicate matter, certainly one requiring much backup data and cool, logical argument.

Use of Supplementary Staffing Patterns. The final staffing pattern may or may not allow for use of supplementary staffing. The justification for these additional staffing patterns is that the regular staffing pattern is based on the "average," the normal situation, and that situation simply does not always pertain.

Emergency staffing and float staffing function on different principles. The emergency staffing pattern describes the redistribution of nursing personnel for an emergency situation. Some fortunate hospitals have extra personnel in the community who can be called in for an emergency situation, but that circumstance is rare. Typically, an emergency staffing pattern rearranges regular staffing for management of the crisis situation. Such an emergency staffing pattern often is devised along with a disaster plan. These documents may be simple or complex; there may be one staffing pattern or alternates designed to meet the contingencies of specific types of disasters. The emergency staffing pattern typically reduces patient care unit staff to the lowest level at which patient safety is assured, freeing staff members for duties elsewhere during the emergency situation.

The float staff pattern consists of a design for regular employees who are not assigned to a specific patient unit but who are regular, either full-time or part-time employees who provide patient care. The float staffing is planned to compensate for two variables: increases in patient activities and absences among the unit-assigned staff members due to illness or other contingencies.

The organization that is unable to maintain a float staff has to have a larger unit-assigned staff. Float staffing, however, enables an institution to "cover for" those units on which the work load is temporarily heavier than the norm. By using a single staff for this purpose (the float staff), there is less need to move unit-assigned personnel so as to balance work load. Movement of unit-assigned personnel is less desirable than use of float staff; this topic will be addressed later in chapter under "Scheduling." The float staff size and composition are determined by data on the institution's total work load variance from the "norm" for the units. In some instances, so as to preserve flexibility of staff, the normal unit staffing pattern will be set to cover the *low normal* work load. Then there is heavy reliance on the float staff.

Most institutions, however, staff for the norm, recognizing that on days when work load is below that norm there will be some "waste" of staff time. Few institutions are able to adjust staffing for periods of decreased activities. Institutions that have a monopoly on hiring of health personnel due to absence of other employing agencies in their area may be able to send employees home when the work load is light. In most instances this is not possible, and the nurse executive does well to have a constructive plan for the use of personnel when such a condition exists. Self-teaching inservice projects are used at such times, and other productive use of employee time can be devised with a little thought.

Use of a float staff is a partial solution to increased activity needs, but it brings its own set of problems. The usual problem with establishing a float staff is finding the right persons for it. An ideal float staff is one staffed with full-time workers who like the challenge of working with different types of patients and in different settings. The problem, of course, is the scarcity of nurses and other workers who enjoy this challenge. The vast majority of workers seem to prefer the stability of working with a known group of patients and staff.

Many institutions, therefore, man a float staff with either part-timers or new personnel waiting for permanent unit positions to become available. Unfortunately, part-timers and new personnel are the workers least likely to succeed in meeting the changing demands of float positions. The institution that desires a good float staff needs to evolve a reward system that recognizes the difficulty of float work.

Another supplementary staffing pattern is on-call staffing. Typically used in operating rooms, this pattern determines how many people of what sort need to be on-call at any given time. Usually on-call staffing is filled with regular employees who receive some remuneration for being on-call whether or not they are called. Such employees often receive further remuneration when they are in fact called.

The on-call pattern has developed more popularity as nursing begins to specialize. Often intensive care units or coronary care units develop an on-call system, formal or informal, in which regular personnel of that unit will be called in emergencies. Usually, this is a scheduling procedure rather than a staffing pattern, however, as the most common "emergency," is the absence of a regular staff member.

Peaks and Valleys in the Work Load. Peaks and valleys in the nursing work load occur on several levels: 1) daily differences in what may be done, 2) irregular peaks and valleys on various days or months, and 3) seasonal, yearly peaks and valleys. Each of these patterns will be examined.

Daily peaks and valleys are caused by the natural flow of events on a patient unit. Hence there may be times when staff are literally unable to proceed with their work because of intervening events. The aim of the unit must be to even out those events insofar as is possible. Otherwise, one needs a larger staff if all the work must be achieved in shorter work periods.

Some unit events are clearly within the control of the nursing division. For example, if a head nurse demands that all patients be bathed between 9:00 A.M. and 11:00 A.M. she is creating her own peak activity period. Examination of the nursing system routines will enable staff to even out many peaks and valleys in the work load. Other events are perceived as outside the control of the nursing division, though that may not necessarily be the case. For example, some nursing divisions have been successful in getting physician staff to stagger their rounds; other nursing divisions have managed to stagger or rearrange visiting hours to fit care needs. In any case, the aim is to establish a constant work flow as this allows for optimal work achievement by minimal nursing staff.

In instances where it is not possible to remove a major peak or valley, the nurse executive should plan for it. Unnecessary events should be eliminated from peak work time periods, and supplementary work or education activities may be planned for the valleys. For example, if mealtimes economically cannot be staggered given the dietary department's budget, then the staff on a unit of primarily "self-care" patients may be given this as their own major mealtime break. (Of course, on a unit with dependent patients the opposite pattern would pertain, and staff would be freed of other tasks at this time to see to feeding needs of patients.)

Another "peaks and valleys" situation occurs in units where patient occupancy rates vary considerably. Unfortunately this condition is more likely to pertain in small specialty units. Such units are short of staff one day and overstaffed the next. Further, since they are specialty units, it is difficult to cover shortages with nurses from other areas. More often, however, the problem of such a unit is overstaffing. For example, one must have a nurse stationed in Labor and Delivery whether or not any patients are immediately in the unit; similarly, the Emergency Room must be ready at hand. In most instances staffing for such a unit simply cannot be cost effective.

One common solution not in the realm of staffing is that of combining services where several hospitals serve a single community. For example, if three hospitals are located in the same small town, they might agree to move all pediatric facilities to one, emergency room functions to another, and obstetric facilities to the third. By having each specialty cater to a larger total population, the waste in staff coverage can be better controlled.

When unpredictable patient occupancy rates occur in nonspecialty units, the problem can be partly cured by float staffing for staff shortages or variable staffing for both staff shortages and oversupply of staff. (Variable staffing will be discussed later in this chapter.) Ironically, the attempt to hold down hospital costs by early discharge of patients may actually be costly if it produces situations where units with low occupancy are manned by a full nursing staff.

In some instances the variance in occupancy rate is a seasonal factor and can be predicted ahead even when it cannot be controlled. For example, a ski town with lodges and tourism expects skiing accidents in winter. In cases of predictable variances, the nurse executive may have to have two or more staffing patterns for a single year. In some situations where tourism is responsible for the increase in patient admissions, the tourist population may increase the nursing population available for hire to fill the heavier staffing needs.

Where nursing moves toward specialization and where variance occurs in the specialty units, it may be difficult to find the staff who can cover such units. One possibility is to encourage nursing staff members to develop two, rather than one, special areas of knowledge and expertise. This is another instance in which variable staffing may be a partial solution.

Planned Alterations in Levels of Care. As nursing moves toward the costing out of nursing services, it is logical to predict that nursing divisions will begin to associate fees charged with level of nursing care received. Certainly, no institution will tolerate a level of care that qualifies as unsafe. Yet it is feasible that levels will be developed, and that the consumer will elect the care level he desires (directly through described material and accompanying fees or indirectly through a choice of insurance coverage which specifies a level of care).

One can imagine a situation where a "luxury unit" has a different staffing pattern from its identical sister unit on an "economy model." Indeed, there might even be a "swing unit" that is staffed for A level care at one time, B level care at another, depending upon the choices of the particular patient body of the moment. While number of staff is not directly correlated with quality of care, it is reasonable to assume that the higher level care will require more staff and a higher ratio of professional staffing.

Some nurses may reject the idea of staffing for level of nursing care. Indeed, they may assert that every patient deserves top quality nursing care. This assertion, in the absence of the resources to deliver it, however, merely produces a disillusioned and angry client. Ultimately nursing will advance as a profession only when the client sees what he is getting for his investment. When this situation comes about, nursing must be prepared to tell the client realistically what services he will receive for what fees. Further, once nursing has specified different levels of care, it must be prepared to deliver on what is promised. This is an ultimate stage in professional accountability.

Obviously, in this case, the diverse staffing patterns would be tied closely to corresponding plans for care. Staffing alone should not be assumed to make the difference in levels of care. Nurses should not fail to note the significance of identifying for the client the level (or levels) of nursing care that he will receive in each institution. Were this to come about—and it is beginning to happen—then the client might select the health care institution on the basis of its nursing, not strictly on the basis of his physician's preference. This change would produce a radical shift of power to nursing. If nursing, as well as medicine, had an effect on whether or not a client selected a given institution, the importance of nursing would be made more visible.

Some nursing divisions already have two staffing plans, one for the normal situation and one for a situation of acute staffing shortage. Again, in this case, the alteration in staffing is tied to an altered care delivery system. (Some places institute such a staffing plan and altered delivery system every weekend.) Unfortunately patients have very little say about this depletion of services today. Certainly, they receive no compensatory adjustment in the fees they pay for nursing services.

Variable Staffing

Variable staffing is an alternate to the permanent staffing pattern. This method does not make assumptions about care units and their patients. In variable staffing, the pattern is determined daily, based upon present input data from patients on each unit. This eliminates the problems that arise when staffing is based on a stagnant predication of patient needs. In this system the staffing pattern of any patient unit may change daily. Here the staffing of the entire institution, rather than of each unit, is held constant; and staff are redistributed on each shift according to the variable staffing calculations. Often computer systems are utilized to determine variable staffing. These calculations usually are based upon patient classification systems or task quantification systems which estimate work load for each patient unit.

Variable staffing combines two elements discussed separately in this chapter: staffing and scheduling. Work hours are scheduled but unit placement is not planned ahead; staffing is planned only as a number of personnel for the whole institution.

Variable staffing is a mathematical solution to the problems of staffing in an uncertain world; but it is not necessarily a solution to the human relations aspect of the staffing problem. Many staff members do not like to participate in a system which regards staff as interchangeable cogs in the big machine. Many prefer to have the constancy of working on a single unit, with a single patient population. Thus the solution to the "wastage" of time by staff relocation may create its own form of wastage in resentful staff or simply in staff who work slower and with less certainty because they are faced with frequent changes of units and patient populations.

The Staffing Plan

It was mentioned earlier that staffing has two components, the staffing pattern, which decides how many staff of what sort are needed on each unit per shift per day, and the staffing plan, the determination of how many people must be hired to deliver on that staffing pattern. Let us look at the staffing plan.

Suppose one were to calculate how many persons needed to be hired to fill a single RN position on a day shift on a given patient care unit. One might make calculations of the following sort:

1. Each RN works a determinable number of days per year.
2. By dividing days worked per nurse by the number of days in a year one derives the number of staff required to fill one positional slot for the year, i.e., on a full-time basis.

Figure 8-2 illustrates such a calculation, using the number of days of vacation, ill time, holidays, and inservice days that are the norm in the hypothetical hospital.

Notice that the mathematical calculation shown in Figure 8-2 is just the beginning of the estimate, not the finish. Several obstacles and problems remain to be solved. First, no one worker would realistically agree to work 65 percent of a full-time job. And if someone did, the payroll and personnel offices would be irate because of the work such an employee would cause them.

Second, even if one found another worker to fill the 65 percent, the work of this employee would complement (and complete) the work of the full-time worker (so the job is filled 100 percent of the time) *only if* the two were never on duty on the same day. Note, however, that the calculation included sick time, an entity that specifically cannot be planned ahead. Further, there is no guarantee that these two employees will use

---

Staffing for One RN Slot on 3 West for a Year (364 days)

I. Deduct days not worked, for total work days for an individual full-time employee

364 days (calculated at an "even" 52 weeks)
− 104 days off (two days off per week × 52 weeks)

260 days remaining
− 10 paid holidays

250 days remaining
− 5 ill days (the institutional norm)

245 days remaining
− 5 paid inservice days (institutional norm)

240 days remaining
− 20 days paid vacation

II. Divide year by number of days worked by a full-time worker, to get number of full-time workers needed to fill the position

220 days remaining = total work days

$$220\overline{)364.00} = 1.65 = \text{RN workers to fill one job}$$

Figure 8-2.   Calculation of Staff Required to Fill a Single Full-Time Position

exactly the correct, normed-out percent of sick days.

Note also that the formula is incomplete in that the 65 percent employee would not actually get the exact prorated number of sick days allowable, vacation days, and so on as the full-time employee. Once again, the formula proves only to give an "estimate" of number of employees.

Such a calculation also may allow one to consider the work of a larger group of nurses together. Suppose for example that a given unit was staffed with three RNs on days, for a total of 1092 work days in a 52 week period (364 days × 3 positions). Here five RNs would appear to be able to fill three positions (220 work days each × 5 RNs) = 1100 days, or slightly more than that required. Notice, however, that a single personnel policy such as "every other weekend off" makes this coverage impossible. Furthermore, the plan would require vacations spread out evenly through the year.

The staffing plan, accordingly, is calculated on a basis of mathematical design plus modification required by policies of the institution and by interdigitation with the scheduling office (whose policies also may impact on what days what workers may be used). At its best, the staffing plan only delivers an approximation of the staffing pattern. Approximation is closer, with more flexibility and shifting of staff from unit to unit, but there are prices to be paid for this approach in terms of human relations and possibly quality of care.

Nor can one come up with a norm for the staffing plan, for example, 1.65 employees per position. Note that this figure would change in another institution which had a different number of holidays, days for vacation, or a different norm for sick time used. Where different categories of workers are entitled to different lengths of vacation, calculations must be done separately for each class of worker.

Calculating a Staffing Plan from Care Hours. Note that in the previous illustration,

the staffing pattern was a given, and the staffing plan was calculated to fill that pattern. It also is possible, where an institution has a good mechanism for estimating patient care hours, to move in the opposite direction—to go from patient care hours per unit per shift, to total number of nursing hours required per year, to number of staff required to deliver those hours (staffing plan), to number of positions required to deliver that staff (staffing pattern).

Suppose, for example, that the institution represented in Figure 8-2 uses the PETO [1] system for patient care units. This is a system easily converted to nursing care hours because each PETO unit equals 7.5 minutes of nursing care. Suppose that 3 West has kept its data and knows that it averages 480 PETO units per shift (days). Then they might do the calculations shown in Figure 8-3 to see what sort of staffing pattern they should have.

Notice that there were some assumptions underlying the calculation in Figure 8-3. First, it was assumed that the 1.65 factor applied to all nursing personnel in this unit; this would not be accurate, for example, if nurses' aides received only two weeks vacation. Furthermore, since the PETO units summarized nursing care given by *all* staff, the final tally represents the *total* employees, not just the RN staff.

Suppose that the PETO units had been given per unit per day rather than per shift. Then the answer would be the staffing for the total 24-hour day, and the nurse executive would have to extrapolate, deciding what percentage of that staff should be distributed on each shift.

The main administrative objective in the staffing plan is one of even distribution of staff. Every event or policy which mitigates against equidistribution of staff makes the staffing plan more difficult to calculate by removing it further from the mathematical model which serves as its base. For example, if unionized staff gain every other weekend off, this will throw off staffing calculations because 50 percent of staff will be off at the same time. This prevents any three-for-one (or five-for-three) sort of arrangement among staff hours. On an every-other-weekend-off plan, one can only provide relief staff on a one-for-one basis, a most costly procedure, and one which does not allow the executive to take advantage of staffing distribution. A nursing executive who agrees to an every-other-weekend-off policy is left with two equally unattractive alternatives: 1) She can use deficient staffing every weekend, allowing the quality of care to drop. Some nurse executives have had the further embarrassment of explaining or trying to explain to their bosses why such a staffing level is not good enough for the rest of the week if it is good enough for two days. 2) The alternate is for the executive to have a staffing plan which calls for enough staff to give quality care on the weekend. This plan will waste money by overstaffing during the week. Some few nurse executives are able to solve this staffing plan problem by having a consistent staffing plan but filling it with part-time, weekend-only workers. Even this is not ideal as a personnel system, but at least it enables the nurse executive to build a rational staffing plan to deliver on a staffing pattern.

A final staffing plan dilemma is whether or not to rotate employees among shifts. Ideally, each shift should be handled separately, but the ideal may not be possible if there are few nurses in a community who voluntarily work the evening or night shifts. Obviously shift work breaks most of the rules nurses teach others concerning one's circadian cycles, but this is a reason outside the domain of the staffing plan. Where workers rotate shifts, it is not possible to derive a staffing plan separate from the

---

480	PETO units per 3 West per one 8-hour shift (days)
× 7.5	minutes of nursing care per PETO unit
3600	minutes of nursing care per 3 West per 8-hour shift
÷ 60	minutes in an hour
60	hours of nursing care per 3 West per 8-hour shift
× 364	days in a 52-week year
21,840	hours of nursing care per 3 West per 8-hour shift per year

On 3 West employees work approximately 220 days per year (see Figure 8-2).

220	days per year per employee per 8-hour shift
× 7	hours (time on duty spent in actual patient care in this particular institution)
1540	hours per employee per 52-week year of patient care

Divide total hours of nursing care required per 3 West per year (on days) by hours given per year per employee to get number of employees needed

21,840	hours of nursing care per 3 West per 8-hour shift per year
÷ 1,540	hours of nursing care per employee per year
14.18	staff members (total) required

To get a staffing pattern, divide total staff members by 1.65, the number of staff required to fill one slot in this particular institution (see Figure 8-2).

14.18	total employees
÷ 1.65	staffing ratio
8.59	employees in the staffing pattern

Figure 8-3.   Deriving a Staffing Pattern from Patient Care Hour Data

scheduling plan. It also makes it difficult to use the shift as the basis for various work load calculations.

SCHEDULING

Scheduling is the final step in the assigning-staffing-scheduling system, the step whereby workers are assigned specific days and specific hours of work. Scheduling tries to approximate the staffing pattern using the resources (people) designated by the staffing plan. Again, the chief goal is balance, distribution of workers evenly throughout the given scheduling period.

Difficult as it is to determine staffing patterns, filling these patterns can be a greater problem. Anyone who tries to fill a given staffing pattern for a given patient unit for seven days per week soon discovers that the seven-day week was created to confound managers. At least this is true in a society in which five-day work weeks predominate. Suppose that one wished to fill two RN positions on one unit for one shift for one year. Continuing the illustration for the hypothetical "3 West" from Figures 8-2 and 8-3, it is necessary to hire 1.65 nurses for one position or 3.30 for two positions. Given that nurses are more likely to apply for full-time, 100-percent positions rather than for 30 percent positions, the closest approximation for these two positions will be three RNs.

When one tries to fit the three nurses into an average week, however, problems arise. (An average week here is taken to be one in which no holidays, vacations, or sick time

occur.) In this arrangement, the following pattern shown in Figure 8-4 emerges.

The pattern reveals the problem that one day per week the unit is overstaffed. There are, of course "solutions" to this problem. One is to credit one staff member's time on the overlap day to inservice education. When this is done, overlapping on several units is made to coincide as to day, so as to be able to collect a large enough group of workers eligible for a planned inservice program. Not all institutions can afford to offer the nurse an inservice day once every three weeks, though the actual total of inservice days is greatly reduced once vacations, holidays, and other interruption days are added to the schedule.

Another solution is to use the overstaffing to solve internal variations in work load. In this procedure, one assures that overstaffed days do not coincide from unit to unit, so the "extra" RN can be transferred to the unit with the heaviest patient activity.

A third solution to the problem of overstaffing is to find a nurse who is interested in working a four-day week. This ideal solution, however, may be difficult to arrange.

Yet another solution to the overstaffing problem is to balance the excess staff scheduling against a deficient staff scheduling pattern. Suppose, for example, that on the same unit four LPNs were filling three positions. Here a deficiency pattern arises, as shown in Figure 8-5.

With four workers for three positions, one deficiency occurs per week. Thus a floor that had the good fortune to have a staffing pat-

X = days worked in the week

RN A	X	X	X	X	X			
RN B			X	X	X	X	X	
RN C	X	X	X			X	X	

Figure 8-4.   Three Nurses Filling Two Staffing Positions

X = days worked in the week

Worker A	X	X	X	X	X		
Worker B			X	X	X	X	X
Worker C	X	X			X	X	X
Worker D	X	X	X	X			X

Figure 8-5.   Four Nurses Filling Three Staffing Positions

tern requiring two RNs and three LPNs per day could minimize losses by seeing that the day with the "extra" RN coincided with the day deficient by one LPN.

Notice that this sample schedule "fit" was attained by having complete freedom for placement of days off. In this pattern, the RN would have every third weekend off, and the LPN would have only one weekend out of every four. This small sample of interplay between staffing and scheduling may give the reader an appreciation of the complexities involved in the process. It should be adequate to demonstrate that hours could be spent in trying to figure out work hours. When the scheduling process is compounded with holidays, vacations, and personal requests, the job becomes mammoth.

Scheduling Formats

There are several basic types of scheduling to ease the complexity of the process. Basic types include block scheduling, cyclical scheduling, and computer scheduling. Each of these represents an improvement on the preceding form, but examples of all three still are in effect today.

In block scheduling, the work schedule for a unit is planned in a "block" of weeks. The term block originally was applied to this scheduling because days to be worked often were blocked together, forming patterns such as that illustrated in Figure 8-6.

Block scheduling often is done for four to eight weeks at a time. It can be calculated without great difficulty, and it has flexibility

X = days worked in the week

Week	RN	M	T	W	Th	F	Sa	Su
I	A			X	X	X	X	X
	B	X	X			X	X	X
	C	X	X	X	X			X
II	A	X	X			X	X	X
	B	X	X	X	X			X
	C			X	X	X	X	X

Figure 8-6.   First Two Weeks of a Block Schedule

in that the next block of time need not necessarily follow the pattern of the preceding block.

Cyclical scheduling is an improvement on block scheduling in that it has repetitive work patterns assigned to personnel. Since each employee has a permanent pattern, he can calculate even months in advance when he will be on duty. A cyclical schedule has a repeated pattern of interweaving schedules. These interlinking parts are a permanent plan, a fixed cycle of, usually, four to six weeks. The employee may have a different schedule for each of the weeks contained in the cycle, but the pattern repeats without change. Some assignment slots within a cycle may be perceived by employees as more desirable than others. Typically the choice of assignment slots is handled on a seniority basis. Figure 8-7 illustrates a cyclical schedule.

There are several things to note in this cycle. First the employee schedules have been meshed so that: 1) there are never less than two RNs on duty, 2) there are never more than two persons (RNs and LPNs considered together) off on the same day, and 3) there is never a day without at least one LPN on duty. These are the factors which dominated the interlinkages of these employee schedules.

In addition to interlinkage factors, the cycles also consider the individual employees insofar as each employee has at least one full weekend off per four-week cycle. Beyond this general principle, it is obvious that some cycles would be likely to be preferred over others. For example, RN 2 actually has two weekends per period (as one cycle joins the next with Saturday and Sunday off). In addition, this schedule never has the nurse working more than five consecutive days. In contrast, RN 4 usually has split days off, and she has one period in which she works eight days in a row. (The only appealing component in this schedule is the three-day weekend between weeks II and III.) Hence a nurse new to the unit would probably be given the fourth rotation pattern, and she would probably bid for a change of schedule if another RN were to leave the unit.

Even though some cycles are less than perfect, nevertheless the employee can plan ahead because the pattern (in this case a four-week pattern) keeps repeating. Moreover, a schedule need only be developed once per staffing pattern. Since it does repeat without change, the only schedules which need attention are those in which exceptions occur, as in a week containing a holiday. Even here, the scheduler is likely merely to modify the basic plan rather than creating a completely new schedule.

Computerized scheduling enables the user

X = days worked in the week

Staff	Week I S	M	T	W	T	F	S	Week II S	M	T	W	T	F	S	Week III S	M	T	W	T	F	S	Week IV S	M	T	W	T	F	S
RN1	X		X	X	X		X	X	X	X			X	X	X	X	X			X	X			X	X	X	X	X
RN 2		X	X		X	X	X	X	X			X	X	X			X	X	X		X	X	X			X	X	X
RN 3	X	X			X	X	X		X	X	X	X		X	X	X			X	X	X	X	X	X	X			X
RN 4	X		X	X		X	X	X		X	X	X	X				X	X	X	X	X	X	X	X			X	X
LPN 1		X	X	X	X	X			X	X	X			X	X	X				X	X	X	X		X	X		X
LPN 2	X	X	X		X		X	X	X	X		X		X	X	X	X			X	X		X	X	X	X		X

Figure 8-7. Cyclical Staffing Pattern

to devise a plan which considers more variables than would be possible for an individual who was trying to interlink schedules by a hand calculation. For example, one might design a computer program for scheduling with the following dictates:

1. Patterns which must be maintained
   a. Miss G goes to school every Friday; she must have that day off.
   b. Mrs. T's religion will not allow her to work on Saturdays; she must have that day off.
2. First priority options where possible
   a. Mr. F must hire a babysitter if he works Tuesday or Wednesday; he would prefer to have these as his days off.
   b. Give every employee one weekend off per four-week period if possible.
   c. Where possible, give an employee two days off together instead of split.
3. Secondary priorities (to be followed if they do not interfere with priority options above)
   a. Preferably do not have an employee work more than six days in a row.
   b. Schedule holiday time off within 10 days of the occurrence of the holiday.

These variables are only a sample of the constraints that may be incorporated into a computer program for scheduling. Note that the computer can combine general directives applicable to all staff with other variables applicable only to individual staff members. Also it can handle those rules which *must* be applied in addition to rules which are assigned different priorities according to their degree of desirability.

There are many instances when staff complain that the computer is less considerate, less successful than a human scheduler. Usually this reflects not so much a computer deficiency as a failure to update the program or make it comprehensive. A computer will consider only those elements which are programmed into its circuits. A poor computer scheduling system indicates a poor programmer.

Centralized versus Decentralized Scheduling

There are many arguments concerning whether centralized or decentralized scheduling is most satisfactory. In centralized scheduling, all work hours for the entire nursing division are planned in a central office by a single scheduler or a staff of schedulers. Decentralized schedules are planned at the unit level, usually by the lead nurse. Either of these systems may use block, cyclical, or computer techniques of scheduling, though it would be rare that head nurses individually would interact with a computer system.

The following arguments are offered in favor of decentralized scheduling by the head nurse. First, the head nurse knows her staff intimately; she is in a better position to meet their individual scheduling needs. Second, because she knows her patients' needs she can respond to them in her scheduling with a sensitivity that someone in a central office cannot have. Further, where there are differences concerning desired work days, the head nurse can get staff members together for negotiation and problem resolution. Also, decentralized scheduling places responsibility right where it belongs—at the functional level. The head nurse is the one who will have to live with the schedule; she should have the right to make it.

Counterarguments identify the problems in a decentralized scheduling mechanism. First, one must recognize that the staff may try to manipulate the head nurse. They may ask for special favors, and she may be afraid not to grant them, especially if the relationship between the head nurse and the staff members is one of close friendship. Hence staff members may try to get the head nurse to put their needs above the needs of the patients. This problem would not occur if scheduling were done by an impartial central scheduler.

A major argument against decentralized scheduling is the massive amount of time that it takes, especially if block scheduling still is used. This means that the head nurse puts a significant amount of her time every month or every six weeks into an essentially mechanical task. Furthermore, there is likely to be more reworking of the schedule since workers are likely to ask for more schedule modifications from a head nurse than from a central scheduler.

Finally, decentralized scheduling never takes into account the whole division. Hence, it might happen that many floors accidentally all select the same night for their shortest coverage. This lack of central planning would make it difficult ever to count on having staff members who could be "pulled" from other, less busy units.

Arguments for central scheduling contain the following lines of reasoning. First, central scheduling is done without personal bias; there will be few claims of discrimination in this system. Central scheduling is likely to use advanced techniques and those formats which allow for a long-term projection of hours. This ultimately is more useful to the employee than weekly or monthly negotiation with the head nurse. In addition, the scheduler, who does this as a full-time job or as a major responsibility, will become skilled in coping with the intricacies of scheduling. It is better to have this work done by one expert than by 20 amateur head nurse schedulers.

Not only does central scheduling save professional nursing time (a non-nurse can easily learn the necessary nursing implications for scheduling), but it allows for coordination over the entire division. Also the scheduler will be in an ideal position to judge how to fill gaps if it becomes necessary to pull personnel because of staff illnesses or changes in patient work load.

Further, a central scheduler is likely to develop efficient systems to deal with personal requests for exceptions or schedule alterations. When this person deals with all the requests of the division, he will probably become less vulnerable to unreasonable or repeated requests. In addition, such a person is likely to build a routine and efficient system for handling such requests. This same notion can be considered a point against central staffing, that the lack of personal relations with staff may make the scheduler insensitive to pressing needs for schedule alterations. If the central scheduler is not skilled in interpersonal relationships, the schedules are likely to become a focus for employee discontent.

Where centralized scheduling is done utilizing a cyclical pattern, the argument can be made that the system takes little or no account of patient work load. Where work load deviations are the rule, perhaps centralized cyclical scheduling is the worst form. However, most new computerized scheduling programs are both centralized and able to consider fluctuations in the patient load. (Of course, if patient work load changes rapidly, from day to day, then no system that schedules work units ahead will suffice without modifications on a daily basis.)

Goals of Scheduling

Regardless of who does the scheduling or what format is used, the goals for scheduling are universal and can be summarized as follows:

1. Achievement of divisional, departmental, and unit objectives, especially those related to patient care
2. Accurate match of unit needs with staff abilities and numbers
3. Maximum use of manpower
4. Equity of treatment to all employees (or equal treatment for all members within a similar job classification)
5. Optimization on use of professional expertise
6. Satisfaction of personnel (both as to hours worked and as to perceived sense of scheduling equity)
7. Maintenance of flexibility to meet care needs while still giving employees maximum ability to know work hours ahead

8. Consideration of unique needs of staff as well as patients

Scheduling Problems

Of the many problems that arise in scheduling, only a few major ones will be addressed in detail here. These include: 1) management of full-time versus part-time employees, 2) use of supplementary personnel, 3) creation of policies that control abuse of sick-time, 4) use of patient acuity or task quantification in scheduling, 5) legal and administrative constraints on scheduling, and 6) irregular-hour scheduling practices.

Full-Time versus Part-Time Employees

Most institutions combine full-time and part-time workers in a nursing division. Where this is the case, it is very important that the nurse executive develop a benefits package for each of these roles that seems equitable to those within the role and to the employees in the alternate time pattern. Some directors, in an attempt to fill position vacancies when full-time staff is scarce, offer disproportionate benefits to part-timers. This may draw part-time staff, but ultimately the nurse executive may lose full-timers if they feel inequitably treated. Many persons work part-time because of constraints in their lives, but if full-timers find themselves working disproportionate numbers of weekends because part-timers are excused, for example, they may feel they are being treated unfairly. Equity may involve pay or benefits instead of preference in hours. Full-timers may be more understanding of some favoritism in hours extended to a part-timer if they know that they have some recompensing factor, such as vacation prorated at a higher level, a higher pay scale, or some other benefit which compensates and equalizes the situation.

Supplementary Personnel and Their Use

Part-time personnel may or may not be seen as supplementary; often they are regular employees in that they work every week just as the full-timers do. Several other groups of supplementary staff are used at times in various institutions: float personnel, "pulled," or transferred, personnel, agency staff, and emergency staff. These personnel are seen as supplementary to the regular staff when vacancies occur (for whatever reason) in the staff or when the work of the regular staff is increased significantly (for whatever reason).

Float staff are persons who routinely are assigned to the most needy unit of whatever sort. (Often the float staff will be excused from rotating to specialized units, though this is not always the case.) Sometime part-timers are given only float positions; in this case the terms "float" and "part-time" are interchangeable. Other institutions place newcomers on float until a regular position on a unit becomes available. As mentioned earlier, float work requires more adjustment and more judgment than a stable unit job, so new people may be the least well prepared for this task.

Where float staff are not available, most institutions balance the work load by "pulling," or transferring, some staff members from units which are overstaffed in relation to the patient work load to other units which need additional workers. This is a policy which maintains managerial flexibility, a necessity in coping with unforeseen emergency situations. However, if used as a routine procedure, pulling creates many difficulties. First, a worker often is resentful when he is pulled from his regular assignment. In being pulled, he faces all the difficulties of the float nurse—having to learn about new patients, new systems, new expectations. Sometimes injury is added to insult when the same worker always is pulled. Some supervisors make the error of always sending the worker who can adjust to a new environment, is most versatile, is smartest. When one examines this practice, it is obvious that the staff member is being punished for excellence in performance—not a practice designed to endear the supervisor to the pulled staff member.

Further, the "pulled" member may find that he is resented on the new unit, and is treated poorly. In addition to his own feeling that he is an interloper, he may be met with hostility or indifference from the very staff that he was sent to relieve of overwork: "Find the supplies yourself, I'm too busy to orient you." "Didn't they teach you anything on 8 North?" To add another burden, the pulled staff member may find that he is assigned some of the more difficult patients on the unit. Ironically, the time when a unit is the least prepared to orient and assist a new member is when the unit is overworked. Hence, it is not surprising that the pulled staff member may meet with less than desirable staff attitudes.

Several things can be done to mitigate this situation. First, staff should not be transferred unless the need for extra staff is acute. In most cases, the overworked unit will be better off if it can alter its work load, perhaps by omitting unnecessary bed changes and skipping some of the other amenities of care. Other institutions get around the "stranger-in-our-midst" syndrome by creating "sister units" in which all members of each staff are systematically oriented to another unit. In this case when pulling is done, it only is done from one unit to the sister unit. The manager gives up some flexibility, but enhances the likelihood that a transferred member will adapt and actually be useful on the new floor.

Agency personnel usually are the least satisfactory supplementary staff. An agency nurse is one who is hired from a nurse-employment agency to work as a staff nurse on a given unit for one or more sequential days, evenings, or nights. Some agency nurses are kept for months, which gives them time to adjust to the institution and their environment, but others may only work one or two days. Since an agency nurse is more costly to the health care institution, she will be replaced with its own staff as soon as possible.

The major problem with agency nurses is their unfamiliarity with the institution, its policies and practices. Since they are only called in emergencies, there seldom is time for an appropriate orientation. A new movement to correct this deficiency is the creation of a shared agency among several institutions. In this way all agency personnel can be oriented to the limited number of hospitals using the personnel. This often increases quality control in that the sponsoring hospitals are likely to build better controls into the processes by which potential employees are screened. (This is not to say that all privately owned agencies are poor in control; some are excellent.)

Agencies tend to attract diverse types of nurses. Some very excellent nurses are drawn to agency employment because life commitments keep them from working hours demanded by the local employing hospitals and institutions. Students working on graduate degrees often fit into this category, and they typically make excellent temporary employees. Agencies also may draw nurses who, for one reason or another, were unsuccessful in holding a full-time position. Further, a "problem nurse" may manage to drift from one agency to another for quite a while before her work reputation catches up with her.

Many nurse executives feel very frustrated by the expansion of agencies. They claim that this growing mode of employment robs the community of nurses who otherwise would seek employment in their institutions. Agency nurses, on the other hand, cite many instances when they tried and were not accepted as employees in the regular health care institution because these institutions had policies which refused positions to nurses who could not work the typical schedules for nursing staff. Hence by their rigid policies, nurse executives have created the opportunity for temporary employment agencies to grow. Further, once agencies are active in an area and have absorbed much of the nursing population, the same institutions may be so desperate that they have no choice but to use agency personnel. Obviously, unless all nurse executives of an area determine together not to employ agency personnel, it will be very difficult for a single hospital to make and carry out such a resolve. Imaginative policies for part-time employees are the logical solution. (But as mentioned earlier, those policies for part-time workers must be such that full-timers are not penalized—but rewarded—for full-time employment.)

Some institutions are fortunate enough to have another source of supplementary personnel: a list of nonworking nurses who will "fill in" for emergencies, heavy vacation times, or other periods when staff is short. As more and more nurses move toward continuous careers rather than interrupted work periods, this source of supplementary personnel will decline.

When no supplementary staff are available in emergencies, the institution may extend its own personnel with double-shifting and overtime. This poses several problems. First, it is extremely expensive, and, second, it pushes staff members beyond normal physiological and psychological limits, decreasing their efficiency and safety.

Where supplementary staff are not available, it becomes critical to average out the work load from unit to unit. If staff cannot be brought in or transferred, then another source of control is patient admissions. When patients rather than staff are considered the mobile factor, then control is established in the admissions office. A patient acuity system or a task quantification system will enable the nursing division to compare work load among units, and patients may be placed accordingly. Such a system requires that there be several units to which each patient potentially may be assigned. Also the admitting nurse or whoever makes such decisions must have enough admission medical information to estimate future patient care needs.

Creating Policies that Discourage Abuse of Ill-Time

Abuse of sick-time is another factor that can ruin a well-planned schedule. Some employees come to perceive sick-time as time that is "owed" to them. Such employees will take sick days whether or not they are ill. Often such practices can be curtailed by good personnel policies concerning chronic absences. In addition, a policy that builds in rewards for failure to use sick-time will discourage much abuse. Some institutions give back a proportion of unused sick days as extra days off. Other institutions allow sick time to accumulate without loss for long periods.

Use of Patient Acuity or Task Quantification in Scheduling

Work load estimates from patient acuity or task quantification systems often are used to make daily alterations in the schedule. As discussed earlier, some workers object to this routine movement of staff according to unit needs. In other cases, work load data are not used routinely to move staff but only when work load deviation is excessive. One problem with regulation by work load is that nurses soon learn to manipulate the system by overweighting unit work load assessments. If the work load data is to play a significant part in staff scheduling, then one must work at developing a system in which nurses cannot or do not manipulate the data unfairly. Use of these systems will be detailed in Chapter 9.

Legal and Administrative Constraints in Scheduling

In devising schedules for nursing staff, the nurse executive and the scheduler(s) need to be aware of laws concerning work time. For example, the Fair Labor Standards Act is a federal law concerning the use of workers, and most states have work laws which must be followed. Such laws usually address such issues as:

1. Minimum number of hours that a worker must have off between shifts
2. Maximum number of days that may be worked without a day off

3. Maximum number of hours within a single shift

Since work laws vary widely from state to state, it is important that the nurse executive review those pertaining in her own state.

The nurse executive also will need to see that personnel policies of her own institution are followed. Of course, she should have major input in the determination of these policies. It is particularly important that no employee labor contracts be negotiated and agreed to until she has reviewed proposals for their impact upon her staffing and scheduling.

Irregular-Hour Scheduling Practices

Periodically 10-hour, 12-hour, or other irregular length shifts come into popularity. One advantage of such a shift is that it often gives the employee three rather than two days off at a time. For some employees this is a great advantage. For others the extra time off is little compensation for the fatigue generated by the longer shift. The 10-hour shift has the disadvantage of not fitting evenly into a 24-hour day, which usually is resolved by having employees work staggered shifts or by compensating with some partial-shift workers. When overlaps do occur on 10-hour shifts, they usually are planned for the peak work hours, but these plans often are costly because they end up increasing the number of required personnel.

While irregular shifts often are popular when they are initiated, the novelty is likely to wear off. The nurse executive should not jump into a major shift-time revision without much thought and testing. It is true that some units and some particular staffs manage better with such schedules. Since these schedules seldom correspond with those of most staff members' mates or children, the nurse executive should not be led into massive shift-time revisions on the basis of enthusiasm of one or two units of staff members who prefer the irregular hours.

SUMMARY

Assigning, staffing, and scheduling of employees are the ways in which the goals of the nursing division are converted into concrete acts by the nurse executive. In these steps, goals are changed from qualitative formulations into quantitative plans. Assigning, staffing, and scheduling cannot be done in isolation from the goals of the nursing division. Because they interact upon each other, moreover, they must be planned as a constellation of activities. Various plans and calculations are offered by numerous authors; many of the best detailed plans are cited in the bibliography of this chapter. The reader is cautioned not to transplant someone else's plan to her own institution, however, without considering the diverse contextual variables that may make a difference in whether or not the application is successful.

REFERENCES

1. Poland, M., et al. PETO: a system for assessing and meeting patient care needs. *Am. J. Nursing,* 70 (7): 1480, 1970.

BIBLIOGRAPHY

Amenta, A.M. Staffing through temporary help agencies. *Supervisor Nurse,* 8(12):19, 1977.

Aydelotte, M.K. Standard I—staffing for quality care. *J.O.N.A.,* 3(2):33, 1973.

Bauer, J. Clinical staffing with a 10-hour day, 4-day work week. *J.O.N.A.,* 1(6):12, 1971.

Berry, V.I., and Reichelt, P.A. Using routinely collected data for staffing decisions. *Hospitals,* 51(22):89, Nov. 16, 1977.

Ciske, K.L. Primary nursing: an organization that promotes professional practice. *J.O.N.A.,* 4(1):28, 1974.

Clark, E.L. A model of nurse staffing for effective patient care. *J.O.N.A.,* 7(2):22, 1977.

Daeffler, R.J. Patients' perception of care under team and primary nursing. *J.O.N.A.,* 5(3):20, 1975.

Dominick, V.M. Automation of nursing staff allocation. *Supervisor Nurse,* 1(6):20, 1970.

Eusanio, P.L. Effective scheduling—the foundation for quality care. *J.O.N.A.,* 8(1):12, 1978.

Felton, G. Body rhythm effects of rotating work shifts. *J.O.N.A.,* 5(3):16, 1975.

Fisher, D.W., and Thomas, E. A "premium day" approach to weekend nurse staffing. *J.O.N.A.*, 4(5):59, 1974.

Fraser, L.P. The restructured work week: one answer to the scheduling dilemma. *J.O.N.A.*, 2(5):12, 1972.

Gahan, L., and Talley, R. A block scheduling system. *J.O.N.A.*, 5(9):39, 1975.

Ganong, J., Ganong, W., and Harrison, E.T. The 12-hour shift: better quality, lower cost. *J.O.N.A.*, 6(2):17, 1976.

Germaine, A. What makes team nursing tick? *J.O.N.A.*, 1(4):46, 1971.

Giovannetti, P. *Patient Classification System and Staffing by Workload Index.* Saskatoon: University of Saskatchewan, 1973.

Hilger, J. Unit management systems. *J.O.N.A.*, 2(1):43, 1972.

Howell, J.P. Cyclical scheduling of nursing personnel. *Hospitals*, 40(2):77, Jan. 16, 1966.

Hubbard, E.D., Clay, N.H., and Coombs, L.B. A proposed system for scheduling nurses. *Hospital Admin.*, 20(4):44, Fall 1975.

Jelinek, R.C., Zinn, T.K., and Brya, J.R. Tell the computer how sick the patients are and it will tell how many nurses they need. *Modern Hospital*, 121(6):81, 1973.

Kelly, P.A., and Lambert, K.L. The effect of a modified team approach on nurse-patient interaction and job satisfaction. *J.O.N.A.*, 8(4):3, 1978.

Knecht, A.A. Innovation on four tower west—why? *Am. J. Nursing*, 73(5):808, 1973.

Kron, T. Team nursing—how viable is it today? *J.O.N.A.*, 1(6):19, 1971.

Levine, E. (Ed.). *Research on Nurse Staffing in Hospitals.* Washington, D.C.: U.S. Department of Health, Education and Welfare, 1972.

McCarthy, D. Primary nursing: its implementation and six month outcome. *J.O.N.A.*, 8(5):29, 1978.

Manthey, M. Primary nursing is alive and well in the hospital. *Am. J. Nursing*, 73(1):83, 1973.

Marram, G. Innovation of four tower west—what happened? *Am. J. Nursing*, 73(5):814, 1973.

Marram, G. The comparative costs of operating a team and a primary nursing unit. *J.O.N.A.*, 6(4):21, 1976.

Mills, R. A simple method for predicting days of increased patient census. *J.O.N.A.*, 7(2):15, 1977.

Norby, R.B., Freund, L.E., and Wagner, B. A nurse staffing system based upon assignment difficulty. *J.O.N.A.*, 7(9):2, 1977.

Ramey, I.G. Eleven steps to proper staffing. *Hospitals*, 47(6):98, March 16, 1973.

Rinker, K.L., Norris, C.L., and Jordan, M.F. Bed and bath teams: one solution to the weekend staffing shortage. *J.O.N.A.*, 5(4):34, 1975.

Ryan, S.M. The modified work week for nursing staff on two pediatric units. *J.O.N.A.*, 5(6):31, 1975.

Ryan, T., Barker, B.L., and Marciante, F.A. A system for determining appropriate nurse staffing. *J.O.N.A.*, 5(5):30, 1975.

Schlegel, M.W. Innovation on four tower west—how? *Am. J. Nursing*, 73(5):811, 1973.

Somers, J.B. Purpose and performance: a system analysis of nurse staffing *J.O.N.A.*, 7(2):4, 1977.

Stinson, S.M., and Hazlett, C.B. Nurse and physician opinion of a modified work week trial. *J.O.N.A.*, 5(7):21, 1975.

Thomas, B. Job satisfaction and float assignments. *J.O.N.A.*, 2(5):51, 1972.

Warstler, M.E. Cyclic work schedules and a nonnurse coordinator of staffing. *J.O.N.A.*, 3(6):45, 1973.

Wicker, I.B., Jr. Team leadership: a process. *Supervisor Nurse*, 1(6):16, 1970.

Williams, M.A. Quantification of direct nursing care activities. *J.O.N.A.*, 7(8):15, 1977.

Zeeger, L.J. Calculating a nurse staffing budget for a 20 bed unit at 100% occupancy. *J.O.N.A.*, 7(2):11, 1977.

Chapter 9   Patient and Staff Classification Systems

Assigning, staffing, and scheduling are not only interdependent systems, but systems that interact with the nursing division's methods of classifying staff and patients. One method of classifying staff is according to job description (discussed in Chapter 6); another is according to level of performance. Such so-called clinical ladders may be constructed for bedside RN staff only or for various types and levels of nursing personnel.

Patients initially are classified by a decision resulting in their placement on one unit versus another, a pediatric unit versus an adult unit, say, or a medical unit versus a surgical unit. Designation of certain geographical areas as units for placement of certain types of patients is a critical, but often unexamined structure for the nursing division. Patients are also classified according to such factors as level of acuity and amount and level of care required. These classification systems are used normatively both to establish long-term staffing patterns and short-term alterations in scheduling.

NURSING STAFF CLASSIFICATION SYSTEMS

Three classification concepts for nursing will be reviewed here: the clinical ladder, the administrative ladder, and the job responsibility scattergram. These will be discussed as they relate to the RN, though principles would be identical for similar classification of other employees.

The Clinical Ladder

The clinical ladder was devised to allow status and rewards to be conferred on the excellent bedside nurse, promoting retention of excellence at the bedside. Hence the clinical ladder offers another mode of nurse advancement besides the administrative route. In a clinical ladder, nurses are ranked or rated from a beginning competency through diverse levels of clinical practice. Some systems have as few as three levels; others have five to seven; a few have even more steps. In some systems, different job titles are associated with the different levels—a good reinforcement since the job title serves as a status symbol; in other systems a number or letter grade follows a common title (Clinical Nurse II, Staff Nurse C). In all the effective systems, salary also is related to classification. Indeed, in a society where money is so closely associated with status, it would be fruitless to try to establish a clinical ladder as an alternate status route if it lacked monetary rewards.

While the system has the potential of keeping the excellent bedside nurse at the bedside, there are several potential problems with the clinical ladder concept. First, it is built on the assumption that there is room within the nursing practice of the institution for all the expertise that a nurse is capable of using. Certainly, it always is true that a nurse may practice "smarter" within the same time period, but if an institution is short-staffed to the point of barely having time for nurses to finish standing treatment and medication orders, one may question whether much advanced practice really is possible. Indeed one may argue that a clinical ladder in such an environment is a waste. Alternately, an argument may be given for needing a clinical ladder even more in such an environment. In any case, the nurse executive must determine the value of a clinical ladder in her particular environment.

Some institutions, particularly in a period of tight finances, are dropping the notion that the nursing division can use all the clinical expertise obtainable. In these cases, often each unit is assessed and given quotas in relation to the clinical ladder levels. For example, 6 North might be judged to merit no more than two Clinical Nurse IV positions. If those positions are already filled, a Clinical Nurse III on 6 North might have to apply to another unit if she were seeking advancement to the next rank.

Such controls on numbers of nurses within each rank may be necessary if an institution is to control its budget tightly. The open-ended system, in which any new nurse may be hired and then ranked based on ability, could create a great unknown in manpower budgeting. Most areas, however, do not need to fear a sudden onslaught of nurses all with advanced abilities although this budgetary nightmare is probably the dream of every nurse executive as she considers quality control for patient care.

Another potential problem with the clinical ladder is the difficulty of creating a fair evaluation system. Nursing performance may be theoretically on different levels, but to establish and describe those levels and to tell where each nurse fits in relation to those levels is a monumental and difficult job.

A third problem is that of deciding whether the clinical ladder should reflect only performance values. Typically the clinical ladder is used to reward both performance and education. The nurse executive who really wants to pay for services delivered will keep her ladder free of credentialism. For example, suppose that the Clinical Nurse V position calls for advanced research. The executive will argue that she cares only that the nurse demonstrate that behavior, not that she have the credential of a master's degree. On the other hand, the nurse executive who uses her clinical ladder as a means to promote and reward advanced education might refuse to promote a nurse to Clinical Nurse V without a master's degree, thereby using the clinical ladder as a mechanism to urge nurses back to school. While an education factor may be built into a clinical ladder as a prerequisite, the ladder will be a poor one if placement on the scale is automatically related to education, with little consideration of performance. Where this is the case, the nurse executive sometimes pays for services not delivered.

Financial compensation (clinical versus administrative) also presents a problem. Although one wants to give status and rewards to excellent clinical nurses, it is a fact that the administrative nurse has greater responsibilities—for staff and for larger patient populations. Hence it is difficult to justify a system where one may make more money for less responsibility, no matter how well performed. This is not an insoluble problem, however, as a coordinative reward system may be devised that judges excellence of administrative performance and rewards that excellence in a similar manner. In such a system, the base pay would reflect larger rewards for administrative positions, but a larger portion of the total salary would be related to merit (ladder placement) than would be the case in another reward system.

Methodologically, creation of a clinical ladder involves several steps. First job descriptions for each level of the ladder must be developed in concrete and highly operational terms. Typically several major categories of nursing performance are defined and addressed on each job description so as to allow comparisons from one level to another. Often systems use some formulation of the steps of the nursing process to serve this function. For example, every job description might address the categories of assessment, planning, implementation, and evaluation. Other systems create their own categories; a system might use care planning, care delivery, coordination with other staff, leadership, research, and contribution to the nursing system. Notice that the latter set of categories brings up a question which inevitably arises in the construction of a clinical ladder, to wit: Where does clinical nursing leave off and management begin? This is a difficult question to answer in nursing since the typical clinical nurse has some responsibility for management within the context of her role. Note that with this set of categories, some components (e.g., conducting research) may not arise at all in the early levels of practice.

Once the key responsibilities have been built into the job descriptions, they serve a secondary purpose: they become the categories for evaluation on the measurement tool(s) which judge clinical rank. Even here the task is not a simple one, for each rank is made up of a constellation of behaviors. One must make decision rules, then, for the behaviors in the constellation. 1) Must the candidate achieve *all* the behaviors listed for this rank? A majority of them? 75 percent? 2) How often must these behaviors be demonstrated? All the time? A majority of the time? 75 percent of the time? 3) Are the measurement tools constructed to show whether the candidate *performs* or *is capable of performing* the behaviors? For example, a candidate might submit three excellent nursing care plans for evaluation by a ranking committee, but this is no assurance that she routinely does care plans when on duty. 4) How does one rank a candidate with a mixed performance, for example, a nurse who performs one-third of the activities on Level II, one-third of the activities on Level III, and yet another third on Level IV? Decisions such as these must be made before a clinical ladder program is instituted.

Procedures of evaluation also must be considered. Who judges the worth of the candidate? An impartial committee of nurses who have not worked with the nurse? Her own peer work group? Her supervisor? In a mixture of judges, what does each contribute, and how is each one's assessment weighted in the final judgment? Who

nominates the candidate in the first place? Is self-nomination required? Must the immediate supervisor recommend the candidate? Is each nurse routinely reevaluated at some specified time interval?

Methods of evaluation present their own set of problems. Is evaluation by means of some test situation such as a nurse's assignment to three difficult patients while under the eyes of a group of evaluators? Or is evaluation based on the ongoing observation of a nurse's daily work by supervisors and peers? By demonstrations? Or by retrospective reviews? What combination of methods will be used?

One also must relate the system to the initiation and continuation of employment. At what rank does a new employee begin when her abilities have not yet been assessed? Does everyone begin at the first level until proved more advanced? Or is the beginning rank estimated via years of experience or education? How soon is a change in rank to be done? How much time is allowed for orientation before ranking judgments are made? For continued employment is routine advancement required? Must one achieve Level II within a year or be fired? Or can one practice at Level I for a lifetime, receiving a Level I salary? The procedures for implementing a clinical ladder are as complicated as is the initial building of the ladder and the construction of the measurement tools. The system will fail unless the decision rules for all these system components are determined in advance.

The clinical ladder is a satisfying concept which is easier to support intellectually than to implement in actuality. The director who wishes to construct such a system must be prepared for the long and hard work involved: a clinical ladder may be very rewarding to both staff and administration, but a good system requires massive effort and continual upkeep.

The Administrative Ladder

Some nursing divisions build parallel clinical and administrative ladders. In this case, a single nurse may have two rankings, one clinical and one adminstrative. Other institutions take an either-or approach; the nurse is ranked either on the clinical ladder or on the administrative ladder. Either approach is defensible. The administrative ladder has several problems unique to its situation. First, it is not possible to pay someone for administrative acumen which is not used in their position. Hence one cannot pay an executive's salary to a charge nurse merely because she has the capability to fill that role were she placed in it. This is unlike the clinical situation, where the nurse is assumed to be able to use all her expertise in her bedside role. The administrative ladder necessarily is tied to the administrative slots available in the given nursing division.

Further, it is difficult to predict the potential for advancement without placing the candidate in the higher role. For example, many excellent head nurses have failed to adapt to the supervisory role. The use of the administrative ladder for assessing advancement potential is somewhat limited. Similarly, although clinical excellence is a prerequisite for an initial management role, in no way does it assure capability in managerial tasks.

Where an individual is ranked simultaneously on both an administrative and a clinical ladder, another complication arises. The long-term administrator often loses some specific clinical skills. For example, one does not expect a director of nursing to be adept in starting intravenous infusions. How, then, is this loss of clinical skills accounted for in the dual ranking system? (Notice that the problem here is one of immediate skill; obviously, the nursing director could regain her clinical skills within a short time, but the use of her time is better put to acquiring additional management skills.)

An administrative ladder implies a ranking of all nursing administrative/managerial positions in relation to one another. This, in itself, raises some problems. Whose position is higher: the evening supervisor who covers more units but superficially or the day supervisor who covers fewer units but in more

detail? The ranking of administrative posts inevitably calls for weighing of factors of depth versus breadth of responsibility or job scope. Notice, that this is a problem because an administrative level is not identical with a specific administrative job.

If administrative levels are to be defined in ways that allow one to differentiate among them meaningfully, a strategy is required. Either one may plan and describe the levels independently and then rank the administrative jobs of the division according to where they fall within the levels, or one may work backwards, cumulating jobs of equivalent responsibility and summarizing them into a level description. The first plan probably is more intellectually satisfying, but the second will pragmatically allow one to relate the administrative levels to the available administrative jobs.

One advantage of having an administrative ladder is that it may be used as a counseling tool for a person who holds a managerial position yet fails to see the full implications of that responsibility. Similarly, such a tool can be used to differentiate management jobs which superficially appear alike, such as the job of a charge nurse of a unit for an eight-hour period versus the job of the head nurse of that unit for an eight-hour period. An administrative ladder would make clear to that charge nurse (were she arguing for equal pay for an equal eight-hour shift) the ways in which her responsibilities are more limited than those of the head nurse.

The Job Responsibility Scattergram

Sometimes it is difficult to compare nursing positions regarding overall responsibility. It may be as difficult to compare two dissimilar managerial positions as it is to compare a clinical position with a managerial position. The job responsibility scattergram enables one to better grasp the significant differences among jobs within a given nursing division. Each institution should designate its own categories for use in a scattergram. Figure 9-1 illustrates the categories I prefer.

RESPONSIBLE FOR	MANAGERIAL TOOLS		
	Self	Staff	Systems
One			
A group	x	x x	x x x x x
A total population	x	x x x x	x x x x x x x x x x x

Figure 9-1.   Job Responsibility Scattergram for a Nurse Executive

RESPONSIBLE FOR	MANAGERIAL TOOLS		
	Self	Staff	Systems
One	x	x	x
A group	x x x	x x x x x x x	x x
A total population	x	x	

Figure 9-2.   Job Responsibility Scattergram for a Head Nurse

In the scattergram, responsibilities are listed in relation to size of group—one-to-one relationships, groups rather than single persons, or multiple groups. Normally these categories would refer to patients, as follows:

1. Single patient. Mr. X as focus (bedside care responsibility)
2. Patient group. Single team of patients (team-leading responsibility) or single type of patients (quality control evaluation), e.g., all diabetics
3. Total population. Several patient groups (supervisor's responsibility) or all patient groups (director's responsibility)

These categories are cross-gridded with the major tools used in meeting responsibilities, for example:

1. Single patient/self. Bedside care by an RN
2. Single patient/staff. Team leader assignment of aide to Mr. X's care
3. Single patient/system. Arranging for home care for Mr. X using a home care health agency

For certain positions, the groups may refer to staff rather than patients. For example, in looking at staff development work, the following illustrations might pertain:

1. Single staff member/self. One-to-one educational consultation by a staff development instructor with a staff nurse
2. A group of staff members/staff. Instructors team teaching a major new procedure to 5 West staff members
3. A total staff population/systems. Staff Development departmental planning for the total program for the year of educational activities

In the scattergram, the greater responsibilities fall toward the lower, righthand box in the diagram. Further, if each "x" represents a key job function, then some jobs will have more total "x's" than others. Hence the staffing coordinator's job functions will fall primarily in the lower righthand area, just like the director's functions. In the case of the coordinator, however, she will have few x's, representing the limited domain of responsibility. Use of the scattergram in this manner, enables one to reflect both scope of the job (number of total x's) and depth of the job (distribution toward lower righthand side). If job scattergrams are superimposed upon each other, their similarities and differences may be easily reviewed.

PATIENT CLASSIFICATION SYSTEMS

Like staff, patients may be classified along various lines of which three will be reviewed here: 1) by placement on a given patient unit, 2) according to acuity, and 3) by assessment through total task quantification systems. Both patient classification and staff classification systems endeavor to make a better match of patient needs and staff delivery of care.

Classification by Placement on a Patient Unit

The placement of patients on given geographical units is a major organizing structure within an institution for health care. It is important for the nurse executive to consider the nature of those placements. Often the nature of the units is dictated by size. For example, a small community hospital may have to mix diverse patient populations simply because it has few geographically distinct units. Even a large institution must select patient populations large enough to fill a given unit; otherwise cost effectiveness will be lost with unfilled beds.

Unit designation usually is a result of past decisions and present power struggles. (Many an institution woos an important cardiologist by promising him "his own unit" for cardiovascular patients.) Unfortunately, nursing seldom is considered in such unit-designating activities. This is not a reflection of logic but of power. Indeed, if one were to assign units rationally, it would be on the basis of nursing, not of medicine. Nursing is a 24-hour-a-day, ongoing activity, while medical care is intermittent, and a short-time unit event. Given this logic, a major aim of the nurse executive should be to gain control of the unit-designating function.

Nursing had control of unit designation in the era of "progressive patient care," when nursing divisions designated units according to type or level of nursing care required. When level was the criteria, there were maximal-care units, medium-care units, and minimal-care units. Indeed, this concept was the start of the intensive care unit (maximal care). A problem with the placement by *level of care* was that the patient was moved from unit to unit as his status changed. This not only caused problems in logistics but also decreased patient satisfaction for just as a patient finally knew all the staff on one unit and felt comfortable with his surroundings, he was moved to another.

When *type of care* rather than level of care was designated, units such as acute-care, convalescent-care, self-care, and teaching units arose. One still sees long-term care units, for example, as an outgrowth of this placement principle.

There is no single principle upon which units should be determined. Many possibilities exist. Fortunately, many of these principles are equally useful to medicine and nursing. Some possibilities include:

1. Similar patient age (pediatric or adolescent units)
2. Similar nursing treatments needed (burn or spinal cord injury units)
3. Similar patient needs (recovery rooms, nursery)
4. Similar medical treatments (surgical units, medical units)
5. Similar medical specialty (genitourinary, gynecologic units)
6. Similar patient behaviors (psychiatry)

Although some of these principles favor nursing and some favor medicine, many represent good compromises. Certainly the nurse executive should be able to sell her proposals for unit designation if she can show that such designation promotes better nursing care. As we move into an age of greater nursing specialization, the control of unit designation will become of even greater significance.

Patient Classification and Task Quantification Systems

Patient classification and task quantification systems are two approaches to the same objective and will be discussed together for the sake of comparison. Both systems aim to make some statement concerning the nurse's work load, though they use different methodologies. In a patient classification system, a judgment of patient needs is established and the patient is classified accordingly in one of several categories. (Some systems use as few as three categories; some as many as nine. Most have four to five groups.) Categories are determined in one of two ways: 1) For some systems each category is described generally, and that description may be reinforced with sample patient cases described. Given these descriptions, the nurse judges which category comes closest to

the patient's status, and he is placed in that category. 2) For some systems, critical indices have been determined, and the indices dictate patient classification. For example, a system may make absolute statements such as: "Any incontinent patient may not be placed lower than Category III." Or a system may classify a patient according to several characteristics considered together, stating: "If a patient has any two of the following conditions, he belongs in Category IV," this statement followed by such characteristics as "immobility," "on intravenous therapy," "unable to bathe self," and so forth. In these systems, not all patient characteristics are considered; only those which have been found to have a significant impact on care level or time are elected for review.

Whether through a summary judgment or a summarization of specific characteristics, patients are sorted into various classifications. Each classification ultimately is associated with a normative number of nursing hours required. Obviously the hours will be different from shift to shift. For example, a patient who is up and about but learning about a new disability (diabetes, for example) may need many nursing hours during the day and virtually none during the night hours. An acutely ill patient, on the other hand, might have need for as much care during the night shift as during the day.

Many patient classification systems actually are patient acuity systems based on how sick the patient is. Acuity alone, however, may fail to reflect nursing hours accurately. In the illustration above, the relatively well diabetic will need many nursing hours to learn self-care for his diabetes. Hence some systems calculate on degree of self-care rather than on acuity. Other systems combine these two factors.

Where a task quantification system is used, the nursing task rather than the patient need is considered. Here all required tasks are summarized on average performance time norms. To calculate total nursing hours required, factors are added to consider indirect nursing time. Again, these systems may attempt to account for every nursing task or only for those which make critical differences. (For example, some systems eliminate items such as "relief of anxiety," assuming they will be addressed while accomplishing a physical task like giving a bath.)

Many nurse executives were dissatisfied with the recommendations that followed the time and motion studies which underlie the task analysis method. Others were satisfied and followed the recommendations whether or not they made sense. Most early studies were designed by non-nurses, and many hospital administrators used the study recommendations to dictate practices to nurse executives. To see what problems were created, one must examine the methods and assumptions followed by the systems analysts who designed the studies and made recommendations.

The methods of these task quantification systems were adapted from studies of other jobs that were primarily mechanical, highly programmed, and physical in nature. Since much of nursing is mindwork rather than handwork, it is not surprising that the methods only captured a part of the nursing work. For example, early studies ignored any nursing that was not evident to the non-nurse and nonmedically trained observer who was timing nursing tasks. Hence a question posed to a patient to elicit information concerning response to a nursing regimen was not even heard by the observer. The studies proceeded with the simplistic notion that "Nursing is the physical tasks that nurses do in the presence of patients."

Although much useful data were gathered in this manner, the problem was that the analysts assumed they were measuring *all* the nursing care that went on. Their subsequent recommendations, which usually affected staffing, often left no time for anything except the physical tasks observed. Another problem was the notion, brought with the analysts from previous non-nursing studies, that each specific task could be assigned to an appropriate level of employee and then done only by that level employee for optimal economy.

Note that with this concept, a throat irrigation might be assigned to the LPN level, with no consideration that *some* throat irrigations might be extremely difficult, requiring an RN because of the patient's particular physiological status. To the early systems analysts, a throat irrigation was "the same" in all cases, and the hospital was cautioned never to pay for a higher level worker to do a lower level task. Notice that this concept of assigning tasks by level of worker not only assumes that all cases of a given task are the same, but it also assumes that workers at a given level are all the same, that they are interchangeable units.

Given these methods and assumptions of the studies, the recommendations were based on an implied method of assignment which parceled out tasks to appropriate level workers. Since this was the "economy model," it was assumed that nurses would function this way. Obviously such a method was counter to all forms of patient-oriented care (as opposed to task-oriented care). Further, there was no consideration of the fact that a patient requiring tasks on many different levels would be faced with a myriad of different staff members daily.

Another problem with the studies soon was recognized. In the other non-nursing studies done by systems analysts, timed tasks occurred in a highly controlled environment, where work could be planned for a given time and done then. Hence, many of the nursing studies assumed that nursing could be managed similarly, and they allowed no time for interruptions in the work flow, for example by visitors to patients, physicians' rounds, or patients simply not being in their rooms on a first attempt to administer some care.

Clearly, the focus on isolation of tasks, assigning tasks to levels, and assuming a controlled work environment—if these are taken as givens—would produce a design for staffing which was understaffing the first time an interruption in the work flow occurred or the first time a task had to be done by a higher-level worker.

What was wrong was not the studies—they produced much rich and usable data. The error was in the assumption that the recommendations from non-nurse analysts should be taken at face value and used as given. These studies often were the nurse executive's first introduction to extensive research methods, and many nurse executives were intimidated by what *must* be "scientific findings." Fortunately, today's nurse executive is better equipped to deal with such research-related problems, and today most time task analysis systems are themselves more sophisticated. They typically include cognitive tasks that were omitted in early studies. Further, they are not used now to dictate assignment systems; nor are they assumed to capture all the work of a nursing unit.

Despite their limitations, task quantification systems do give an excellent rough average of the amount of work to be done on a unit (or for a given patient). When these studies are used in the appropriate manner, they are excellent tools for planning the delivery of nursing care.

For task quantification systems, it is common to create some form of "patient care unit." In the PETO system, for example a PCU equals 7.5 minutes[1]. Other systems may use time norms directly without creating an intervening unit of measurement. The nurse executive must be aware of how the time norms are set for her system. Typically they are norms of what *is* done, not what *ought* to be done. If the real and the desired performance vary greatly, the present time norms may need to be reviewed. Also, the nurse executive should be careful about "borrowing" time norms established in another institution. It would not be surprising to find that time norms differed from place to place; differences might reflect variations in patient acuity as well as differences in equipment and supplies used.

Whether time norms are cumulated per patient or per nursing unit depends upon the use to which they are put. For example, these norms may be used in calculating staffing needs, revising scheduling, setting individual patient fees, in determining supply and equipment needs, or in developing trend data over time. (The same uses apply to patient acuity or patient needs systems.) Not only may data be collected per patient or per patient floor, but it also may be collected per 24-hour time period or per shift. Again, the intended use of the data dictates how often it must be obtained.

Whatever the system that is used to collect data, it should meet the following criteria: 1) simplicity and speed of data collection, 2) accuracy versus ability to manipulate data to one's own ends, and 3) reliability and validity of the format used. Accurate patient or task data enable the nurse executive to relate patient need and nursing care delivery. Such data also will reveal instances where a constant patient population (number) has increasing or decreasing needs for nursing services. Indeed, many nurse executives claim that today's average patient is sicker than was the case five to ten years ago. Patient or task data enable one to support such claims in defending proposed budgets or staffing plans.

SUMMARY

Both patients and staff may be classified for various purposes: staffing, scheduling, assigning fees, rewarding advanced clinical practices, collecting data on changes in the health care delivery system. Classification systems are useful if they are reliable, valid, and easy to administer. They allow one to compare interinstitutional data and to account for differences. Such systems increase the data base upon which the nurse executive may build and make decisions.

REFERENCES

1. Poland, M., et al. PETO: a system for assessing and meeting patient care needs. *Am. J. Nursing,* 70(7):1480, 1970.

BIBLIOGRAPHY

Anderson, M.I., and Denyes, M.J. A ladder for clinical advancement in nursing practice: implementation. *J.O.N.A.,* 5(2):16, 1975.

Bracken, R.L., and Christman, L. An incentive program designed to develop and reward clinical competence. *J.O.N.A.,* 7(3):8, 1977.

Colavecchio, R., Tescher, B., and Scalzi, C. A clinical ladder for nursing practice. *J.O.N.A.,* 4(5):54, 1974.

Daubert, E.A. Patient classification systems and outcome criteria. *Nursing Outlook,* 27(7):450, 1979.

Giovannetti, P. Understanding patient classification systems. *J.O.N.A.,* 9(2):4, 1979.

Haynor, P. Career ladder—back to the bedside. *Supervisor Nurse,* 9(2):33, 1978.

Kissinger, C.L. Community nursing administration: quantifying nursing utilization. *J.O.N.A.,* 3(5):42, 1973.

Miller, R. Career ladder program: a problem-solving device. *J.O.N.A.,* 5(5):27, 1975.

Nelson, C.A., and Arford, P.H. Strategy for clinical advancement. *J.O.N.A.,* 7(4):46, 1977.

Norby, R.B., Freund, L.E., and Wagner, B. A nurse staffing system based upon assignment difficulty. *J.O.N.A.,* 7(9):2, 1977.

Roehrl, R.K. Patient classification: a pilot test. *Supervisor Nurse,* 10(2):21, 1979.

Tescher, B.E., and Colavecchio, R. Definition of a standard for clinical nursing practice. *J.O.N.A.,* 7(3):32, 1977.

Wandelt, M.A. and Steward, D.S. *Slater Nursing Competencies Rating Scale.* New York: Appleton-Century-Crofts, 1975.

Zimmer, M.J. Rationale for a ladder for clinical advancement. *J.O.N.A.,* 2(6):18, 1972.

Earlier the elements which structure nursing management were likened to the two types of structures that organize a chess game: 1) the structure of the chess board itself, a structure that constrains and directs space, and 2) the "rules" for moving each playing piece, that is, the structures that constrain and direct events. Elements already discussed in this book (functions, organization charts, assignments, staffing plans, schedules, and classification systems) may be compared to the first type of structure; they set the scene (structure and space) on which the game will be enacted. The policies, procedures, and practices discussed in this chapter may be compared to the second type of structure, the rules for moving pieces, for they constrain and direct specific events. Policies, procedures, and practices are all rules of one sort or another which together determine the nursing systems of the division. These systems should be revised periodically for logistic efficiency, safety, and effectiveness. Often the nurse executive is made more aware of her own nursing systems by reviewing systems used by others. Professional interchange among peer nurse executives is helpful. Nursing systems will be reviewed in detail in Chaper 21.

POLICIES AND PROCEDURES

There are many different meanings given to the term policy. As used in this chapter, policy means a guideline that has been formalized by administrative authority and directs action to some purpose. A policy system is the total constellation of events and rules related to that policy. There are three major components in a policy system: 1) a purpose, 2) a policy rule, and 3) a written directive on actions to follow in implementing the rule, i.e., a procedure. A procedure also is a formalized guideline, but a second-level one; it details the means to be used to achieve the ends specified in the purpose and delineated further in the policy. The procedure may or may not allow discretion in application of a policy statement. A procedure specifies the way in which a policy is to be implemented if the mode of implementation is to be restricted. Hence many policy statements, but not all, are accompanied by procedures. To best reflect their function, procedures are referred to here as action directives.

Policies and action directives contrast with practices in that practices are the actual and habitual behaviors of organization personnel. Policies and procedures are prescribed, but practice, prescribed or not, is what is actually done. Practices are the behavior patterns that are maintained and followed. A practice may address behaviors prescribed in a policy or it may address behaviors which have not been addressed in policy.

Policy Systems

The components of a policy system are demonstrated in the following illustration. Suppose an institution has a policy that no new employee will be granted vacation time for the first year of employment. Such a policy rule requires a written directive on actions to be followed, for the policy itself is still flexible enough for multiple interpretations. For example, is the end of the eleventh month or the end of the twelfth month considered as completion of a year's employment? Does the policy refer to all vacation time or only to vacation time with pay? Does this policy mean that the new employee earns no vacation time at all during the first year, or simply that he must take the earned vacation during the second year?

Clearly this policy needs an action directive if diverse managers are to apply it consistently. Typically both policies and action directives (together or separately) are recorded in a "policy book" and are referred to as policies. The common use of the term *policy* for both policy statements and action directives is misleading. Managers tend to fuse these two components in their thinking, but they are distinct entities.

The same policy about vacation time can be contrasted with the purpose for which it was formulated. Simply by examining the policy statement one cannot determine the purpose for which it was derived. Without knowing the circumstances under which the rule was created, there is no way to determine the purpose.

One is led to an observation of the peculiar relations among the three components of a policy system: there is no way to derive the other two components from any one given component of a policy system. For any given purpose, many different policy statements could be derived. For example, even an apparently simple purpose of establishing racial equality in hiring practices could lead to several contradictory policies such as 1) hiring on a quota system designed to reflect local population percentages, 2) hiring on a system that gives certain compensatory advantages to minority candidates, or 3) evaluation of candidates' qualifications without reference to race.

Nor is one able to deduce the purpose from the policy. For example, if a company has a policy of evaluating candidates without reference to race, there is no assurance that the purpose is one of racial equality. The purpose may be simply to get the candidate with the best qualifications for each job, or it may be one of having policies that qualify the institution for desired federal funds.

Similarly, for any given policy statement,

any number of different action directives can be devised, and an action directive may or may not be successful in implementing the policy for which it was drafted. Many action directives have effects far different from that intended by the creator.

The components of a policy system can be differentiated from each other by the means with which they are evaluated. Fig. 10-1 illustrates this point.

Unanticipated Outcomes.

An interesting aspect revealed in the chart is that unrelated (and usually unanticipated) results may occur when an action directive is effected. Such results may be beneficial or detrimental to the functions of the division.

Detrimental effects can follow action directives by several ways. The first occurs when the original purpose is covert, unknown, or forgotten. Most of the negative effects occur when an action directive "stays on the books" long after the purpose it served has disappeared. One sees instances of this problem every day. Take, for example, staff members still assigned to 10:45 A.M. lunches, a practice started because the "old cafeteria" could not handle the full employee load over regular lunch hours. This practice, of course, continues even though a new and efficient cafeteria has long since replaced the old one. If no one remembers why the 10:45 lunches were begun in the first place, then it's difficult to calculate the effects of a proposed change in the time schedule. Thus the 10:45 system is likely to go on forever, even though it is burdensome to employees and disruptive of the morning work.

The reason even courageous administrators fear to change a policy once it has been established is that no one can anticipate all the possible effects of a proposed change. One effect that *can* be anticipated is that someone will object to the change, even of a clearly detrimental directive. For example, at least one group of workers will fight for maintenance of the 10:45 A.M. lunch hour.

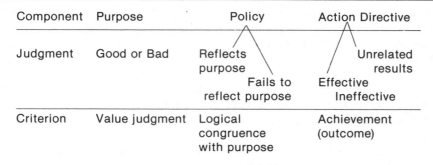

Component	Purpose	Policy	Action Directive
Judgment	Good or Bad	Reflects purpose / Fails to reflect purpose	Unrelated results / Effective Ineffective
Criterion	Value judgment	Logical congruence with purpose	Achievement (outcome)

Figure 10-1. Components of a Policy System

If all a person knows about a directive is that it cured some problems of the past—and it must have, otherwise no one would have bothered to make such a directive—it is not surprising that the nurse administrator hesitates to change it and possibly institute an unknown problem.

A change in or creation of an action directive has not only the potential for reinstituting past problems, but also the potential of creating new and unanticipated negative effects. There is no way that all such effects may be foreseen because most negative effects occur in areas totally unrelated to the directive's purpose.

Nevertheless, risking some unanticipated negative effects seems a better alternative than continuing apparently meaningless old policies or managing without a policy where one is clearly needed. Given this situation, two rules for drafting and implementing action directives are evident: 1) Test any new directive on a small population (one unit) before applying it throughout the institution. 2) Identify the purpose and the policy in the document containing the action directive. Later, these inclusions can be used in measuring the effectiveness of the action directive or in determining the need for its continuation.

Perspectives on Policy

There are many and contradictory perspectives on policy and the function it performs in organizations. Moore, for example, identifies the following working assumption in her writing on the subject: "policies are required in areas in which actions have been delegated to individuals who are not equipped to process the relevant information needed to make enlightened decisions about these actions"[1]. Thus Moore sees policy as a substitute for decision making.

This view can be contrasted with Perrow's view, "our Policy Document, Standing Orders and Directives, causes people to assume the precise opposite of the real situation, i.e., that this extant written policy will deprive them of the right to make decisions. In fact, it is only by delineating the areas of 'freedom' in this way that a subordinate knows when he can make decisions. The absence of written policy leaves him in a position where any decision he takes, however apparently trivial, may infringe (upon) an unstated policy and produce a reprimand"[2].

Perrow stresses the positive aspects of policy. In this vein he notes that every department protects its autonomy by establishing rules. In addition, he says that rules are great scapegoats, for one can cite "the rule" when having to hand down an unpleasant decision or take an unpleasant action. Another function of a good rule, says Perrow, is that of deciding between two choices where no clear advantage can be perceived between the two alternatives.

Perrow offers some excellent insights on the organismic nature of rules. He notes that the sources of rules are either past adjustments or present searches for stability. He finds changes in rules to be incremental rather than substitutional. Thus the "red tape" takes on a growth of its own; it becomes the memory of the organization.

Many persons think that cutting back rules increases organizational efficiency. Perrow disagrees with this generalization and attempts to identify those situations in which rules can be reduced successfully. One such situation exists where a high degree of mechanization is possible. Perrow notes that machines are bundles of "built-in" rules; hence external rules can be decreased. It is interesting to note that he considers professionals to be like machines in this sense; they also have the "built-in" rules and thus need fewer external ones.

Another situation that allows for reduction in rules is high uniformity in personnel. A good example of this is the difference in the number of rules necessary to regulate a nursing faculty group as compared with a nursing service group. Clearly a faculty group is comparatively homogeneous, consisting of similarly educated persons with like value systems. A nursing service group, however, has diverse persons from different life situations and with different educations and different values. Clearly the nursing service group will need more rules than the faculty group.

A third factor that allows for reduction in rules is found in the nature of the work. If the product is very simple and the transformation from raw to finished product is uncomplicated, there is little need for rules. At the opposite extreme, if the product is exotic and highly individualized, it is not possible to have exacting rules. Here one might compare the number of rules in a coronary care unit to those in a medical-surgical unit. Typically the coronary care unit will have more written policies because its "product" is more uniform and easier to predict than is that of the medical-surgical unit.

One can summarize Perrow's stand by his observation that rules do exist in any situation and that if they are written the areas of freedom are delineated. They tell a subordinate what decision he *can* make. In response to negative views of policy formation, Perrow notes that the problem is not rules; indeed, effective rules are not noticed. The problem is *bad* rules, and they should be changed.

Formulating Nursing Policy

Content of Policies

Several questions must be considered when formulating nursing policy: How does nursing policy relate to other institutional policy statements? What content should be included in a manual? How specific should policy statements and action directives be? How should policy statements be worded? What are the mechanics of creating a usable policy manual? What content belongs in nursing policy statements?

It is important to understand how nursing policy relates to other administrative policy. Policy established at higher organizational levels should not be contradicted by nursing policy, but nursing policy need not be limited to areas covered under these general policies. The nursing division is expected to establish its own policies on the operational level.

One area in which problems commonly occur is in the interaction between a personnel division and a nursing division. If the operational nature of policy making is kept in mind, such problems tend to clear. As a condition of hire, for example, a personnel division may have a policy that all employees of a particular job classification receive four weeks vacation yearly. Unless she cares to challenge the policy at a higher organizational level, the nurse executive is bound by this commitment. On the other hand, the personnel division has no right to direct the nurse executive in operational application of the policy. The nurse executive has the right to make further restrictions on when and under what conditions that vacation time is given, as long as it is in fact given. Thus, the method of implementing administrative policies remains the operational prerogative of the nurse executive.

A special instance in policy formulation is that of the coordinated policy. This policy represents an agreement between two divisions as to some aspect of their relationship with each other. Nursing and Medical Records, for example, may have agreed on a routine for the handling of readmission charts. Validation of such policy requires consent and signature of both division heads on the published action directive. In this example the policy requires the signatures of the nurse executive and of the director of the division controlling medical records. The nursing manual may be planned so as to integrate or to separate such coordinated policies.

Selection of content is an important factor in formulating a policy manual. When should a policy statement be made? One answer is that a policy should be established when its creation solves a problem that recurrently affects the work of the division. This answer alone, however, is not adequate, for policy should describe the total scope of the division's autonomous responsibility, not just the problem areas.

Sometimes it is difficult to identify all relevant areas for autonomous policy formulation. The nurse executive's problem is that she is too close to the division, unless she herself is a new employee. It is difficult to discern discrete divisional activities when one is already adjusted to these behavior patterns. The behaviors become habituated and no longer come to conscious attention. Just as it might be difficult to describe what one does when driving a car, so it becomes difficult to *see* the activities a nursing division routinely performs if one is habituated to these activities. It is these divisional patterns that should be captured in policy statements.

Two measures can be used to identify content gaps in policy. One system is to ask new employees to carefully log those questions for which there is no policy statement and

for which they have to rely on word-of-mouth information. These logs are useful sources for locating gaps. Another measure is to carefully categorize the policy manual into a comprehensive topical arrangement. Each topic can then be studied for omissions.

Two types of policy exist, and they require different formulation. Policy meant to give facilitating information often requires detailed action directives. For example, if the nurse needs to find out the policy for renting a piece of equipment not available in the home institution, she needs to know precise facts. Indeed, such a document needs to be "heavy" on procedure and "light" on policy. Similarly, if she needs to know nursing's responsibility (as opposed to the laboratory's responsibility) for an unusual test, she needs exact information.

The second type of policy is one used as a basis for administrative problem solving. Policies for the second purpose need action directives that establish boundaries, reference points, and guidelines without limiting the nurse manager's ability to use judgment. If a policy is too exacting, a nurse manager may find that she is forced to make an unfair or less than desirable decision upon occasion. For example, a nurse executive might find herself unable to finance the needed education of a coronary care nurse if a tuition policy is written with only college credit courses in mind. Thus action directives guiding management decisions should leave room for unanticipated qualifications and conditions that are in the spirit of the original policy statement. If the manager is thrust into a lock-step procedure for every occasion there is little need for management at all.

Policy Format

Another major question concerns the format for the nursing policy statement and action directive. The chief criteria for policy format selection are simplicity and utility. If the policies structured are complex and difficult to follow, the manual will not be used. There is no one ideal format for policies, but a few principles can be given:

1. If possible the title of the policy should use the most common terminology (for easy location).
2. A brief description of the policy should be set out at the top of the document so that the reader can rapidly tell if it contains the desired information (without having to read the entire action directive).
3. Objectives (purposes) for the policy should be stated on the action directive. This is important for periodic manual review. If the policy no longer meets the original objectives, it will be apparent, and the policy (or the action directive) can be discontinued.
4. A code system should be used to enable the reader to find related policy and procedural statements.
5. All policies should be authenticated by date and by the nurse executive's signature.

Pagination of policies is a potential problem area. Some manuals are constructed with all policies placed in alphabetic order by title, with page numbers assigned in sequence. This system represents two problems in use of the manual: 1) If one cannot guess the correct title of the desired policy, there is no way to locate it except to read the entire index until the particular policy comes up. 2) Every new policy that is added to the manual, if placed in alphabetic order, requires new pagination for the rest of the manual.

It is easier to locate material and to add new policies if the content of the manual is divided into mutually exclusive sections or subsections, each of which has its own pagination. In this way the reader need consult only a small area of the index to find the policy he seeks. A cross-indexing system will facilitate policy location also.

There are some common variations that are found in policy format. 1) Some institutions intermix institutional and nursing policies in a single manual. There are both advantages and disadvantages in this practice. The employee only has to deal with one manual, but it may be so extensive as to make it more difficult to locate specific policies. 2) Some institutions separate policies and procedures into two manuals. (The nursing procedure book is one instance of this practice which is peculiar to nursing.) Again, where the practice is applied to all policy statements, there are advantages and disadvantages. The policy book usually is terse and easy to use, but one must seek out cross-indexed procedures frequently.

Also, the mechanics of creating and maintaining a nursing policy manual should be reviewed. The manual should be constructed so that policies can be removed readily or added to appropriate sections of the book. A simple loose-leaf notebook fits this criterion. In addition, a plan should be evolved for periodic review and updating of the contents.

It is important that outdated copies of policies that have been revised be thoroughly destroyed (except, perhaps, for a historical copy in nursing division files). Nothing is more frustrating to a staff member than to follow what appears to be the most recent policy, only to find out that it was superceded but not replaced in the manual. Furthermore, staff members should be instructed to disregard undated and unsigned (unauthorized) policies; such pieces of paper only confuse an already complex system. Finally, a policy manual is only as useful as it is accessible; up-to-date copies should be available to all nursing staff.

PRACTICES

Practices may or may not implement policies. In a legal age, it is important to see, however, that policies and practices do not conflict. Indeed, in court or arbitration cases, employees are likely to be held to the common practice, not to the published policy, when the two differ. This can make employee discipline a problem. This issue will be further reviewed in Chapter 23.

Many practices arise separate from those issues discussed in policies. Practices which disrupt the work of the division may need to be controlled through creation of new policies. However, the nurse executive needs to be careful to examine such practices first and to ask what purposes they serve. Some practices grow up in compensation for poor work systems. Most practices are meeting *some* need, so critical inquiry should take place before a practice is countermanded.

All new policies need to be widely displayed, but it is particularly important to ensure that all employees have seen a new policy which will have wide impact on a present practice. In a contested case, the nurse executive may have to prove that the employee not only had the opportunity to become familiar with the new policy but that the conditions were created so that he *necessarily* was made familiar with it.

SUMMARY

Policies, procedures, and practices define the events of the nursing division. Together they comprise the rule structures of the organization. Policies serve several purposes; they 1) provide information, 2) guide decision making, 3) substitute for some decision making, 4) define and limit roles with relation to decision making, 5) create standard operating procedures among organizational units, 6) solve recurrent problems, 7) eliminate likely areas for conflict, and 8) make choices among equally attractive alternatives. Procedures detail the way in which policies are to be carried out if a specific means is to be preferred. Practices include all behaviors, those created by policy decisions and those arising by habit or tradition or general problem-solving behavior.

REFERENCES

1. Moore, J.A. JCAH standard III: policies—guidelines for action. *J.O.N.A.*, 2(3):30, 1972.
2. Perrow, C. *Complex Organizations*. Glenview, Ill.: Scott, Foresman, 1972, p. 27.

BIBLIOGRAPHY

Casanova, G. Developing and writing policy. *Supervisor Nurse*, 3(4):62, 1972.
Feldman, J., and Hundert, M. Determining nursing policies by use of the nursing home simulation model. *J.O.N.A.,* 7(4):35, 1977.

Part III

Processes of Nursing Management

Part III of this book reviews the intellectual, personal, and technological processes which the nurse executive and other nurse managers apply to the daily tasks of administration. Chapter 11 looks at the basic thought processes used by the nurse executive, comparing decision-making and problem-solving processes. Quantitative and qualitative methodologies for deciding are explored. The relationship of decisions and goals is discussed as is the psychological element of deciding.

Chapter 12 explores basic communication processes and communication skills specific to a managerial role. These skills include running meetings, media appearances, and effective committee participation. Chapter 13 reviews the nurse executive's basic strategies for management, stressing change theory, conflict theory, and theories of power and politics. These and other diverse bodies of administrative knowledge are examined.

Chapter 14 examines role theory as a strategic tool of the nurse executive. Role theory is discussed as it relates to alternate conceptualizations of the managerial process, such as managerial or worker skills, activities, styles, and personality traits. The major managerial literature on administration is reviewed briefly, and administrative theories are compared and contrasted. Role theory is viewed as an active managerial tactic. The selected management role is considered as it relates to the nurse executive's skills and to the characteristics of her organization and division.

Chapters 15–17 explore the role characteristics and problems of the head nurse, supervisor, and clinical specialist. Environmental constraints upon performance of these roles are identified and discussed.

The processes of nursing *administration* complement the *organization* of her division by the nurse executive. Part II identified those principles by which the nurse executive organizes her division and thereby contributes to the organization of the total institution. Part III identifies those principles and theories which the nurse executive uses in organizing her own time and efforts. Together, organization and administration represent major components of the nursing management effort.

Chapter 11

Thought Processes for Management Decisions

The nurse executive, unlike the sociologist, does not simply theorize; her aim is not just to understand and explain phenomena. The nurse executive combines thought and action; she is paid to think, decide, and enact her decisions. Without action, a nurse executive is ineffective. But actions must be based on intelligent decisions, which in turn must be based on appropriate assumptions about the world, patients/clients, health, and nursing. This chapter concerns the thought processes which the nurse executive uses in making decisions about goals, means, and problems in her division.

PROBLEM-SOLVING AND GOAL-SETTING ACTIVITIES

The activities of the nurse executive typically divide evenly between two major intellectual tasks: problem solving and goal setting. Problem solving, as used here, refers to removal of immediate obstacles and impediments within or affecting the nursing division, that is, eliminating obstructions to the work flow of the division. When a nurse executive has taken on a division that is in trouble, she may need to spend a disproportionate time at first in problem solving.

Goal setting involves both envisioning the long-range goals of professional nursing and identifying more immediate nursing goals for the nursing division itself. Whereas problem solving focuses on removal of an obstacle, goal setting focuses on achievement of a defined objective. Despite their different focus problem solving and goal setting are not entirely separate. In problem solving, for example, an obstacle only becomes a problem because it blocks move-

ment toward some goal, whether that goal be well defined, intuited, or merely some ill-perceived direction of movement.

Similarly, one may or may not encounter problems in achieving the goals one sets. Most plans for goal achievement are designed to solve, eliminate, or prevent the occurrence of problems. Although these intellectual activities may interweave, the focus is clear in each case: in problem solving the intent of the agent is to remove an impediment; in goal setting the intent is to purposely set about achievement of carefully selected, specific objectives.

In nursing care delivery, these two contrasting approaches are reflected in problem-oriented charting (which implies problem-oriented thought in care delivery) and in the so-called nursing process. In problem-oriented charting, the nurse cannot even write her notes about a patient except in relation to a given patient problem. Obviously this recording system forces the nurse to *think about* the patient in a certain way, that is, to think about him in relation to his problems. In contrast, the nursing process begins the relationship with the patient by a nursing assessment. This assessment is not initiated by the perception of a problem, instead, the assessment is the first step in determining goals for care. (A nursing diagnosis is an interim step between assessment and goal determination.) While problem-oriented charting and thinking focus on resolution of the patient's problem, the nursing process focuses on the achievement of nursing goals set within the process itself.

From a managerial perspective, the nurse executive cannot afford to select either problem solving or goal setting as her entire focus; she must be sensitive to and recognize problems in her division, and she must be able to lead by establishing goals and directing her organization toward their accomplishment.

LIMITATIONS IN LITERATURE ON MANAGERIAL DECISION

It is interesting to note that most managerial literature on thought processes focus exclusively on decision making, a phase of both problem solving and goal setting. Decision making reflects the necessity for a manager to exhibit both thought and action, for a decision is the critical point where thought leads to action. Much of the management literature is incomplete, however, its inadequacy stemming from two discrete though often intermixed sources: 1) Where *only* the *decision* element of thought is considered, much of the significant thought process that precedes and follows the decision is lost. 2) Many management texts on decision making focus exclusively on quantified decision-making techniques and on the sort of decisions that lend themselves to this type of management. The first deficiency is addressed here by comparing decision making with problem solving; comparing it to the larger concept of goal setting would have been equally satisfactory in pointing out the limitations of the typical decision-making model. To illustrate the second deficiency of the literature, quantified decision making is examined and compared to other decision-making tactics for dealing with various types of problems.

DECISION MAKING VERSUS PROBLEM SOLVING

Most books on management include a chapter on decision making. Levey and Loomba give the following definition: "A decision is the conclusion of a process by which one chooses among available alternatives for the purpose of achieving a set of desired objectives. Decision making involves all the thinking and activities that are required to produce a choice among alternative courses of action; it is the central activity of all human beings."[1] The focus in this definition is the concept of choice: selecting from among a specified set of alternatives to fit a given purpose. The term *alternatives* is used loosely in this chapter to denote two or more options in a choice set. While the term *option* is more suitable, alternative is more commonly used in the managerial literature.

Decision-making literature typically focuses on how one chooses among alternative "solutions"; it creates systems for rational comparison of options so as to pick the best one. This single act, choosing, may be compared to Simon's model of deciding. He lists the following components[2]:

1. Intelligence activity. Searching the environment for conditions calling for decisions.
2. Design activity. Inventing or developing and analyzing courses of action.
3. Choice activity. Selecting among alternatives.
4. Review activity. Evaluating the outcome.

In the choice-focused model of decision making, certain limitations arise.

1. There is little examination of the problem for which these givens *are* alternatives.
2. It is assumed that one logically *knows* of what the alternatives consist (that they are "knowable" in advance).
3. It is assumed that *all* alternatives can be considered (that they are finite in number).
4. It is assumed that the results of each alternative can be predicted accurately.

Most of the illustrated problems in choice-focused management literature are problems of inventory, equipment selection, or other relatively simple, unsubtle situations. For problems of such simplicity, the possible alternatives may be finite, known, with predictable outcomes. If one tries to decide a simple nursing management question by this way, however, the weakness of such techniques becomes apparent. Suppose, for example, that a nurse executive asks what sort of assignment system should be used in the newborn nursery:

1. One may ask if there really is any need for an assignment system at all. One begins to examine the problem for which assignment systems are proposed as solutions.
2. Some traditional assignment systems are known, but new alternatives could be created, depending upon the initiative and imagination of the staff.
3. To any number of assignment systems suggested, one could add others if prompted (radically different systems or systems combining in different ways the elements offered in the original alternatives).
4. One might predict results of hypothetical systems, but they would have to be confirmed or disconfirmed by actual testing.

The narrow focus upon the choice element may be contrasted with Dewey's concept of problem solving[3]. In problem solving, the focus is on how the problem is cast and on the process of deciding versus focus on the choice element. Problem solving generally follows the following sequence: An "itch" or perceived obstacle gets the attention of the problem solver. He surveys, explores, or interacts with the environment of the obstacle to try to understand it. He formulates some initial statement of the problem (describes the nature of the obstacle). Based on this tentative formulation, he again surveys the environment. (What constitutes a related environment changes as the problem definition is evolved.) Based on this survey, he further refines and delimits the problem. He goes back and forth from survey (interaction with the environment) to problem definition and back to survey as many times as necessary, until the problem definition is concrete. He conjures up one or more tentative solutions for the problem.

These solutions begin to present themselves as the problem becomes refined; this step is not actually a separate activity from problem definition. Indeed, the way the problem is constituted virtually dictates how solutions will be sought. He picks the one solution he thinks will be the "best bet" and tests it out. If this solution fails, he may try another one from his previous list, one that has occurred to him in the midst of this testing, or he may determine to start anew with a redefinition of the problem.

Note that in this conception the problem exists when it is perceived; it is not "out there." It is the agent's definition of the situation as problematic that makes it so. He coins the problem, gives it form and substance. The way he casts the problem will dictate what solutions are considered. His creativity and vision, or lack of them, will dictate how many solutions are conceived as well as how the problem is interpreted.

The problem-solving process begins long before the decision-making stage—it begins when a person senses that an existing situation needs to be clarified. It begins before the person can say what that problem situation really is.

Nor is decision making the final stage in problem solving. A decision is not the resolution of a problem. Problem solving is a process that extends beyond a finite decision to the state in which the original problematic situation is resolved. It is not completed until all the decisions and changes necessary to solve the problem have been effected and the problem no longer exists.

Defining the Problem

The most important part of problem solving is defining the problem. What problems the nurse executive "sees" will determine what solutions, or changes, are introduced into the nursing organization. Unfortunately, there are many ready-made solutions simply looking for problems. The nurse executive regularly encounters persons who claim to have the solution to her problems. Hawkers of solutions come in many forms: businessmen trying to sell a particular management course to an organization, other nurse executives who are sure that "their" solution will work for everyone else's problems, consultants with particular packages to sell, and fads that appear from year to year, such as T-groups for employees, job enrichment programs, or attitude training.

With "solutions" pressing from all sides, it is not surprising that the nurse executive is tempted to reach out and grab one. Later, when the results of that solution are found to wear off after a short period, the nurse executive condemns the solution as ineffective. The truth, of course, is that solutions are effective only when applied to the right problems.

The real danger in ready-made solutions is that they dictate what the nurse executive sees as problems. They create artificial problems or, worse yet, they distort her perception of real problems.

Careful diagnosis of problems must precede any consideration of solutions. Take, for example, the nurse executive who calls in a psychologist as a consultant to investigate a prevalent interpersonal hostility between the RNs and LPNs in her organization. The nurse executive may not realize that she has closed off problem definition. She thinks she has called in an expert to help her *define* the problem, but this is wrong, for she has called in an expert of a particular kind. Psychologists can be expected to come up with psychological interpretations of problems. Thus the nurse executive has already defined the problem as a psychological one simply by the act of calling in a psychologist.

Suppose that the source of the problem is organizational, that the LPNs resent being used to fill RN roles and functions at a drastically reduced salary. One can anticipate that the psychologist's efforts will ease the interpersonal problem temporarily, but the underlying problem will eventually rear its head again.

The most critical step in problem solving, therefore, is that first step in which the nurse

executive classifies the problem, for the classification will direct the solutions sought. The nurse administrator should learn to suspend premature classification of any problem. There are several principles that will help her avoid premature classification. The nurse executive should insist on knowing all the relevant facts before diagnosing any problem. This principle has become an overworked cliché in nursing literature. The disadvantage inherent in the principle is twofold: 1) knowing the principle does not help a person know when he actually has at hand all the relevant facts, and 2) the method by which a person picks out what is "relevant" is dictated by his tentative diagnosis of the problem.

In the example of the LPNs' hostility to RNs, the director assumed that "psychological facts" were needed to explain a problem in interpersonal relations. If the director had recognized this underlying assumption, she might have broadened her search to include other kinds of facts.

The simplest way for the nurse executive to identify assumptions that limit the search for facts is to ask herself, "Why have I picked out these as the important facts?" A thoughtful answer to this question will help her to recognize the limitations she has put on her definition of the problem.

There is no easy way to determine whether one has all the relevant facts, but a pragmatic suggestion can be made: the nurse executive should not rely on a uniform source of information in seeking the facts. Hearing from four supervisors about a supervisor-head nurse problem provides multiple input, but it still uses a uniform source of information. One would have to interview those on the head nurse side of the argument to derive a balanced view of the "facts."

The second principle for averting premature classification is that of recognizing that most problems are not problems of fact but of interpretation. If the nurse executive can separate facts and interpretations of facts in her thinking, she will not make the mistake of acting on the first interpretation as if it were a factual reality. The nurse executive should make herself aware of the diverse interpretations of facts before classifying them into a statement of the problem.

The third principle for averting premature classification of a problem is to make a systematic investigation of the scope of each presented problem. Is the problem one in its own right, or is it merely a symptom of a problem broader in scope? Accurate assessment of the scope of a problem will determine if the nurse executive addresses her efforts to finding a lasting solution to problems or just to plugging holes in leaky dikes.

The foregoing issues are lost in a decision-making model, for it begins and ends with the selection of an alternative. For this element (choice among alternatives), problem-solving and decision-making models share principles and problems.

Choosing among Alternatives

One principle in choosing among alternatives is first to see that alternatives exist. Unfortunately, this is a principle that has become a cliché. Those who "follow the rules" typically draw up a few straw men, alternatives that easily can be discarded so as to get on with implementing the originally proposed solution. This process clearly defeats the purpose of identifying alternatives. All alternatives must be viable ones whose merits deserve serious consideration, and their identification is a step needed to keep the nurse executive flexible and open to the potentialities present in each situation. If the nurse executive's final decision invariably corresponds with the solution she proposed initially it is unlikely that she is generating realistic alternatives.

Failing to generate viable alternatives is not the only possible defect in this stage of deciding. Some situations offer an insufficient range of feasible alternatives. Of course, one must always question whether a lack of alternatives accurately represents the environment of the problem or merely lack of ingenuity on the part of the decision maker.

An even more complex situation is the one in which there are unlimited potential alternatives. In this instance the nurse executive must utilize some categorization in order to select a representative but feasible number of alternatives for consideration. In instances when these alternatives can be stated in quantitive terms, it may be possible to utilize computer programming, thereby comparing a greater number of alternatives than could be constructed by a single reasoning person.

Specific methods of choosing among alternatives will be discussed in the section on decision methodology in this chapter. In some cases, where prospective evaluation is seen as the mode of choosing, evaluation and choice coincide. These cases will be discussed now.

Criteria for Assessing Choices

The evaluation of a decision can be accomplished in several ways:

1. Evaluation of the anticipated outcome for each alternative, called prospective evaluation
2. Evaluation of the actual outcome of the decision as it relates to predetermined criteria
3. Evaluation of the decision process itself

Much decision-making literature relies upon a before-the-fact evaluation of the outcome for each alternative; obviously such literature assumes that it is possible to predict outcomes with accuracy. Problem-solving models tend to consider the wider scope of evaluation methods.

Criteria for assessing outcomes either prospectively or retrospectively, often are preset as the objectives for the situation. For example, in a change of assignment system, the nurse executive might have predetermined the following criteria: increased patient satisfaction, increased staff satisfaction, improved quality control results, and economic savings. One of the factors that makes evaluation difficult is that few decisions can be weighed in relation to a single value, like a 20 percent increase in output. In most situations, there are several criteria for judgment, and one seeks the alternative that best satisfies all criteria. Seldom is a situation so ideal that a single alternative ranks highest on all set criteria, hence one usually must determine what is the best constellation of values that one can achieve. For example, one must decide whether to select an alternative with some loss of staff satisfaction but a great economic savings, or whether to select one with less economic gain but greater patient satisfaction. Often one is forced to weigh incommensurables, multiple values, in a single decision.

In situations of this sort, it is seldom possible to *maximize* one's gains, to have the greatest amount of all values involved. Typically, one settles for *optimizing*, getting a decision which seems to represent the best balance of gains among several values. Some decision makers are content with *sufficing*, taking a decision which at least meets the minimum goals set for the decision in the first place. (The word "satisficing" is sometimes used instead of sufficing.) In sufficing, the decision maker terminates his search with the first alternative that fits his predetermined criteria, and thus he may settle for a minimally suitable answer as long as it "gets by." Policy formulation based on sufficing behavior has been termed *incrementalism*. In this method, any policy is adopted as long as it is better than the one that preceded it; policies improve over time, even though no single policy gets the attention it deserves when it is enacted.

Another set of criteria useful in a management situation is a comparison of alternatives as they relate to goals, structures, and technologies. (See Figure 11-1.) A proposed alteration in any one of these aspects may be assessed by its compatibility with the other two aspects of the model.

Structures are the systems that regulate and control activities. They include the systems of communication in the organization, the ways in which authority and responsibility are distributed, the ways in

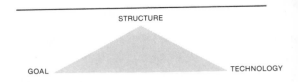

Figure 11-1 Model for Evaluating Proposed Alternative Actions

which assignments are made, and the patterns that regulate the work flow. Structures are patterned relations that coordinate and control the work; they are the patterns by which people interact with one another.

Technology concerns the equipment and instruments required for getting the work done. The programs and processes for using the equipment and instruments are included in the concept of technology. Many aspects of nursing require a high level of technology, as in coronary care units. Other aspects of nursing, such as maintenance care of the senile patient, require a lower level of technological skills.

Goals are the objectives of the work performed. They represent the desired outcome of a particular process, and they are the anticipated effects of a concerted and coordinated plan of action.

The foregoing model can be entered at any one of its three components, depending upon what alternatives are to be assessed. Take, for example, a nurse executive who is trying to determine a realistic level of patient care for her institution, a goal. She might ask, "Given this organization's structure (staffing patterns, assignment systems) and technology (technological skills of the staff and available support equipment), what level of patient care is the highest realistic level of care to which one can aspire?"

Suppose the decision has to do with structure instead. One such problem might be stated as follows: given a *goal* of reaching all obstetric clinic patients with birth control information, and given the *technologic* capacity (nurses with the right information and the right teaching techniques), how should clinic appointments and clinic management be structured?

The model that compares goals, structures, and technologies easily picks up disjunctions between components of a proposed system. Some examples of disjunctions follow:

Case 1

1. Goal. The nurse administrator sets a goal of distributing detailed monthly budget reports to each head nurse for each patient unit.
2. Structure. The accounting department does not charge supplies on a patient unit basis due to scarcity of personnel for this paperwork. Instead, the department simply charges supplies to a general budget category of "medical-surgical nursing units."
3. Technology. The accounting department has the knowledge necessary to do the task. Technically the accountants are trained to do the requested task and they have the necessary equipment, such as calculators.
4. Disjunction. The structure is unable to support the proposed goal.

Case 2

1. Goal. The inservice department wants its education to be based on individually prescribed instruction via audiovisual instructional units.
2. Structure. An audiovisual laboratory is constructed with enough space and hours per day for all employees to use the required programs.
3. Technology. All types of audiovisual hardware are available in adequate numbers, but the faculty is unable to find or produce software programs to cover all required areas of study.
4. Disjunction. The technology cannot support the goal.

Case 3

1. Goal. The inservice department plans to educate selected staff nurses for part-time relief in the coronary care unit.
2. Structure. The nurses are sent to a well-organized course in coronary care at another health agency.

3. Technology. The course teaches the nurses utilizing monitors and equipment unlike that used in the home institution. When the nurses return to the home institution, they are unable to use the institution's equipment.
4. Disjunction. The selected structure is incompatible with the technology.

Sometimes a nurse executive is pressed to accept a particular goal, structure, or technology on its individual merits. Salesmen, for example, will stress the advantages of their equipment, and proponents of particular nursing care systems will encourage the nurse executive to change her structures to stay "contemporary." If the nurse executive considers such proposed changes in the light of the goal, structure, and technology model, she will be able to make a decision that is not influenced overly by the appeal of one component of the model.

Obviously any criteria which may be applied prospectively to anticipated outcomes may be applied retrospectively to actual outcomes. Lack of correspondence between anticipated and real outcomes may mean either an unrealistic prior assessment or a situation that simply was too complex and unpredictable to be accurately forecast.

Janis and Mann note the ultimate impossibility of comparing the results of an implemented alternative to the results of an alternative that was never tried[4]. Therefore, they recommend that one evaluate the decision process itself rather than the alternatives or their outcomes. They suggest the following criteria:

1. Were a wide range of alternatives canvassed?
2. Were the full range of objectives and values to be fulfilled canvassed?
3. Were the costs weighed—positively, negatively, and in relation to the consequences for each alternative?
4. Was there a search for new information concerning each alternative and for new alternatives?

5. Was new information assimilated and subjected to expert judgment?
6. Were the consequences of all alternatives reexamined before a final decision was made?
7. Were provisions made to implement courses of action for each contingency, each risk in the decision?

Clearly, there are many ways to look at the phenomenon of deciding. One may look at the decision maker. Who decides? What sources do they use? What is the nature of the situation that occasions a decision? What is the nature of the problem itself—is it complex or simple, programmed or unstructured? What are the possible courses of action? What are the processes of decision? What elements are predictable? What elements cannot be predicted? What methods may be used to facilitate deciding?

METHODS OF DECISION MAKING

Differences in ways of making decisions reflect two divergent approaches to the subject: some authors explain and devise methods for deciding by examining the characteristics of the alternatives and their consequences, whereas others explain decision methods by studying the decision maker himself. The first approach looks for rational laws and rules, relying primarily on mathematical techniques. The second approach focuses upon the psychology of human behavior. These schools present very different recommendations and conclusions, primarily because human behavior is not always rational and not all decision situations are capable of being settled rationally, or quantitatively. Each school has its advantages and limitations.

Quantitative Decision Making

Quantitative decision making relies heavily on such tools as computer simulations, linear programming, decision trees, probability theory, queuing theory, payoff tables, and other techniques for dealing with quantifiable data. Clearly, this mode of decision making is very useful when applied to appropriate problems: scheduling length of time for clinic visits, planning operating room schedules, ordering supplies, planning the staffing and scheduling patterns. In other words, the quantitative techniques of management science are perfect tools for use in a situation whose elements can be easily and naturally quantified.

In order for a decision situation to be appropriate for quantitative decision making it must meet the following criteria:

1. The problem must be stated in quantitative terms.
2. Relations among all significant variables must allow mathematical manipulations.
3. Results of actions must be predictable and measurable.

Notice that such rules make certain unstated assumptions about the nature of the decision-making situation. The first assumption is that reductionism (focus upon the parts, the variables) is the way to make decisions, rather than focus upon the whole. The decision-making world in this model has no room for a gestalt perception. The second assumption is that the decision-making situation can be simplified, that all the significant variables can be identified. The situation is considered one in which clarity prevails, with no chance that an unforeseen element will enter into the outcome. A final assumption is that one can reasonably quantify most variables, or at least assign mathematical values to them.

Where absolute values do not pertain, quantitative measures are devised in terms of probability theory. Hence, decision-making rules are determined for three states: 1) decision making under *certainty*, the state in which all outcomes of all alternatives can be accurately predicted; 2) decision making under *risk*, the state in which at least probabilities can be established concerning outcomes; and 3) decision making under *uncer-*

tainty, when no probabilities can be established. In determining the degree of prediction possible, variables are assessed on two dimensions: whether or not they can be controlled by the decision maker and whether or not their values (quantifications) can be known, absolutely, in some degree of probability, or not at all.

The objective of the mathematical manipulations in most cases is to reveal the decision which offers the least possible risk—to determine the "safest" decision. Certainly the careful measurement of each factor, the methodical weighing of each possible outcome, is conducive to a cautious approach to management decisions.

Psychological Approach to Decision Making

The psychological approach to decision making need not be perceived as in conflict with quantitative decision making. In fact, there is room for quantitative decision making within the psychological approach. Since quantitative decision making was devised by man, its existence proves it is within his psychological and intellectual boundaries. The problem, so one might argue from the psychological approach, is that focus on a set of devices for decision making does not get to the heart of decision making itself, which can be done only by looking at how real people (in this case, managers) actually make decisions in real decision-making situations.

Simon did just that, studying managers as they went about making decisions in the context of their work[5]. He found that the typical decision-making tactic bore little resemblance to the highly prescribed, rationalized processes used in quantitative decision making. Simon notes the poor quality of organizational decision-making practices. He finds that managers tend to classify problems along established dimensions and make only a limited search for alternatives. Most managers construct a simplified model of the real problem situation, built on past experience and a par-

ticularized view of the present problem stimulus. Decisions usually are made with incomplete knowledge of the consequences of the selected alternatives, and not all possible alternatives are considered. The manager, says Simon, mostly uses solutions that he has used in the past; the typical manager has a limited number of rules, programs, and actions that direct his decision making.

Simon notes that most managers do not seek ideal solutions but only those that will suffice. The manager usually settles for the first satisfactory solution that is structured. Seldom are new answers offered; at most mild innovations are proposed.

This sad report on the state of the art of decision making should make the nurse executive sensitive to deficiencies in her own decision processes, for it reflects some realities of the typical problem situation. Man is "intendedly rational," Simon notes. Yet in most situations the material for rational decision making may be absent and it may not be possible to obtain knowledge of the consequences of a decision before it is enacted. Further, Simon notes that most alternatives cannot be exhaustive for few situations are so simple as to have limited alternatives. And, indeed, even where it is possible to obtain with time more information concerning both outcomes and alternatives, the time needed may be so long as to make the subsequent decision useless. Hence the manager must act and decide in a real world, not in the best of all possible, imaginable worlds.

Considerations such as these make sufficing decisions or decision by incrementalism more understandable. Given the realities, is there any advice that may be offered to a nurse executive? One suggestion is that real-life decision making may be improved by retrospective study of previous decisions. This may be done by reviewing the major decisions made by the manager in the previous year. Any division's immediate status depends heavily on a few decisions of the past. These can be analyzed by identifying which decisions had the greatest impact on the division and by analyzing the results of those decisions as compared to the anticipated results when the decisions were made.

In the retrospective analysis, both of these activities may yield surprising results. For example, the nurse executive may find that the most critical decisions were not always seen as important at the time they were made. The analysis will tell her whether or not she is astute at recognizing critical issues. In comparing actual results of decisions to the results that were anticipated, the nurse executive will obtain a measure of her predictive power. One of the best ways to learn good decision making is by such careful analysis of post decision-making results.

The nurse executive also may wish to examine organizational decisions to consider delegating authority for decision making. For example, does she spend her time making decisions which should have been made at the supervisory level? Do her head nurses make decisions which should have been the responsibility of professionally prepared staff nurses? If decisions are not made at appropriate levels in the nursing division, the nurse executive is not getting what she pays for.

There are tactics the nurse executive can use in teaching subordinate staff to assume responsibility for decision making. Suppose a supervisor brings a problem to the executive for solution. If the director believes that the problem falls within the domain of supervisory work, she should not give an immediate answer; she should not reinforce dereliction of responsibility for decision making. Instead, she might ask the supervisor to suggest alternative solutions and to evaluate their potential. She might have to push the reluctant supervisor to a choice among alternatives. If the supervisor is literally unable to propose reasonable approaches and to assess their potential outcomes, then the director will need to consider whether or not such a person belongs in such a responsible position. If a nurse executive does have to make a decision for a supervisor in a given instance, she should tell that person that she believes the decision should have been made on the supervisory

level. At times apparent inability to make decisions on the part of subordinates may reflect unclear job boundaries rather than real inability. Decision power must be clearly granted and described. The supervisor who is unable to recognize the appropriate level for her own decision making is a danger. Either she will make decisions which should have been referred up the chain of command or she will waste time making decisions that should have been made by her own subordinates.

Objectives of Decision Tactics

The psychological approach to decision making also looks at the makeup and managerial intentions of the decision maker. Mintzberg illustrates three basic managerial intentions (strategies) which would impact upon the nature of decisions made by an executive[6]. An *entrepreneurial* strategy is one that contains an active search for new opportunities; it is characterized by proactive dramatic leaps forward in the face of uncertainty. This entrepreneurial manager will see opportunities for decisions where other managers would find no problems. Such a manager is more interested in a "big win" than in "minimizing loss" and hence would seldom be satisfied with quantified, cautious approaches. This is the manager who incorporates vision into decision making.

An *adaptive* strategy, in contrast, tends to use reactive deciding and remedial actions in an attempt to reduce conflict with the environment. The user of such an approach might very well use incrementalism in making decisions waiting for feedback from the environment before making another change. Here most decisions would be cautious; only mild innovation would be likely.

A *planning* strategy, unlike the adaptive strategy, is forward looking. The planner, unlike the entrepreneur, however, will make no dramatic leaps in the dark. Anticipatory decision making relies heavily on quantitative techniques. Rational goals are set with systematic plans for achievement in the planning strategy, which stresses rationalism and minimizing risks.

Obviously, the decisions of the nurse executive will be different depending upon whether she has an entrepreneurial, adaptive, or planning set in her decision making. The particularly adept executive is able to vary her strategies, selecting the strategy appropriate to the nature of the particular problem at hand. The executive who can bridge these strategies probably also can bridge the gap between quantitative and psychological approaches to decision making.

Misapplication of Methods

Unfortunately, many managers with strong educational backgrounds in quantitative techniques advocate their usage for *all* problems, all decisions. In such instances the results may be ridiculous or misleading. Consider the actual instance of the nurse executive who decided to fill an important nursing administrative post by quantification techniques. First she determined the chief characteristics that the position incumbent should have; then she weighted those components according to their relative importance. She developed a "grading system" for the tool and then interviewed candidates, carefully marking each candidate on each characteristic, cumulating a "final score" for each hopeful. Peculiarly, the candidate with the highest score was one who had not impressed the nurse executive in the interview. Nevertheless, convinced of the omniscience of mathematic technique, the nurse executive hired the woman. Not surprisingly, this new employee had to be dismissed before she had been in the job for three months. The nurse executive then hired a "low scorer" who *had* impressed her in interview, and that person has now functioned in the position successfully for several years. The point to be made by this illustration is that quantification techniques are limited when applied to a complex or subtle issue. It is spurious applications of this sort that lead

some executives to mistrust quantification technology. The fault is not in the technology, however, but in the application of the technology in an inappropriate situation.

BASIC APPROACHES TO INTELLECTUAL TASKS

Whatever the problem or issue at hand, there are several approaches which may be used by the nurse executive in reasoning and reaching conclusions. The effective executive probably is skilled in using several approaches and fitting the approach to the nature of the task at hand. One approach, problem solving, has been elaborated upon in this chapter. A systems approach is a second possibility. Here a problem, issue, or set of facts is reviewed and seen as a set of interacting components. The focus is upon the parts and their interrelations. Such an approach is useful in handling situations which naturally call for the development of integrated systems. For example, a systems approach will be useful in devising a scheduling plan, a personnel file system, a disaster plan. In each of these illustrations, there is a need for careful consideration of how each component relates to every other component in the total system. A systems approach is detailed in Chapter 21. Since a systems approach looks at a phenomenon in terms of its components (variables) and their interrelations, a systems model often is compatible with quantitative decision-making techniques.

An operational approach is a third possibility in dealing with issues and problems whereby thinking focuses upon making finer and finer discriminations within the subject matter. Differential diagnosis, wherein one possibility and then another are systematically eliminated, is a good example of the approach in medicine. Decision making uses an operational tactic in the elimination-by-aspect approach[7]. Here alternatives are determined and then eliminated by application of criteria. The decision maker continues to think up criteria until all choice has been eliminated. Figure 11-2 illustrates this point. Note that the criteria are personal and not elaborated in the way that they might be if this were a formal operation rather than an interpersonal one.

Vroom and Yetton also use an operational approach to decision making when they differentiate out decision styles according to who participates in the decision, in what way, and what information is used in the decision making[8]. La Monica and Finch apply this model to nursing management situations[9].

A final approach to problems and issues is the dialectical one. The nurse executive uses this approach when it is necessary to synthesize diverse elements rather than to differentiate among them. For example, two nurse researchers investigating sensory deprivation and loneliness, respectively, might come to the conclusion that both of the concepts studied actually were illustrations of some overarching principle, such as isolation. In management, a participative approach to decision making may result in movement by a dialectical process.

The nurse executive, then, has an array of intellectual tools to bring to the task of decision making or problem solving. She may use an approach aimed at determining and resolving problems presented in a situation; she may consider the situational elements as they relate to each other through a systems model; she may differentiate and clarify the issue by discriminating among its elements; or she may seek a synthesis which assimilates the elements of the problem. The effective nurse executive keeps her response options open, using the intellectual approach to the situation which seems most productive in a given case. Indeed, she may consider several approaches to the same problem until she discovers which has the greatest potential.

SUMMARY

Management literature which examines the thought processes of executives tends to focus upon the act of decision. This is a logical perspective in that deciding links thought and action, and this is the function of the managerial role. Nevertheless, this perspective is limited and omits other critical aspects of thought within the managerial situation. The nurse executive needs to be aware of the larger context in which decision making takes place as well as to develop expertise in using decision-making techniques and applying them judiciously to problem situations.

Candidates for Associate Director								
Personal Criteria of Nurse Executive		A	B	C	D	E	F	G
(applied to all qualified candidates with "favorable" interview results)	Cooperative versus conflict-producing approach	yes	no	yes	yes	no	yes	yes
	Supervisory staff also liked them	yes		no	yes		no	yes
	Makes a smart appearance	yes			yes			no
	Brings an "outside" perspective	yes			no			

Figure 11–2. Elimination-by-Aspects Approach to Decision Making

REFERENCES

1. Levey, S., and Loomba, N.P. *Health Care Administration—A Managerial Perspective.* Philadelphia: J.B. Lippincott, 1973, p. 169.
2. Simon, H.A. *The New Science of Management Decision* (rev. ed.) Englewood Cliffs, N.J.: Prentice-Hall, 1977, p. 41.
3. Dewey, J. *Democracy and Education.* New York: The Free Press, Macmillan, 1966, p. 150.
4. Janis, I.L., and Mann, L. *Decision Making: A Psychological Analysis of Conflict, Choice, and Commitment.* New York: The Free Press of Macmillan, 1977, p. 11.
5. Simon, H.A., *Administrative Behavior.* New York: Macmillan, 1957, pp. 79–109.
6. Mintzberg, H. Strategy-making in three modes. *Calif. Management Rev.,* 16(2):44–53, 1973.
7. Janis, I.L., and Mann, L., 1977, p. 31.
8. Vroom, V.H., and Yetton, P. *Leadership and Decision-Making.* Pittsburgh: University of Pittsburgh Press, 1973, p. 13.
9. La Monica, E., and Finch, F.E. Managerial decision making. *J.O.N.A.,* 7(5):20, 1977.

BIBLIOGRAPHY

Aylesworth, T.G., and Reagan, G.M. *Teaching for Thinking.* Garden City, N.Y.: Doubleday, 1969.

Boehm, G.A.W., Shaping decisions with systems analysis. *Harvard Business Rev.,* 54(4):91, 1976

Bursk, E.C., and Chapman, J.F. (Eds.) *New Decision-Making Tools for Managers.* New York: Mentor, 1963.

Church, C.W. *Systems Approach.* New York: Dell, 1968.

Daniel, W.W., and Terrell, S.A. Introduction to decision analysis. *J.O.N.A.,* 8(5):20, 1978.

del Bueno, D.J. Need to know versus nice to know. *J.O.N.A.,* 6(8):6, 1976.

Erickson, E.H., and Borgmeyer, V. Simulated decision-making experience via case analysis. *J.O.N.A.,* 9(5):10, 1979.

Gordon, G., and Pressman, I. *Quantitative Decision-Making for Business.* Englewood Cliffs, N.J.: Prentice-Hall, 1978.

Heenan, D.A., and Aldleman, R.B. Quantitative techniques for today's decision makers. *Harvard Business Rev.,* 54(3):32, 1976.

McKenney, J.L., and Keen, P.G.W. How managers' minds work. *Harvard Business Rev.,* 52(3):79, 1974.

Mintzberg, H. Planning on the left side and managing on the right. *Harvard Business Rev.,* 54(4):49, 1976.

Mintzberg, H., Raisinghani, D., and Théoret, A. The structure of unstructured decision processes. *Am. Sci. Quart.,* 21(2):246, 1976.

Nadler, G. *Work Systems Design: The Ideals Concept.* Homewood, Ill.: Richard D. Irwin, 1967.

Oncken, W., Jr., and Wass, D.L. Management time: who's got the monkey? *Harvard Business Rev.,* 52(6):75, 1974.

Rosen, H., and Marella, M. Basic quantitative thinking for nurse managers. *J.O.N.A.,* 7:5(6): 1977.

Taylor, A.G. Decision making in nursing: an analytical approach. *J.O.N.A.,* 8(11):22, 1978.

Wong, P., Doyle, M., and Straus, D. Problem solving through "process management." *J.O.N.A.,* 5(1):37, 1975.

Chapter 12

Communications in Nursing Management

Knowledge of communications theory is essential since the nurse executive affects her health care institution primarily through others. In this chapter a general communications model will be offered and its application in nursing executive management will be considered, together with related topics of special interest to the nurse executive— institutional relationships, the successful management of meetings, and media appearances.

THE COMMUNICATIONS MODEL

An understanding of communication theory begins with an analysis of the functional unit of communication. The simple components of any single communicated interchange to be identified and examined are shown in Figure 12-1.

The system in its simplest terms consists of a sender with certain goals. He encodes those goals (translates them into symbols) to form a message. That message is transmitted via some medium (audiovisual-sensory input system) to the intended receiver. Upon its sensory intake, the receiver decodes the message (interprets the symbols) and responds to its perceived content. How he interprets the message and how he responds to the content he perceives are influenced by his own goals in relation to the sender and in relation to the message's subject matter. When the response includes communication feedback to the sender, the receiver assumes the sender role and the communication cycle begins again.

The Function of Communication

The sender always communicates for some purpose, to have some effect upon the receiver. Common purposes include: to inform, to entertain, to inquire, to persuade, to command. The goal may be to evoke a particular attitude or a particular behavior, verbal or actional.

The success of a communication is usually judged in terms of the goal-response relationship. Organizations usually define a good communication as one in which the goal of the sender was attained. This definition, however, has a limited perspective because it assumes that only the goals of the sender have relevance in receiver's response. The receiver may have goals of his own which modify his response to the message. This consideration leads some authors to define a good communication as one in which both sender and receiver achieve goal satisfaction.

The Structure of Communication

Communications can take place in two ways, by direct action and through symbols. A pat on the back or an opening of a door might be examples of direct communication. Even such actions, however, are subject to misinterpretation. Most communication is of the symbolic type. Verbal communication is the most common form, words standing for meanings. When symbolic communication is used, the degree of common understanding achieved between sender and receiver

153

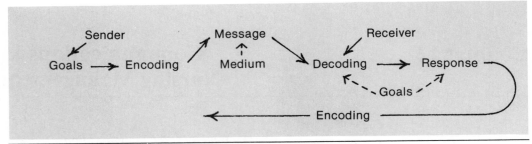

Figure 12-1.   The Communications Paradigm

depends on whether they both interpret the words or other symbols in the same way. For example, telling the man-in-the-street to do something "stat" would not produce the same effect as using that term with a nurse. Of course the man-in-the-street might pick up the meaning of stat from the speaker's direct communications, such as the urgency in the voice of the speaker or the apparent seriousness of the situation. The point is that some form of common understanding of the symbols used must be reached between sender and receiver if communication is to take place.

The act of putting meaning into a symbolic form is called *encoding,* and the act of extracting meaning from symbols is called *decoding.* The degree of agreement between the message sent and the message received will depend on the degree to which the symbols have the same meaning for the two parties. In the model shown in Figure 12-1, arrows branch from the goals of the receiver toward both the decoding and the response, indicating that goals can affect not only the receiver's response but even his interpretation of what is being conveyed to him.

The Methods of Communication

There are many different methods for communication: talking, writing, showing, and all the various possible combinations for sensory input. These sensory messages can then be delivered face-to-face or by the communications medium of choice. Media have their own particular effects upon the

message. Consider, for example, the delivery of the same message face-to-face or by letter, by film, or by slides. Effects such as closeness, distance, warmth, and coolness add overtones of meaning to the message.

These then are the primary components of a functional communications system: sender, goals, encoding, message, media, decoding, receiver, goals, and response. Both the parts and the relations of the parts are important in analyzing or constructing a communication.

THE NURSE EXECUTIVE AS SENDER AND RECEIVER OF COMMUNICATIONS

In the role of sender, the nurse executive's underlying personal, cultural, and professional biases direct her goals and her way of encoding messages. She must recognize that the receiver also has personal and cultural biases that color his decoding activity. When the nurse executive's biases are different from those of the receiver, she must allow for such differences. She needs to encode in symbols that have the same meaning to the receiver as to herself. Failure to use clearly understood symbols is probably the most common sender problem in communication.

Another sender problem is the general failure to communicate to all who need to know. For any communication instituting a change in policy, practice, or procedure, the nurse executive should carefully identify all individuals who need to receive the message. The executive needs to consider not only the face value of the message but the implications it may have, not only for her staff members, but for other departments of the institution. Poor personnel relations are bound to follow if changes are instituted without proper communication.

Not all communication problems are sender problems; many are problems of message reception.

Selectivity

People tend to see or hear messages in which they are interested and to miss messages in which they are disinterested. This mechanism is called *selective attention*. Selective perception is another factor; with this phenomenon, the receiver selects those parts of the message that conform with his desires or expectations. Such picking and choosing can cause either incomplete or distorted interpretation of the message.

Anticipation of Content

Some persons assume that they have grasped the essence of a message before really hearing it out or reading it carefully. These persons tend to tune out the message because they think they already know what is being communicated.

Thinking ahead into the Sender Role

Some persons become so enamoured of their upcoming response to the message, they tend to be mentally formulating their answer rather than really digesting the message. Persons who think ahead into the sender role also are often guilty of interrupting the speaker and responding to incomplete messages.

Receiving Skills

Receiving skills are seldom given sufficient attention. Conscientious effort should be made to apply such basic listening techniques as the following:

1. Give the speaker your full attention; try to hear what he is saying, not what you expect him to say.
2. Do not interrupt or begin to mentally formulate your answer until he has finished his statement.
3. Listen for both facts and feelings. What has the speaker said, and how does he feel about it?
4. Tell the speaker what you think he has said; see if that is really what he meant.
5. Use questions to clarify meanings.
6. Suspend judgment until the speaker finishes talking.

Reading skills should follow similar patterns.

1. Read for what the author says, not what you expect him to say.
2. Periodically summarize in your own words what the author is saying and doing. What structures is he building? Where is he leading?

The nurse executive must be a sensitive message receiver because of the nature of her job. At times, messages to her may be somewhat distorted, due to the attempts of her staff to please. Her receptivity to messages must be such that staff do not feel inhibited when delivering unfavorable reports.

MESSAGE CONTENT

The message itself is, of course, the most important factor the nurse executive must consider. In a face-to-face communication, clarity is usually attained by immediate feedback and interaction between at least two individuals. The nurse executive, however, does much of her communication in written form, and such immediate corrective feedback is not possible. Before publication, messages should be carefully checked for clarity of meaning, accuracy of content, and completeness of detail. The nurse executive who has problems with written communication may find it useful to have her messages read before publication, by a disinterested party who can suggest needed revisions. Usually self-disciplined message evaluation satisfactorily serves the purpose and the writer can revise her own communications.

ORGANIZATIONAL COMMUNICATIONS

Communication Forms

Any nurse executive finds that a great percentage of her time is spent in communications of one sort or another. Communication forms useful for analysis of organization communications are listed in Figure 12-2. This taxonomy has two axes; the first one runs from the one-to-one relationship through the one-to-many. It is important that the nurse executive use discretion in selecting options on this axis. A common error is communicating content that should be reserved for the one-to-one relationship in the one-to-many situation. Discipline of an employee in front of her peers, for example, is seldom an appropriate form. Nor is it appropriate to waste the time of a group of persons to discuss issues pertinent to only one or a few members.

Another defect exists where the nurse executive chronically communicates to some of her immediate staff to the exclusion of others. The nurse executive must be extremely careful not to penalize some staff members by accidental withholding of necessary information. Some executives use a weekly newsletter for top administrative staff to avert such accidental omissions.

The one-to-small group situation is a communications form that is most useful when the communication affects the group as a whole rather than as individuals. This provides for clarification, feedback, and reinforcement immediately within the group that will have to function with the same understanding of the message.

The second axis of the communications taxonomy has two poles, face-to-face and mediated communications. A mediated communication is any form presented through some device, such as films, slides, or tapes. It is possible to combine mediated presentations with face-to-face communication, for example by showing a movie and then having a group discussion of its content.

Here again selection depends on the goals of the communicator. Person-to-person communication has advantages such as forcing the receiver's attention to the issue, providing immediate feedback and clarification, and allowing the message to be adapted to a specific audience. Mediated forms also have their advantages: The message can be given to different groups with no alteration in the

Sender-Audience Relationship	Science	Communication Mode	
		Face-to-Face	Mediated
One-to-one	Interpersonal relations	Conversation	Correspondence
One-to-small group	Small group dynamics	Meetings, task forces	Films, tapes, slides
One-to-many	Rhetoric	Speech making	Mass media: radio, television, flyers

Figure 12-2.   Forms of Communication

presentation or meaning. Appealing to more than one sense (combining visual and audio) may be more vivid than mere speech. The mediated form allows a complex idea to be edited and tested until the presentation has optimal clarity. The mediated communication has the effect of formalizing and recording a decision. Mediated forms can be retrieved for future reference to the subject.

Some communications are most effective when combining the two processes: face-to-face communication followed by written reiteration of the message.

When communications require specific actions on the part of the recipient, it is effective to follow face-to-face communication with a written reiteration of the message. It is also possible that several alternative modes may be viable for any one communication. Policy change may be announced at a mass staff meeting, or it may be published in a general memo, or it may be discussed with small groups (one unit at a time). Selection of the proper mode of communication can be very important in effective leadership.

Factors to be considered in selecting a mode of communication include the message content and the anticipated audience response. An additional Christmas bonus may easily be announced in a printed memo; anticipated lay-offs announced in this manner would not only be insensitive but would represent the worst of strategies.

Some questions to consider in selecting a communications mode are the following:

1. Is the message easy to understand or does it need a mechanism for feedback? Is the feedback need immediate or will delayed response be adequate?
2. Who is the audience? Will the message reach all who need to know?
3. What is the audience's anticipated response? What is the intensity of the issue? Will it cause a change in routine practices?
4. What need is there for formal documenting of the message? Is the content proper for a policy statement, procedure statement, memo, or other form?

5. What are the abilities of the nurse administrator? With which mode of communication is she most comfortable and most adept?

Directional Flow

Another factor to consider when discussing communications in an organization is directional flow. Communications are necessarily influenced by the hierarchical structure of an organization. Communication lines between the nurse executive and all relevant persons in or closely associated with the organization can be visualized as in Figure 12-3.

It is usually easier for the nurse executive to evolve outgoing communications than incoming communications, for outgoing communications are perceived as more directly under her control. If the nurse executive learns to express herself and to consider "who needs to know" for all communications, her outgoing messages have likelihood of success. There are, however, many ways in which she can foster good incoming communications. For example, many nurse executives use the mechanism of the weekly report to gain information from their own supervisors and head nurses. A format for a weekly report can be created in such a way as to encourage staff to include the information most needed by the nurse executive. The nurse executive should carefully examine both the written and the informal parts of her communication system in order to assure that it facilitates incoming as well as outgoing communications. (See Chapter 27.)

Institutional Relationships

The effect of group membership is another factor that has an impact upon organizational communication. Many of the nurse executive's communications are directed toward groups rather than toward individuals. Even when a communication is directed to an individual, he still reacts on the basis of his group memberships.

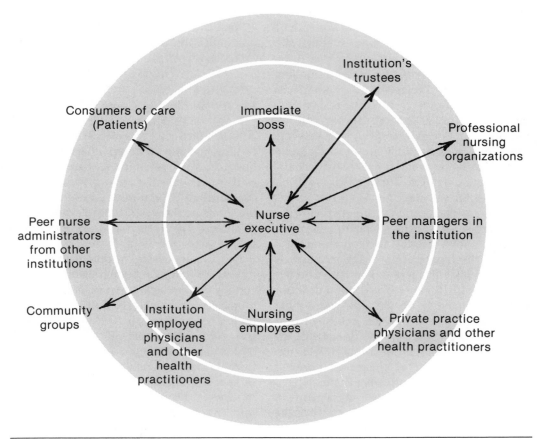

Figure 12-3.   Communication Lines in Nursing Management

Blumer, in his description of symbolic interactionism, notes that all things derive their meanings out of social interaction[1]. Human beings act toward things on the basis of the meanings those things have for them, and those meanings are social products. For Blumer, even a physical object is a symbol and a social creation; its meaning comes from the society, not from the object itself.

This concept has important implications for the nurse administrator. Because work groups are also social groups, the administrator must consider group responses to her messages as well as individual responses. The group places a certain meaning on a communication and there is pressure on individual members to conform to the group interpretation. In many instances it is more productive for the executive to deal directly with group feelings and reactions than to focus on the members as individuals.

An interesting traditional means of communicating with groups is the administrative nursing rounds. In these rounds, the nurse executive visits selected patient care units, views and evaluates the care of selected patients and talks at random to staff members. The nurse executive seldom takes time for the prolonged and formal evaluation necessary to produce accurate care samplings; this is not the purpose of administrative rounds. Instead they serve the important purpose of letting the staff members see the boss. The mere periodic presence of the "boss" on the working unit has the effect of decreasing the employee's perceived distance between himself and the boss and gives the nurse executive several advantages. It assists in the implementation of her policies, because the employees are more apt to identify with the director's goals when she is personally known. Her physical presence can act to increase discipline where needed because the employees feel that the executive really knows what is going on. The executive's presence is a symbolic means of communicating her authority.

Figure 12-3 indicates the major communication links that the nurse executive must address in her role performance. These communication links will *all* require attention, but there may be a different balance from administrator to administrator in the amount of time devoted to each relationship. For example, in a major health care institution the major nurse executive, often a vice-president of the organization, may focus on communications upward in the administrative hierarchy and outward, while the four or five directors of nursing who report to her devote more time to downward relationships. The importance of upward and outward relationships will be discussed in Chapter 13, which looks at nurses' acquisition of power. Clearly, these are the relationships that give entrée to power.

In general, the more communication links that the nurse executive is able to form, the greater will be her power and her ability to get things done. Knowledge is power, and extension of the executive's network of communications will extend her information power; when she knows the values, interests, and modes of operation of these groups and individuals with whom she must deal, then she is better prepared for negotiations with them.

GROUPS IN MEETINGS

The nurse executive typically finds herself directing many types of meetings. The abilities needed for this function vary depending upon the type of meeting. For example, for a major, formal meeting of a large group or assembly, it is essential that the nurse executive know the procedures to be followed. Large groups can function only when detailed procedures exist; there simply is not time for all to participate, and with large numbers consensus would be very difficult to reach. Usually this means that the nurse executive must know parliamentary procedure. Indeed, she should become expert in parliamentary procedure if she is to succeed in situations of this sort. One's personal input in presiding over large groups is minimal compared to the leadership one can offer in small groups, but such a meeting can be destroyed by a leader who is unsure who has the floor, what motions can be made, or how to use her prerogatives as chairman.

Sometimes a nurse executive will address a large group on an informal basis. For example, she may set up several large meetings with the nursing staff to present to them the status of a major institutional change. Here procedure is not the major factor; the major skill required here is the ability to address and respond to a public.

Managing Committees

Much communication of the nursing division is done through committee work. Here the director needs two sorts of skills. She needs to be able to create and structure committees that will achieve their objectives, as well as to run committee meetings successfully.

The term *committee* is used here as a general term to describe a relatively stable group which meets periodically for an identified purpose or purposes, has official status and sanction of the nursing organization, and has some established mechanism for maintaining and selecting members as well as for recommending or implementing its group decisions. Unless a specific kind of committee is indicated, the term *committee* can be assumed to refer to all kinds of committees and formal groups.

In determining the types of committees she needs, the nurse executive should first examine the objectives and functions of her division to decide which objectives and functions can be best met through committees and which can be best handled by other means.

Committee structures are preferable for two kinds of situations: those requiring multiple input for goal attainment and those in which diverse representation facilitates implementation of proposed activities. There are many reasons that multiple input might be required. Some problems require the combined knowledge of various specialists for solution. Other problems require multiple input about how proposed solutions will affect the environment in which they will be implemented. Still other problems simply need brainstorming and reasoned interaction for reaching the most satisfactory solution. Diverse representation on a committee also may help in project implementation, lending legitimacy to projects and encouraging acceptance of solutions because of the democratic appeal.

The nurse executive must also be aware of the limitations of committees. Many projects are better assigned to a single individual than to a committee. Projects that require complex research and planning are better given to a single individual who can become familiar with and sensitive to each aspect of the project and its effect upon other aspects of the project.

Nor should a committee be used to supplant the authority and responsibility of line managers. Committees are not designed to handle most day-to-day decisions. Indeed, the splintered responsibility in a committee makes it easy to avoid such decision making. Committees are better able to handle the larger issues, such as major policy changes or long-term divisional plans. When, because of the committee structure, a manager cannot take direct action in a situation impeding work flow, then the committee is handling the wrong kind of activity.

Thus in designing committee structure, the nurse executive determines what goals and functions best can be handled by committees, decides what committees will exist, and examines the relationship of the committees to each other. It is impossible to evaluate any one committee without considering its relationship to the rest of the nursing organization. Some questions the executive may use as guidelines in evaluating committee structure and function are the following:

1. Are there adequate committee structures to enable the division to reach its goals? Are there any obvious omissions?
2. Does each committee fill a vital need that is not within the scope of any other committee? Does each committee have a clear reason for existing?
3. Are the purposes of the nursing committees consistent with the avowed divisional definition of and philosophy of nursing?
4. Is the total number of committees logical for the size of the nursing division and the thrust of its objectives?

Committee Power

The first consideration in examining the effectiveness of any single committee is the degree of power delegated to the group. It is important that the group be given enough authority to fulfill its objective. It is not logical, for example, to expect a committee to evaluate nursing care unless it is given the power to institute evaluation processes on the nursing units. A committee should not have to rely on persuasion if its directive is to produce action. Even intracommittee factors may be important. Does the committee, for example, have the power to delegate assignments to members?

Giving the committee enough authority to do its assigned job is one power issue. Another is the committee's ability to implement its decisions. The executive may give a committee power to recommend or power to decide. She may give a committee one standing level of power, or she may state power options relevant to specific issues and assignments. Where the nurse executive chooses to adjust the power to fit the assignment, it is important that the committee members clearly understand their powers in each case.

The next power question is, What does it mean to say that a committee has "decided"? There are two major forms of decision making by committee: majority rule and consensus. The executive may deal only with consensus decisions or be content with majority decisions. She may wish to adjust the degree of unanimity required to the problem situation. Once more, it is important that committee members be given a clear directive.

Committee Membership

The committee should be viewed primarily as a means of getting work done, not as a means of meeting status needs, a popularity contest, or an exercise in democratic process. There is no logic in appointing a member to a committee if one can predict him to be noncontributive to the committee's objectives. One should "play the best odds" by appointing persons most likely to do a good job. This focus is one of the reasons design groups are often more creative and productive than committees based on organizational position. Executives must also be cautious against overuse of the same reliable people on all committees. When such participants become a select group, to the exclusion of others, an obstructive "we-they" syndrome may occur.

In selecting members for a particular committee, the executive also must consider "who needs to know" in the implementation phase. One often sees such catastrophic events as a group of higher-level employees planning a change for a lower-level group without any representation from the latter. Representatives should usually be included from the group that is to implement any proposed change. There will be times, however, when confidentiality at a selected management level is needed, particularly in early planning stages for major divisional changes. In those instances, the executive must use discretion in determining appropriate committee membership.

A committee should consist of the smallest number of persons who can meet the committee's objectives. To do otherwise is to misuse human resources. Committee membership can be controlled on large projects by creating a small stable force for the total work, giving them the option to call in others as needed at various stages of the project development. When a person is asked to join a committee for this type of interim membership, the duration of, and reason for, his participation should be made clear to him.

Committee Feedback Mechanisms

Another important facet of committee effectiveness is its structure for feedback to and from nonmembers and administration. If, for example, the committee project is a long one which is expected ultimately to bring about a change in nursing education or nursing practice, it may be wise to publish periodic status reports to the nursing groups that will be involved in the change. These reports will serve to create interest in the project as well as to prevent the resentment that arises when a plan suddenly materializes full blown and ready to be implemented.

Periodic status reports also are useful for the nurse executive because they let her know the direction, rate of progress, and general productivity of the committee. In addition, requiring periodic status reports as opposed to mere minutes of meetings forces committee members to return their attention to the original goals and to evaluate progress toward those goals.

In addition to creating communication channels *from* committees, it is important to create channels *to* committees whereby organization members who feel that they have something to offer can submit ideas and suggestions. Creating input channels helps to build general acceptance for committee recommendations and decisions.

Committee Productivity

The nurse executive is responsible for seeing that optimal use is made of staff time.

Nowhere is there more danger of unproductive use of time than in committee work. When, for example, ten supervisors sit around a table for two hours and accomplish nothing, the cost in salaries for those two hours may be hundreds of dollars. The administrator therefore cannot allow chronically unproductive committees to continue to exist simply because the participants enjoy the meetings. When a committee is unproductive (comparing committee man-hours to committee output) the cause must be found.

Often a committee is unproductive because it does not really need to exist. This occurs when its objectives are either not attainable or not important at the particular time. When the objectives of a committee are judged valid, but the committee is still unproductive, then it is trying to do the job with the wrong people. A committee leader without appropriate skills may be the problem. A second possibility is an incompatible mix of members, incompatible in regard to the objectives of the committee, not necessarily incompatible in their interpersonal relations with one another.

Since design groups are single-purpose entities, it is easier for the nurse executive to calculate timing factors for them. She can decide at the start how much time she is willing to invest on a particular task. Design group members can be given a deadline.

Release time for committee participants is another important timing consideration. Two factors enter decisions in this area: how much involvement the committee work will require and how each person's normal job tasks are distributed. Projects have been known to fail because of resentment felt by those carrying excessively heavy work loads for task force or committee members. Also, if committee participation is just another duty added to an already busy schedule, participation may suffer.

Committee Functions

The nurse executive may find it useful to examine the output of each committee through a taxonomy of committee functions like the following one:

Functions in Relation to Projects	Functions in Relation to Committee Members
Problem solving	Communicating
Researching	Expressing
Standard setting	Compromising
Designing	Harmonizing
Implementing	Consensus taking
Monitoring	Reasoning
Evaluating	Socializing

Functions in Relation to Others

Communicating
Educating
Recommending
Clarifying
Summarizing
Encouraging

Such a taxonomy can be useful in committee evaluation. For example, suppose the nurse executive finds a committee in which all functions are socializing activities among members. The nurse executive may need to question the value of such a committee to her organization, since it neither advances project work nor extends services to those outside the committee membership.

Committee Leadership Skills

Basic Rules

There are a few basic rules which will help the nurse executive run committee meetings. Some rules concern preparation for the meetings; others direct the leader's activity during the meeting. Preparation rules are simple and self-explanatory.

I. Preparation of the physical environment
    A. Comfort should be assured by:
        1. Adequate ventilation, light, and heating

2. Comfortable seating
3. Good visual arrangements
4. Adequate space for the writing or reference materials of each participant

B. Convenience for participants can be assured by:
  1. Supplying paper, pencils, name cards, if indicated
  2. Minimizing interruptions
    a. Informing the telephone operator of who is in the meeting and who will take messages
    b. Marking all entry doors to signify what meeting is in progress
  3. Preparing and checking-out all necessary audiovisual aids
  4. Supplying agendas and documents to be discussed. (Do not assume that everyone will remember to bring his original copy.)

II. Preparation of participants
A. Distribute detailed agendas long enough in advance for necessary preparation or research
B. Distribute for advance preparation any documents to be approved or analyzed
C. Indicate any materials that the participant should bring to the meeting

III. Leader preparation
A. Prepare an agenda which clearly indicates the purpose and content of the meeting
B. Review the status of all agenda topics to date
C. Gather all necessary background information and supportive data on agenda topics
D. Determine who need to be invited as resource persons based upon agenda topics
E. Prepare a list of critical questions that can stimulate committee interaction on agenda topics

F. Prepare such handouts or audiovisual presentations as will facilitate committee understanding of topics
G. Prepare a strategy or strategies for handling the meeting

The leadership activities *during* a meeting must also be considered. The leader has two functions to fulfill during a meeting: structuring the business to be done and directing and controlling members' behavior. These will be separated for discussion though it is not always so easy to tell where one leaves off and the other begins in an actual meeting.

Structuring the Business to Be Done

This function will be considered as it applies to a single-purpose meeting. The same principles would apply for each segment in a multipurpose meeting. In structuring the business, the leader should plan to start each topic with an orientation phase which includes a brief review of past actions and decisions on the topic (if the topic is not new) and a clear statement of what is to be accomplished with regard to that topic in this particular meeting. Once the objectives are so stated, the leader usually turns the action over to the committee members. The leader should prepare a lead-in question or suggestion for this purpose.

The primary duty of the leader during the meeting is to keep the committee to its task. This requires that the leader remind the group of its objectives when the conversation strays. Another tactic is the periodic use of short summaries of committee progress during the meeting. The leader must also be cautious not to rush groups into premature decisions in overzealous pursuance of the meeting's objectives.

At the meeting's termination, it is the responsibility of the leader to summarize what has occurred during committee interaction. The leader identifies the decisions reached and reviews the responsibilities accepted.

The structuring of the business to be done varies with the type of communication desired from the meeting. Several communication options exist. Some meetings aim at information transmittal. The simplest form is that in which the leader merely wishes to inform the group of something, basically a one-way communication. There may be some slight communication flow from the group to the leader concerning parts of his message that were unclear or incomplete, but essentially the meeting remains in the control of the leader.

In contrast with this "tell" meeting, the "sell" meeting is one in which the leader is anxious not only to inform but to convince the group of the worth of his particular idea. When persuasion is the intent, the meeting should be allowed to develop into a three-way interaction. This means that after the leader explains his idea to the group, he allows them to pose questions and give their reactions. In addition, he allows time for the members to discuss the proposal with each other.

A third type of information transmittal meeting is the one in which the leader wants information from group members concerning a particular topic. In this case, there is a simple one-way flow of information from each member to the leader.

Meetings not intended for information transmittal are usually focused on decision reaching. Several different levels can be identified in the decision-reaching meeting. "Brainstorming" is the simplest form, because the communication flow is one-way, from each member to the leader. In the brainstorming session, judgment of ideas is suspended; the purpose is to collect as wide a variety of tentative solutions as possible in a short time. Since there is no judgment placed on the suggestions of the members at the time, there is no need for a two-way communication.

The advice-seeking meeting is the next level of decision reaching. In this meeting, the leader wants to gather the opinions and judgments of committee members on an issue. Under strict control, the advice-seeking meeting may also be a one-way flow from each committee member to the leader. More often such opinions and judgments create interactions between committee members, and it is likely that the leader will find these interactions a useful part of the advice giving.

The highest level of decision reaching is that in which the members are asked to work together to arrive at a single best solution to the presented problem. This problem-solving meeting involves three-way interactions between and among leader and group members. Problem solving is the most complex meeting activity; it is also the most time-consuming.

One of the most important leadership activities in structuring the committee's business is to make clear to committee members the communications purpose of the meeting. When the leader fails to do this, most people act on the supposition that problem solving is required. This is wasteful of committee time if the leader is not interested in having the committee come to the decision. Moreover, when a committee does expend the time to reach a decision, members are resentful if their solution is ignored.

Directing and Controlling Human Behavior

The leader's second function during meetings is the directing and controlling of human behavior. This function will be discussed in relation to the problem-solving meeting since this is the activity that involves the most complex human behaviors. The leader has two objectives in relation to his role: he wants to maintain his position of control while still encouraging active interchange among members.

Part of directing behavior is done by the leader in setting the tone of the meeting. At the start of the meeting, the leader sets the stage for free interaction by seeing that members are acquainted. If members of the committee do not know each other, the leader makes the introductions. Introductions include enough about each member to let the others know what talents and knowledge he brings to the group for its defined purpose. Until the members get to know each other, the leader facilitates interaction by directing questions to appropriate individuals.

When the leader is dealing with a familiar committee group, she has a different set of problems. She needs to think about the reaction patterns of individual members and about anticipated interactions among members. For the counterproductive reactions that can be predicted, the leader can develop controlling strategies, ready for use should those behaviors appear during the session.

The leader both maintains control and promotes interaction by seeing that each member contributes to the work of the committee. This usually involves some degree of supression of overactive members and drawing out of timid or reticent members. Another control mechanism the leader uses is restatement and redirection. She rephrases a contribution from a member and uses it as a pivot for changing the direction of the conversation. This is particularly important when a committee has overworked one section of the problem and should be moving on to another piece of the topic.

The functions of the leader during the committee meeting can be summarized in four functions: 1) focusing the issue, 2) refocusing when conversation strays, 3) changing the focus when an issue has been covered adequately, and 4) recapping the status of each issue, the decisions made, and the commitments for action.

The best way for the nurse executive to develop expertise at running meetings is to allow time immediately after each meeting for analyzing her performance. In the analysis, she should focus on two questions: Did I meet my objectives for the meeting, i.e., did I really get the business done? Did I facilitate appropriate interactions among members and divert unproductive interactions?

In summary, standing committees and design groups represent functional units working toward defined ends. Committees must be seen as investments of human resources. Thus a division that has committees working in more directions than it can accommodate in terms of actual institutional change is wasting its resources. Similarly, it is a waste of human resources to use 20 committee members where five can do the same job. The nurse executive should remember that a committee is not created for the sake of its members, but that its members are selected on the basis of their potential contribution to the goals of the committee.

The Nurse Executive as Committee Member

In addition to responsibility for committee leadership, the nurse executive often is a committee member. For example, she serves on the executive committee (by whatever name) that manages the main affairs of the institution that employs her. She may be on some committees created by the institution's board of directors, and she probably serves on numerous professional organization committees. The nurse executive cannot be less prepared for the meetings of these committees because she is a member rather than their leader. Indeed, in meetings with peers, whether organizational or professional, or with superordinates, she had better do her homework and be prepared to be an active participant.

One's participation in meetings often sets the tone for how others regard the nursing directorship and its incumbent. Further, it is not infrequently the case that the nurse executive may be the only female on such committees. It is important that she establish herself as a serious manager in such situations. Consider the following experience of a new nurse executive in an institution that was building a new hospital. A meeting had been called for all vice presidents and medical directors concerning distribution of space (for offices, laboratories, and other purposes) that would be available in the old building. This was the new nurse executive's first contact with many of her peers in the organization. When she arrived at the meeting, the "gentlemen" all commented upon how considerate it was of the nursing division to supply them with such a beautiful female committee member. (Indeed, this nurse executive did happen to be a beauty.) She just smiled although fully aware that this was an attempt to dismiss her by putting her in the "cute little girl" category.

When the corporate president asked the members each to voice their space requirements and requests, each of the men made a speech indicating that he needed all the space available because of his present lack of space. None was prepared to elaborate beyond the cry demanding "all of it." The new nurse executive was the last addressed; the others apparently assumed that she might not have a request since she was new to the institution. Instead, she was prepared with specific, written plans for the amount of floor footage desired for each specific space need, including a rationale for the estimation of floor space required for each projected area. The corporate president then asked each committee member to go back and prepare appropriate and justified requests "just like nursing." As the new nurse executive was leaving the meeting, she accidentally heard one of the members comment to another, "Gee, she was pretty when she came in, but did you notice that she got ugly as the meeting went on?" This, clearly, is one director who will not again have her femininity used against her by her peers. She had recognized that she would need to do her "homework" even better than the rest in order to promote the understanding that the nursing division not only was important but was a managerial unit in the true sense of the word.

MEDIA APPEARANCES

Many directors in nursing divisions fail to recognize their responsibility for maintaining the visibility of their organizational unit within and outside of the institution. To maintain this visibility requires that the nurse executive be adept at use of the media of mass communication. The nurse executive should be able to use the written media—professional publications and popular communication with the public at large. This requires that she develop both writing skills and knowledge of the communication vehicles which may be interested in publishing her work. Obviously, publication also requires that one have something of value to say. No amount of writing skill can assure that one will be published if the author has no fresh ideas, projects, or research to share, or no innovative methods or approaches. One would hope that a nurse so lacking in development would not be appointed (or accept) an executive position.

If the nurse executive has plenty of ideas but lacks the writing skills, help is available. Most communities offer writing courses of one sort or another, and many nursing groups periodically offer this sort of assistance to would-be authors. Indeed, most hospitals have at least one accomplished writer in the public relations department. This person can be a big help to a nurse executive. The greatest help for a would-be author, however, is simply practice with corrective feedback from a good critic. Writing is never a pleasant task, even for those who appear to do it effortlessly. That apparently effortless piece probably took more work than did the more labored seeming piece by another author.

The nurse executive also must learn to address large crowds (or unseen crowds via television or radio). Again, there are courses available on public speaking. Improvement comes with practice in this area too. A few brief rules may help the novice: 1) Be conscious of your voice characteristics; listen to tapes of your presentations to cultivate a pleasant and full speaking voice. 2) Don't read papers; learn instead to speak from notes. Be conscious of your effect on a crowd; speak as if you are enthusiastic about and committed to the ideas you are presenting. 3) Plan your presentation to suit the audience. Don't present a professional paper to a lay audience; fit the level of complexity of the subject matter to the average audience member and his level of understanding about the subject. 4) Develop a sense of timing. You should neither rush nor belabor a presentation. Until you learn to pace yourself, you may want to prepare some secondary material which may be inserted or deleted near the end of your presentation if the timing is off.

Interviews are more complex modes of mass media interaction. In an interview, much of the control is in the hands of the person who is interviewing you. It is important, therefore, to have an agreement ahead as to what will be covered in an interview. Plan your answers ahead for those questions which you have been given, or for those questions which you anticipate will be asked. Don't feel that you must answer each question as it has been put to you. If a question needs to be rephrased to be fair, feel free to point this out. Some reporters will try "trick questions," questions that will put you in a bad light however you answer them. Even though you do not wish to be tricked into answering the wrong question, you must be careful to answer fair questions even if they are tough ones. Where there are problems, you will do better to be forthright concerning them. Don't look as if you are trying to hedge; your credibility must be maintained in the interview.

If an interview is for publication rather than for immediate broadcast, request a copy of the final interview before publication so as to correct any errors in fact. Most reporters will not change the "slant" of their article to please you, but at least you will know what to expect. Don't hesitate to request publication of a "rejoinder" if a reporter really misinterprets your statements or quotes you inaccurately or out of context. Finally, unless you already have a close relationship with that reporter, never assume that any part of a discussion with a reporter will be "off the record." (Many of us have been "burned badly," at least once on this issue.)

Remember that you always are seen as the representative of your institution and your division. Theoretically, one should be able to speak as an individual, as a citizen apart from the managerial role one holds. In truth most people who hear you speak will not make this intellectual separation even if you announce that you are speaking strictly as a private citizen.

SUMMARY

In organizational communication, the nurse executive may find it useful to see herself as a center of a communications network. Much of her time is spent in one or another form of communication, a fact which causes some analysts to claim that all organization problems are really communication breakdown problems, a view that ignores the existence of many real problems of other types. Nevertheless, there is a partial truth to this perspective. Certainly, the nurse executive can eliminate many unnecessary problems by appropriate use of communications and communication techniques. Further, she can advance the visibility and effectiveness of her division if she is able to communicate its goals and actions to others in a meaningful way.

REFERENCES

1. Blumer, H. *Symbolic Interactionism—Perspective and Method.* Englewood Cliffs, N.J.: Prentice-Hall, 1969.

BIBLIOGRAPHY

Blau, P.M. *Exchange and Power in Social Life.* New York: Wiley, 1964.

Brunner, N.A. Communications in nursing service administration. *J.O.N.A.*, 7(8):29, 1977.

Burger, C. How to meet the press. *Harvard Business Rev.,* 53(4):62, 1975.

Cooper, S. Committees that work. *J.O.N.A.*, 3(1):30, 1973.

Culbertson, R.A. The governing body and the nursing administrator: an emerging relationship. *J.O.N.A.*, 9(2):11, 1979.

Davis, A.J. Body talk. *Supervisor Nurse,* 9(6):36, 1978.

Elliott, T.G., Everly, G.S., Jr., and Everly, G.S. Communication: a program design. *Supervisor Nurse,* 10(2):12, 1979.

Golde, R.A. Are your meetings like this one? *Harvard Business Rev.,* 50(1):68, 1972.

Harriman, B. Up and down the communications ladder. *Harvard Business Rev.,* 52(5):143, 1974.

Holle, M.L. Public relations in nursing service. *Supervisor Nurse,* 6(7):32, 1975.

Mueller, R.K. The hidden agenda. *Harvard Business Rev.,* 55(5):40, 1977.

Newman, R.G. Case of the questionable communiques. *Harvard Business Rev.,* 53(6):26, 1975.

Rosendahl, P.L. The verbal side of effective communication. *J.O.N.A.,* 4(5):41, 1974.

Thibaut, J.W., and Kelley, H.H. *The Social Psychology of Groups.* New York: Wiley, 1959.

Webber, J.B., and Dula, M.A. Effective planning committees for hospitals. *Harvard Business Rev.,* 52(3):133, 1974.

Welch, L.B., and Welch, C.W. Making press interviews work for you. *J.O.N.A.,* 9(5):48, 1979.

Chapter 13

Continuity, Change, and Modes of Change

This chapter examines the continuity-change cycle as a means of management in nursing. It then examines modes of initiating change such as management by objectives, assertiveness techniques, use of power and politics. Fads in modes of change will be considered as they relate to nursing management.

CONTINUITY AND CHANGE

Continuity and change are two halves of a complementary system in the management of a nursing organization. Continuity is represented in the traditions and status quo patterns of behavior, policies, and states of affairs. Change is represented in the upheavals, flux, and ongoing adaptation processes. Continuity for its own sake is meaningless. Yet, traditions that accomplish goals—maintenance of sterile fields, for example—must be valued and sustained. Similarly, change for its own sake is meaningless. Change has value only when it is instituted to accomplish some defined end.

Initiation of Change

Two stimuli of change are the setting of a goal and the identification of a problem. The commonly used system of management by objectives (MBO) is an example of the first type of initiator. It requires that the nurse manager set clearly defined goals for her division, department, or unit. Where the goals reflect ends not totally achieved by the present organizational system, the necessity for change is evident. Hence MBO is, by design, a change-oriented system of management, whether used by a whole institution or by a single patient unit.

Similarly, a problem-oriented approach to management creates change because each problem identified points to a failure in the present system. Where a problem is the stimulus to change, the objective is resolution rather than goal achievement. Nevertheless, a problem-oriented approach is change-oriented. This holds whether it is applied to the whole nursing department or to the derivation of care of a single patient.

In nursing one often finds these dual initiators of change working concurrently. A nursing department may set a goal to establish a new patient teaching program (MBO) while simultaneously devising plans to cope with a high incidence of patient injuries from falls (problem-oriented response).

Whether initiated by setting goals or by identifying a problem, change always is a *means* to some other *end,* never an end in itself.

Problems or losses inevitably occur when change is seen as valuable for its own sake. Unfortunately, nursing is not immune to this pattern. Nurses and nursing organizations often hop on bandwagons for no justifiable reason. For instance, a few years ago when education in the care of the dying was popular, it became a program topic among diverse groups, even those functioning in well-care settings. Superficially, it seems a harmless pattern, an educational change for its own sake. When one considers the opportunity costs, however, the price becomes evident. Had the nurses from well-care settings invested that time in learning nursing care that would profit their clients, thousands of hours of improved patient care might have followed. Change unrelated to extant problems or goals is pernicious because it robs us of time and effort which could be directed to improving nursing practice.

Continuity-Change Cycle

Change and continuity are related to each other in the pattern shown in Figure 13-1. The paradox of the continuity-change cycle is that the ultimate objective of change is continuity, that is, its opposite. When a change achieves its objective, then one aims for a new state of continuity. Indeed, a change cannot be adequately evaluated until it has reached the state of continuity. For example, one cannot tell if a new bladder training program works until it has been applied consistently for a large number of patients. The error of age is tradition for its own sake, accomplished by inertia; the error of youth is rapid, goalless change for its own sake, without stabilization or evaulation. It is essential to know which is needed—change or continuity—when, and why. Both must be judged by their success in relation to the desired ends.

Why all the literature about change implementation but little about maintenance of continuity? One possible explanation is that the literature reflects a false bias of our times—in favor of change rather than of a proper balance between change and continuity. As the profession grows in its ability to evaluate its own activities and in the use of research processes, nursing will come to an appropriate equilibrium, with needs for continuity assuming equal importance with needs for change.

Another explanation for the literature's emphasis is that change reflects a procedural issue. Admittedly, it is harder to generate innovation than to maintain a status quo, thus there may be more relevance in discussing change than continuity.

One must also note in passing a human tendency to prefer change to continuity. Whether this relates to simple boredom or to attempts at self-actualization is difficult to determine. Clearly, there are some nurse executives who enjoy a situation only so long as it needs radical change. Such executives usually move on to another position once a division has been stabilized. Some few executives meet their personal needs for change at the expense of the institution, changing well-functioning systems simply for the sake of change.

Since personal needs for change may vary, they will not be considered here as criteria for organizational change. Indeed, one person's natural pace of change is another person's stimulus overload. Attempts at self-renewal through institutional change will not be considered as valid in this discussion.

Types of Change

In looking at the process of implementing change, there is a grammatical problem. The single word *change* is used in two different ways. First, it indicates *the change itself,* the content of the future continuity, the new system of activities or events presently being

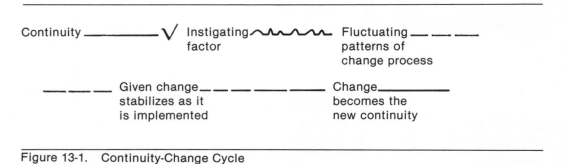

Figure 13-1.   Continuity-Change Cycle

installed. The same word, change, also refers to the *process* of bringing about that new entity, the events involved in terminating the old system of activities and establishing the new ones.

It is useful to differentiate between these two types of change even though both are involved in any alteration process. For purposes of discussion, the first type will be called the *activity plan*. It consists of activities and events specifically designed to reach a stated goal or to solve a particular problem. For example, an activity plan might be a new medication distribution system (means) designed to decrease medication errors (end).

The second type of change will be called the *strategic plan*. It consists of activities and events designed to prepare the environment for acceptance of the activity plan. That environment may be physical, psychological, organizational, or some combination of these factors. For the previous illustration, the strategic plan might include education of the staff in using the new medication system, attempts to win positive attitudes from the staff and others toward the new system, institution of administrative rewards or punishments for compliance/noncompliance with the new method. Thus, the strategic plan is one step further removed from the final objective (to decrease medication errors); yet it is still a vital means in accomplishing that end.

In implementing a change, it is important to consider the activity and strategic plans separately. Failure in either aspect could mean an unsuccessful change process. An excellent activity plan may fail because the strategic plan offends people with power. Similarly, an excellent strategic plan cannot compensate for an activity plan incapable of achieving its purported ends.

Implementation of Change

Since both activity and strategic plans are designed according to the nature of a specific aim or issue, they cannot be successful in im-plementing change if the goal is inappropriate or the problem is misdiagnosed. Assuming the goal or problem was well-conceived, the following principles assist in construction of activity and strategic plans.

Activity Plans

The most important consideration in implementing an activity plan is recognizing the need for one. Some head nurses assume that their task is complete once they have identified objectives for their patient units. But objectives do not magically accomplish themselves; objectives are achieved through the use of carefully designed activity plans, telling who will do what, when, where, and how.

In designing an activity plan, it is paramount to appraise several logical choices of action. These potential plans should be well-developed and debated to assure that ultimately the superior one is selected. Activity plans are only the means, and there may be many different ways to reach the same end. There is no assurance that the first one conceived will be the best; comparison and debate provide a safety check and a selection mechanism.

A means should never be selected without an end in view. Many nursing departments have made this mistake, purchasing equipment or audiovisual software without first considering the needs and goals of their particular department.

The activity plan may be simple or complex, depending upon the nature of the goal or problem. Even a relatively simple decision, such as deciding to keep charts in the patients' rooms, requires a fairly complex plan. It must answer basic questions such as: Where in the room will the chart be kept? What writing surfaces are available for making entries? How will charts be protected from the eyes of nosy visitors? Who will add extra sheets and when? How will physicians write and indicate new orders? Is any material to be kept confidential and how? The plan should identify all the chart-related events involved in the change.

When an activity plan requires integration of many diverse activities, a flowchart may assist in master planning. A flowchart identifies each event and sequences it in relation to others in the plan. In essence, however it is designed, an activity plan operationalizes the stated policy change.

In addition to determining what events and activities must take place, one also must determine what resources will be needed. These may be material, human, or organizational. Material resources include equipment, supplies, and facilities; human resources comprise manpower, specialized knowledge, and specialized abilities; organizational resources entail those multiple systems which pattern and interrelate the work. A change associated with one type of resource usually affects the other two. To illustrate, installation of nurse-server cabinets in patients' rooms (a modification in material resources) may require a change in human resources (a reduction in personnel) or a change in organizational resources (a new assignment system).

Costs of resources needed for a given change are often projected in a budget plan. This plan must include start-up costs for a change is usually more expensive initially than after full implementation because of extra demands during the early phase. Such start-up charges as for additional staff education hours, original cost of equipment, or supplementary staffing must be anticipated until the new system settles into "routine." Hence both start-up and full-operating costs should be projected.

If necessary resources are not available, the change process should stop. Nothing is more discouraging to the staff than to see a favored change fail because it has not received this requisite support, and it is folly to think that good intentions alone accomplish change. Executives often miscalculate human, material, and organizational resources. Common administrative myths about resources include the following:

1. If one or two people attend a three-day workshop, they will develop enough facility with a new plan to successfully begin organizationwide institution of that plan.
2. A new plan can be implemented on the basis of inservice education alone, without designing administrative rules, policies, and procedures to support the plan.
3. A new plan can be successfully instituted in the entire organization without first testing it to work out the "bugs."
4. People take seriously and follow the "do better" memo: "There will be no more eating in the nurses' stations," "Colored headbands are not to be worn with uniforms," "Lunch times are to be strictly limited to 30 minutes," when it is not accompanied by a planned administrative control system.
5. A good plan will work even though the organization can invest only half as many workers as the plan requires.

The activity plan is a logistic design for a change, determining the necessary movement of people, supplies, and equipment to achieve a particular end. The logistics must encompass the change itself and also its environment. The necessary environment is determined by the nature of the change. For example, a change which gives head nurses 24-hour responsibility for patient units requires both internal and environmental logistic alterations. Internal logistics would require specific plans for managing: 1) decisions and task determination in the absence of the head nurse; 2) decisions regarding the staff on all three shifts; 3) the use and distribution of the head nurse's own hours on duty over the three shifts; and 4) the nature of changed relationships with her subordinate managers (charge nurses). Environmental logistics would include plans for administering altered evening and night supervisor responsibilities and personnel salary scales (financial recompense for a revised managerial role).

Where an adjustment in the surrounding environment is required, the logistics of that secondary aspect must be specified if the change is to be successful. Planning the logistics of how a proposed change is to interact with other organizational systems is crucial. Responsibility for each activity plan component should be placed with specific staff members; an order to everybody is an order for which no one feels responsible.

An important factor in the change process is the time frame needed for implementation of a new activity plan. Generally, the larger the institution the longer the process of change. The nurse executive who moves from one institution to another of a different size needs to adapt to a different pace of change. The time frame for change also is affected by the complexity of the proposed plan, the amount of educational inservice required, and the number of persons involved. The multiplicity of variables involved prevents the reduction of timing factors to a simple formula, but the nurse executive should be sensitive to appropriate pacing for change in her institution.

The implementation of an activity plan follows these stages:

1. *Information.* This step is conducted on a "need to know basis" or on a larger scale, seeking response to the plan from those who may not be intimately involved in the actual change.
2. *Education.* Preparatory training sessions are held for those persons whose activities will be altered.
3. *Administration.* Plans are made for any administrative changes required to support the total project; education alone is never adequate. The administrative structures must be modified to uphold and maintain the change.
4. *Testing.* Where possible, an activity plan is tested on a small unit before it is installed organizationwide. Trial periods help resolve any of the inevitable glitches. Strict enforcement of the plan is necessary during the pilot project if it is to be judged on its own merits.
5. *Evaluation.* The plan is judged on the basis of its trial period. Preestablished, appropriate criteria are used for this assessment.
6. *Adaptation.* Revisions are made in the basic activity plan based upon the test

and evaluation phases. Reevaluation follows the implementation of these adaptations.
7. *Adoption.* The activity plan in its revised form is implemented throughout the organization. Further testing on this larger scale may be indicated for any extensive changes.

Where a change is individual and voluntarily initiated, the stages are slightly different than those of an organizationally imposed change. Stages of voluntary acceptancy are the following:

1. Awareness of the new idea, practice, or system
2. Interest in it as evidenced in the seeking of more information concerning the change
3. Evaluation through sifting of information in light of existing conditions
4. Mental trial of the new ideal, practice, or system
5. Actual trial, ideally in a limited circumstance
6. Adoption and integration of the change into the ongoing operation.

Again, these stages represent the steps by which a change naturally evolves. In making an organization change, the nurse administrator may choose either to accelerate this natural process by use of informational and propaganda techniques or to enforce the desired behavior, bypassing the stages of acceptance.

Strategic Plans

The strategic plan is designed to remove any barriers to the implementation of the activity plan. Those barriers, to name just a few, may be psychological, financial, physical, legal, or political. Although resistance will differ for every change, each anticipated barrier requires a counterplan if change is to be effective. Strategic plans will be examined for two types of barriers: psychological and political.

Psychological barriers may stem simply from the fact that change, beneficial or not, requires human adjustment, and poses a threat to each person touched by it. The following questions are asked by virtually any person facing a potential change:

1. Role-related
   Will it alter my role in the organization?
   Will I have more tasks? Fewer? Different?
   Will I have more power and status? Less? Different?
   Will I have more freedom or less, or freedom in different work contexts?
2. Hygiene-related
   Will my salary be affected?
   Will my work environment be modified? For better or worse?
   Will the conveniences/inconveniences of my position be altered?
3. Futurity-related
   Will it impair my future job security?
   Will it impair/advance my future earning power?
   Will it impair/advance my opportunities for promotion?

In strategic planning, it is important to calculate in advance who will be discomfited by the answers to these questions. Then one can seek ways to ameliorate their resistance or at least to be prepared to face it squarely.

In trying to make change as smoothly as possible, the nurse executive may ask herself the following questions:

1. Who will resist the change and why? What can be done to ameliorate their displeasure? Are there some minor modifications to the plan that could make a difference to a large number of dissenters?
2. What is the basis for the displeasure of dissenters? Does the plan affect their self-interest? Or is the objection caused by some perceived defect in the plan itself? If the latter, carefully consider their complaint.
3. Does resistance rest upon inadequate knowledge of the plan itself, its purposes, or its implications? If so, aim for clarity and better communication.
4. Is the resistance simply the resistance of inertia—the resistance to change just because it is change?

Since much resistance arises through misinformation, opposition often can be reduced simply by a campaign to distribute explicit information lucidly describing the change and its implications for involved personnel. This may curtail unnecessary resistance, leaving only that which is inherent to the change itself. In managing the resistance of subordinate staff, always consider both attitudes and behavior. Where possible, create positive attitudes toward the change before it is implemented. For some cases, however, that positive attitude is not likely to occur. Many head nurses have been unsuccessful, for example, in changing attitudes toward the completion of nursing care plans. The nurse manager may decide to enforce the change before worrying about attitudes. In this instance, cognitive dissonance works in favor of the change. The theory of cognitive dissonance asserts that when a person is required to demonstrate a given behavior consistently, his attitudinal patterns are apt to become favorable to the enforced behavior. In essence, a person's required action resolves the conflict between his behavior and his attitudes. Thus, staff nurses who are forced to complete nursing care plans may soon rationalize the desirability of the plans.

A deciding factor in choosing between the two approaches, modifying attitudes or modifying behavior, may be the time factor. Acceptance of a new idea takes time. Less time is needed for group acceptance of ideas that fit the existing attitudes and goals of the group. These attitudes include not only the value systems of the individuals but the institution's value system. Each institution has its own little areas of pride: "We may not have everything here, but we certainly are tops at. . . ." If the desired administrative change involves considerable conflict with individual or institutional values, neither persuasion nor propaganda may be effective.

In dealing with the resistance the nurse administrator will be aided by a knowledge of the typical stages of resistance. Stages will be identified for the typical situation in which a change is first considered and publicized and then instituted by executive order:

1. Undifferentiated resistance comes from various sources.
2. Pro and con sides line up, developing their stands in reasoned arguments or slogans.
3. Direct conflict takes place between the two sides.
4. Those favoring the change come into power as the executive institutes the change.
5. Old adversaries begin the stages of acceptance.
6. Few adversaries are to be found; most people do not recall that they ever opposed the change.

The nurse executive should not let herself be tricked into making premature and ineffective responses to resistance. Such ineffective responses include defensive self-justification, advice giving ("What I would do if I were you . . ."), premature persuasion ("Later, you'll see it my way"), censoring or meeting opposition with disapproval, and punishing.

Accepting that resistance is inevitable, the nurse executive wisely performs a "force field" analysis for a proposed change, identifying and predicting all the driving and restraining forces. Calculation of this balance of forces gives an idea of how much work will be involved in effecting the change. Change may be facilitated by moves that decrease the restraining forces or by moves that increase the driving forces. In estimating the forces, the nurse executive will consider the numbers and status of persons on each side; administrative and other forms of power held by each side; the im-

mediate and the prolonged resistance which may be anticipated; the costs involved in maintaining the given position, such as loss of esteem, friendships, position.

From a force field analysis, the executive should have a good idea whether or not a change actually is possible; whether it is worth the effort required; whether it will create enemies, disruption, or hard feelings that will counter its benefits; whether it will require extensive efforts for its maintenance.

The nurse executive's power to counter opposing forces ranges from persuasion to influence to force. Persuasion can appeal to reason, emotion, or both. It is not the tool of the executive exclusively, but the executive has more communication channels to use for persuasion than does any other person in her division. Influence is a stronger force; it is persuasion independent of arguing a cause. Here it is the opinion of the individual that carries weight, because of the esteem in which that person is held. Although influence is not necessarily assured with position, it is very likely that the nurse executive will have influence equal to or greater than others of her staff. Force, the last alternative, is available in the form of the formalized powers of the executive's organizational position. This is an option which belongs to the executive in greater degree than to any of her staff. The nurse executive should try to use the lowest-level power or combination of powers that can do the job adequately and thus must have an accurate perception of her own ability to influence and persuade.

Politics of Change

Resistance of a political nature is different from that labeled psychological. Although political opposition may be directed toward the change's content, it usually emphasizes the effect on the status and resources of a particular group or department. To illustrate, certain departments of a health care institution may object to a proposed change which would shift status and resources from their departments to nursing. An objection of this character is inclined to be strong regardless of the change's beneficial aspects for patients or the institution as a whole.

Political resistance can clarify the nature of goals in an organization. Ostensibly, everyone in a health care institution shares the same goal of delivering quality care to patients. This does not, however, prevent different groups from establishing their own ambitions and their own small dynasties within the organization. The nurse manager who fails to recognize these variances is not likely to be effective in implementing modifications that affect other groups or departments. A campaign which merely iterates the merits of the proposed change will not gain support from groups whose goals diverge from the nurse manager's.

The nurse manager, therefore, must learn to use other means of persuasion. She must learn to be an effective politician and to fight when confrontation is unavoidable.

The politician's tactics are quite different from those of the person relying upon the justice of her cause. First, the art of compromise must be accepted as a valid mode of operation. The nurse manager ultimately may succeed through a series of partial wins where an "all or nothing" position might never prevail.

Similarly, "trade-offs" may garner the necessary support: the nurse executive supports some cause of another person in exchange for support of her own proposed change. The formation of appropriate coalitions with other power groups is another way to circumvent a strong opponent.

One characteristic of a political maneuver is that it creates obligations. Favors are given and expected in return. For some nurses this action mode opposes the absolutes of the nursing ethos. Nursing literature tends to be written in absolutes such as *total* nursing care, *optimal* return to health. A realistic approach will help the nurse appreciate that partial service is better than none at all, and partial wins are a step toward final achievement of a goal.

In nursing, one often forgets or fails to consider important potential support groups:

1. Upward. The board of trustees, one's own boss
2. Collateral. Other division heads, other professionals outside the nursing division
3. Outward. Patients, community groups, legislators, other groups of professional nurses

The nurse executive must be careful to pick her issues when appealing to external groups. She cannot ring these doorbells too often or she loses credibility.

A political assessment of a proposed change views the issue in light of degree of opposition to be expected. Opposition may range from none at all to long-lasting and strong opposition in the following degrees:

1. No opposition evident
2. Opposition that may actually be "won over" to your side
3. Opposition that will tolerate your change and give no resistance though not actually accepting the change positively
4. Opposition that complies with the change only because of authority, remaining intellectually or emotively opposed to the change
5. Opposition that is firm and resists the change overtly or covertly

When overt opposition to a change is anticipated, another tactic is called for. The best advice for this situation comes not from nursing literature or from change theory, but from the expert strategists in the art of warfare. Hart's axioms of strategy give a flavor of this literature:

1. *Adjust your end to your means.* In determining your object, clear sight and cool calculation should prevail. It is folly "to bite off more than you can chew," and the beginning of military wisdom is a sense of what is possible . . .
2. *Keep your object always in mind,* while adapting your plan to circumstances.

Realize that there are more ways than one of gaining an object . . .

3. *Choose the line (or course) of least expectation.* Try to put yourself in the enemy's shoes, and think what course it is least probable he will foresee or forestall.

4. *Exploit the line of least resistance*—so long as it can lead you to any objective which would contribute to your underlying object . . .

5. *Take a line of operation which offers alternative objectives . . .* to assure the chance of gaining one objective at least—whichever he guards least . . .

6. *Ensure that both plan and dispositions are flexible—adaptable to circumstances . . .*

7. *Do not throw your weight into a stroke whilst your opponent is on guard . . .*

8. *Do not renew an attack along the same line (or in the same form) after it has once failed.*[1]

Thus strategic planning involves many different tactics. Dependent upon the nature of resistances offered to the change, various modes of cooperation and conflict may be used. Strategic planning employs whatever means are required to prepare the environment for acceptance of the change (as represented in the activity plan).

Implementing Action and Strategy Plans

What, then, are the steps that the nurse executive can take in implementing a change? The first is to set up good communications. Everyone who needs to know about the change should be identified, including the opinion leaders. The advantage of the change over what it replaces should be spelled out. Both the informational and emotional aspects of the change should be reviewed. The executive should allow time for those affected by the change to discuss it among themselves. It should be possible for those who oppose the change to voice their objections. Letting persons who will be affected participate in the change planning and change process is useful.

In the implementation process, the nurse executive should remember that an order to everyone is an order to no one. Some executives put out orders in general memos that are quickly filed in the wastebasket or placed on a bulletin board to be ignored. To be effective, a communication must clearly state who is to do what, at what time, and in what way. In addition, the administrator must be prepared to provide follow-up to ensure that such communication is implemented.

When the nurse executive expects strong resistance to a particular change, she can take extra steps to ensure the successful implementation of that change. In instances such as this, she should begin with a clear understanding that control rather than persuasion will be the primary implementation tool. Nevertheless, a few steps short of control can be used toward winning staff support. Use of an independent change agent may be successful. With this scheme, a resource person from outside the organization and with no personal bias may be called in to act as a catalyst in the change process. A similar effect may be attained by use of a design group from within the organization. If a group such as this is to monitor and lead the change process, the selection of members is a critical factor. The design group should consist of knowledgeable and strong leaders in favor of the proposed change. Other members may be persons who are undecided about the issue. Even those who are against the plan but who are openminded and objective can be good task force members. The latter two groups provide a realistic control on group planning, and the executive has to reserve the right to remove any members who assume outright obstructionist roles.

Another system for attaining staff acquiescence is to assure members that they will have an opportunity to evaluate the new plan after it has been in effect for a determined period of time. When a nurse executive makes this commitment, there are four essential agreements to be made:

1. The trial period must be long enough for

the system to become functional and have a fair chance to succeed.

2. The staff must agree to cooperate fully in putting the plan into effect. There can be no half efforts or mere biding of time, waiting for the trial period to end.

3. The nurse executive must stick to her agreement and hold the evaluation session when and as planned.

4. There must be a clear understanding from the start as to whether the nurse executive is to be bound by the decision of the evaluation committee or whether she is merely to consider the committee's recommendations in her final decision.

When none of the suggested measures are going to work in instituting a change, then the nurse executive must rely strictly on the power and control vested in her administrative office. In such instances she must be prepared for a possible power conflict. She does well to consider what kind of support she can expect from her own boss if her staff simply says "No." Should she decide to institute the change, it is important that she indicate that she means business. She dare not waver, seem unsure, or yield any ground. She must set absolute performance standards to be maintained; she must set time limits for action; and she must be willing to take strong action against those who fail to comply with the directive. She also must make certain that the issue is important enough to justify such measures.

Implementing change is only the first step for the nurse executive. She must plan for follow-up if she expects the change to be maintained. She also must be on the lookout for unexpected consequences. No matter how well a change is planned, it is always possible that it may bring about unanticipated outcomes. Part of follow-up on any change project involves a thorough evaluation based on objective criteria derived from the goals and objectives of the change project. One of the most important administrative talents is the ability to deal honestly with the knowledge that a change project was a mistake. The executive

naturally has a great investment in change projects she has originated or supported. She must be very careful that her vested interest does not blind her to the demerits of a plan once it is put into action.

Most change projects, however, if well planned and well executed, will be accepted with surprising rapidity. Often, by the time the trial period is over, the participants have so adapted to the new system that they will resist a return to the old way.

Evaluating Change and Continuity

In evaluating a specific change, one first evaluates the goal or problem which the change addressed. Given an infinite set of identifiable goals and problems, was this particular one worth the investment of resources and energy required to achieve or solve it? Was a more worthy project overlooked when this one was selected for attention? Assessment of the project's inherent worth is the first step in a full evaluation plan. This should be accomplished before a decision is made concerning institution of change.

Since change is only a means, it can only be evaluated by its contribution to the desired end. The next step in evaluation, therefore, is to measure how appropriately the end is achieved. Quantifying information requires a reference point against which the new results are pitted. Baseline data must be collected prior to the establishment of the change; one must evaluate conditions prior to change. Later one cannot judge success if there are no baseline data on which to compare the new state. Unfortunately, this critical step is often omitted. Nurses will institute a primary care assignment system to "improve nursing care" without identifying in just what way care is to be improved. No measure is taken of how the present system (such as the team method) is performing. Hence, after the primary care system has been installed, there is no plausible way of judging its superiority over the old system, except by that rough, and possibly inaccurate, estimate made by the staff happiness quotient.

In addition to evaluating the primary operationalized goals for a change, one also should evaluate other affected indices. For instance, a change to primary care nursing may have as its goal improved patient health states. These outcomes will be measured (before and after the change) by quality control tools devised for that purpose. One might also collect data on indices such as staff satisfaction, incident/error occurrence, number of staff required, and nature and number of nursing orders written. Again, these indices are collected both before and after institution of change.

What criteria are used to assess a change? Every assessment should consider effectiveness, efficiency, and satisfaction. A given change (means) is *effective* if it achieves the desired end; it is ineffective to the degree that it fails. A change is *efficient* if it achieves the desired end in the most economical way, conserving time, money and other resources. A change is inefficient if any alternative could have achieved the same result with less expenditure. A change is *satisfying* if the important reference groups (patients, nurses, others) are content or pleased with the alteration. It is dissatisfying to the degree that preference for the previous system (or alternative, untried change patterns) persists.

In conjunction with evaluating the content of the change, one should also assess its process. What energies and resources were required to reach the end by this means? Was it worth the price? Was completion of the continuity-change cycle reached with a minimum of trouble, confusion, and resentment? If the change solved one problem (or reached one goal) did it create new ones—foreseen or unforeseen—in so doing? Were they bigger or smaller problems than the original one?

A final point should be made concerning evaluation of change. Though evaluation follows soon after implementation, it is critical that final assessment not be made until a state of equilibrium has been achieved, when the change is perceived as the new continuity. At that time all the artificial supports or detractions have been removed, and only then the old continuity state can be compared fairly to the new one.

Where change is perceived as an end in itself, continuity is never achieved. Though one may have a sense of advancement in such a setting, one never knows for certain whether superior nursing has resulted. Thus continuity and change must be kept in proper balance. Both must be seen as means to other ends, and their success requires an evaluation of their achievements.

MODES OF CHANGE

It is interesting to review the nursing literature for an historical perspective on change. For many years there was a heavy focus on change itself; more recently, the literature has concentrated instead on the modes of achieving change.

Initially nursing management literature stressed change itself. Change was discussed divorced from the subject matter to which it was to be applied; it was viewed as a process. The focus was primarily psychological and descriptive of how people act in change situations; it did not prescribe how people should be manipulated to act. It had the sociological onlooker's perspective rather than the active perspective of the manager. Change was accepted as a good, implicitly.

The first major application of change to be discussed in the nursing literature was management by objectives. Prescription rather than description prevailed, but change was viewed primarily as a logistic system, a cool and rational activity plan for the achievement of predetermined goals. In MBO, little, if any, attention is given to strategic planning. It is *assumed* that the construction of a good activity plan is adequate preparation. The existence of an active opposition seldom, if ever, is considered.

MBO is goal-directed, uses rational techniques such as flowcharts, path analysis, and quantitative methods to establish a logical plan to achieve a goal. The focus is on the steps inherent in the goal achievement itself. Note here that the focus (as compared to the ''change'' literature) has switched from a descriptive to a prescriptive one, and from a psychological to a logistic concentration.

After long-lasting attention to MBO, nursing literature on change modes turned to assertiveness training and conflict theory. The literature on getting one's way by assertive behavior moves away from the logistic arena to a psychological one. Here many techniques are offered to the nurse manager, ranging from the steady repetition of one's position to the art of saying ''no.'' In the assertiveness literature, unlike MBO, there is a sense of opposition. One's primary opponent is *oneself,* and one's own inability to deviate from the expectations of others.

Assertiveness management training deals primarily with the nurse manager herself, making her conscious of when her rights are abridged and helping her to reduce the ''followership instinct'' if she has it. Following the psychological motif divorced from the specific work objectives, assertiveness training focuses on the nurse herself rather than on any logistics of a situation.

Conflict theory has different premises than assertiveness training. Opposition is considered external, not internal. Opposition is real, and attention must be given to eliminating it, defeating it, or using it in some productive manner. The conflict literature combines the psychological and logistic means to combat the opposition. The stress is on processes rather than substantive issues of conflict. Since conflict theory comprises a major thrust in the change-related literature, it will be reviewed in some detail later in this chapter.

After a major period in which nursing literature concentrated on conflict theory, attention switched to politics and political processes, the art of promoting one's own ends through use of available resources. This literature, while incorporating the notion of opposition, is more complex and subtle, narrowing in on the achievement of a goal (like MBO) rather than focusing only on opposition to the goal (like conflict theory). Here indifference as well as opposition becomes a facet of the total panorama of achieving one's ends. Focus in political theory is:

1. On the ends (like MBO, unlike conflict theory);
2. On strategic planning rather than on activity planning (unlike MBO, like conflict theory); thus politics stresses *both* ends and means.
3. On indifference as well as on opposition to the goal. Various publics are considered as they line up pro, con, and indifferent to the objective.

It is surprising that the nursing literature has failed to draw from the most comprehensive body of literature—that on warfare theory. Indeed, warfare theory is the only body of knowledge that:

1. Considers the ends in view;
2. Develops an activity plan to reach those ends;
3. Develops a strategic plan to achieve those ends;
4. Considers both logistic and psychological factors.

Much recent nursing literature combines the domains of politics and power or looks at power exclusively. This literature reflects the obvious: the need for power in order for political moves to be effective. Modes of achieving power usually are discussed apart from the subject matter to which power is applied, that is, apart from goal-content. Power literature focuses upon both psychological and logistic mechanisms. Since power and politics are dominant in today's nursing management literature, these elements will be reviewed in detail later in this chapter.

Given the present focus on power and politics, we can hope only that the future will bring a concentration on ''statesmanship,'' on goal-related use of power. The focus on power is meaningless until it is attached to goals, yet to date, most of the nursing literature views power as an end in itself—not as a means to some other end. Statesmanship and vision in nursing would correct this perspective.

Conflict Theory

Conflict theory recognizes that one man's goal is another man's anathema. It recognizes that legitimate differences can exist, especially in the organizational setting. Conflict theory implies opposition.

Conflict theory as it applies to organizations incorporates many elements. First, one may examine the *subject matter* of organizational conflicts. The subject matter of conflict may be: 1) disagreement as to goals—absolute disagreement or disagreements as to priorities among goals; 2) disagreements concerning the methods to be used to achieve goals—technical or moral arguments may enter here; 3) disagreements as to the "facts of a case"; 4) disagreements as to how certain facts are to be interpreted; or 5) differences concerning values or ideologies—e.g., the accounting department's goals versus nursing's goals.

Conflict theory also reflects various views on the virtue (or vice) of disagreement. Those who claim that conflict in various degrees is good, cite the following reasons: conflict promotes thinking and creative problem solving. Conflict clarifies issues and lets undermining problems rise to the surface. Conflict improves production by creating a useful level of tension and competition. Those who reject conflict as beneficial cite the following reasons: Conflict promotes partialities; workers take on the objectives of the small work unit versus the broad goals of the whole institution. Conflict creates distance and distrust among workers. Conflict holds the potential of denigrating and demeaning certain workers when they are on "losing" sides. Conflict produces high levels of tension, which are inhibitive of productive work.

Some managers who believe that conflict is beneficial purposefully create tension among their staff; most managers prefer to prevent or resolve conflicts that arise. A manager might reflect either of these positions or yet a third alternative: that conflict is inevitable in the organizational setting, and the manager's job is to manage its resolution.

Managers also differ in what they attribute to be the primary sources of conflict. Often cited are three potential sources: human shortcomings, interpersonal failure, and the nature of an organization (not of the people in it). These sources are frequently offered as opposing theories. What notion of the source of conflict is held by the nurse executive will affect how she goes about resolving conflicts. (The rest of this discussion will assume that the resolution of conflict, rather than the creation of it, is the aim of the nurse executive. This, clearly, is the more popular interpretation.)

The nurse executive may play many different parts in a given conflict; she may be participant, explicator, mediator, or judge of the conflict. Each of these positions will be reviewed briefly.

As a participant in a conflict, the nurse executive first determines what is the real issue at hand. Is it a question of fact or of how a fact is to be interpreted? Is it a question of conflicting values? Of means? Or ends? Surprisingly, people often are found to "argue" when their positions are not really in contradiction. Hence the first task in any apparent conflict is to lay clear the subject matter and the differences among opponents on that subject matter. In organizations, many conflicts are due to role differences. The business manager necessarily gives more credence to finance than does someone in a direct service role. These differences are inherent in the roles they perform for the organization. A conflict that is related to role can be mitigated if each party is able to recognize the role impact for himself and the other; this will defuse the issue by depersonalizing it.

Whatever the issue, the nurse executive should strive to depersonalize the argument.

Keep to the issues, not to the personalities of the parties to the conflict. The nurse executive should watch to see that feelings do not intervene in the argument in such a way as to cut off productive search for a solution. Additionally, the nurse executive may elect the mode in which she wishes to respond to the issue. Schmidt identifies five modes: competing, accommodating, avoiding, compromising, and collaborating[2]. He defines competing as being all out to win; accommodating as letting the other party achieve what is important to him so as to preserve the relationship; avoiding as the mode in which the conflict is not faced; compromising as a case in which each party settles for "half a loaf"; and collaborating as the ideal solution in which the parties accept each other's goals, and both come away with a win.

Schmidt diagrams these modes of response in relation to two dimensions: assertiveness and cooperativeness. These are shown in Figure 13-2, in which yet other modes of response have been added.

The added modes on the chart are probably self-explanatory. Forcing occurs when conflict is consciously pushed and the opponent is not allowed to use a mode of withdrawal or avoidance. Smoothing is a mechanism by which one party attempts to deny that there really is a conflict. Withdrawal is a form of avoidance instituted after first joining the issue. Negotiation is a mode in which both parties agree to reach agreement by give and take on various issues which will never be resolved by consensus. Often negotiation becomes a structured, formal procedure.

The choice of mode of response to conflict should depend upon the nature and the seriousness of the subject matter under conflict. But no matter the mode the nurse executive will maintain control of the mode of response only so long as she maintains a cool head in the discussions.

When the nurse executive is explicator in a conflict between other parties, she tries to help the parties clarify the issues, and she acts to defuse personal attacks if they occur. As mediator, the executive aims to bring the conflict to a close by getting the parties to reach some form of agreement. She may assess the ability of each party to "give," and she may suggest compromise positions. As judge, she performs a different function,

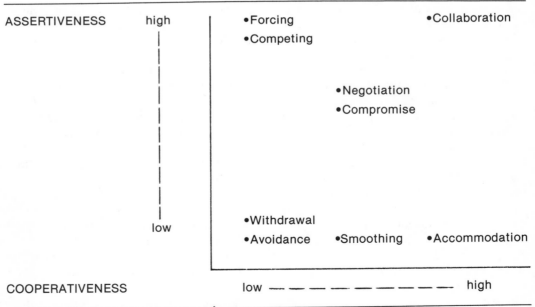

Figure 13-2.   Modes of Handling Conflict (Adapted from Schmidt)

hearing both sides and pronouncing a decision. That decision may be in favor of one participant or it may be a compromise. In any case, when she plays this role, the final decision remains hers alone.

The nurse executive must be careful not to act as if she is mediating when, in fact, she intends to play the judge. For example, a nurse executive might try to mediate but then refuse to accept the compromise arrived at by the two opponents, thereby losing all credibility with the conflicting parties. She must be careful to define her neutral, third-party role in any conflict and then to stick to it.

To resolve conflict it is always best to look forward rather than looking backward, looking to place blame. If the nurse executive can promote an orientation towards the future regarding resolution of conflicts, she is likely to become an effective negotiator as well as a successful participant when conflicts do occur.

Power and Politics

Power and politics often are discussed together in the nursing literature or joined in the term, power-politics. The reason may be the difficulty in distinguishing them. Both are vehicles for achieving one's ends, and both do so through manipulation of others. Even though power and politics are means to other ends, for some persons power becomes an end in itself. Power and politics also interact: the powerful have more ways in which to exert political clout, and political success is one means by which one acquires power. Both power and politics focus upon strategy for achieving one's end rather than on the activity plan itself.

What distinctions, then, can be made between power and politics? Here power will be discussed as a *state* and politics as a *process*. Power is that state in which one is *able* to manipulate others; politics is the process through which one *attempts* (successfully or unsuccessfully) to manipulate others. Indeed, one could say that politics (influence—

dynamic) is not required where power (absolute—static) already exists. Power, however, is seldom absolute for the power holder; it varies in degree from situation to situation. And successful political attempts are one source of cumulation of power. For simplicity let us consider these concepts separately at first.

Power

Among the many perspectives from which to examine power are its sources, its relation to status, and states that contribute to power acquisition.

Sources. Power often is viewed as an interpersonal, dyadic relationship in which one party has control over another in some aspect. This perspective is predominant in the psychological literature. The one-to-one power relationship is a good place to begin understanding power, for the structure of the one-to-one relationship pertains in formal and informal groups also.

Power is a dyadic relationship, based on both the strengths of the powerholder and the dependencies of the followers. No matter what his strengths, a power holder cannot exist without someone else over whom he holds power. Jacobson defines power by noting that the dependency of B upon A is proportional to B's motivational investment in the goals mediated by A[3]. Power is inversely proportional to the availability of these goals to B outside the A-B relationship. Thus power can be seen as an interpersonal relationship. There is no such thing as power outside the context of a relationship. Jacobson also notes that a statement of power is incomplete when it fails to include the cost to A of attempting to influence B.

The principles of power relations can be clarified by some examples. The first principle is: The dependency of B upon A is proportional to B's motivational investment in the goals mediated by A. Suppose A is a head nurse and B and C are staff nurses.

Goals mediated by A include possible raises and interesting work assignments. If B really does not care what assignments she gets or whether she gets a raise, then she is much less dependent upon A than is C, who is counting on that raise to pay for her new car. Nurse A will have far more power to make C write out her care plans, for example, than she will to make B write hers.

The second principle is: Power is inversely proportional to the availability of these goals to B outside the A-B relationship. If A is the only faculty member who knows how to produce videotapes, and B wants to learn this skill, then A can exert much more power over B than she could if other faculty members were available to teach B the desired skill.

The third principle is: A statement of power must take into account the cost to A of attempting to influence B. Head Nurse A may have the power to suspend Staff Nurse B for reporting on duty late for the third time in a month. She may, however, not want to go through all the paperwork involved and the hostility she anticipates would follow from B.

Sources of dependency are multiple. A common example is one in which A has skills that B needs or wants to learn. If A is the only source of this learning, then B's dependency on A is increased. A's power over B lasts, in this case, only so long as he still has some knowledge that B wishes to attain. This is one of the costs of power arising from the skill source; one attains power by acting as the teacher, but once he has taught all he knows to the other, he has "used up" his source of power. Skills are not the only source of power. Many power holders arise due to their abilities in handling interpersonal relations of groups. Where all workers have similar skills, this is often the source of power. Power holders who arise because of their skill in interpersonal relations have ability to persuade, manipulate, inspire, or a combination of these. A third source of power is that bestowed by organizational authority. This power holder has the greatest number of tools at his disposal, for his power base is absolute. If he fails to persuade, manipulate, or inspire, he can resort to use of administrative dictate.

The nurse executive must be aware of power plays made by staff members. A typical power play is that based on learned skill. It is not uncommon for older employees to withhold necessary teaching from new employees in attempts to retain superior status. Older employees may refuse to teach the new employee procedural tasks or they may refuse to teach "the ropes," the unwritten code of systems and practices that get the work done in a particular institution. Moves such as these need to be countered by authority moves from the executive. Such moves are typical of lower-level employees, who have little power and therefore guard the small quantum zealously.

One power-equalizing move that can be found at any level in the organization is withdrawal. The employee who uses this technique recognizes that when he withdraws from the dependency role, the power of his boss is negated. Withdrawal of mass followership clearly eliminates the leader. When the nurse executive has the power of an organizational position, however, the only complete withdrawal of the subordinate is resignation. Subtle partial withdrawals are more typical of the subordinate who is trying to equalize power. The employee who assumes an attitude of "I'll put in my eight hours" is likely to frustrate the manager. Most employees who try this type of withdrawal manage to fill minimum job requirements, thereby maximizing job security with minimal dependency upon their boss.

Withdrawal is indeed the power play that costs the manager the most effort to resolve. To counter a withdrawal move requires that the manager reassert goals the employee cannot ignore. Usually these goals are position, salary, and job retention. When a supervisor or head nurse uses withdrawal, the simplest solution is the reduction of the individual to a staff assignment. Many institutions have union contracts, but few contracts guarantee a management position.

When withdrawal occurs in a staff

member protected by a contract, the process of removing the individual requires careful documentation of any actions that fail to meet those defined minimum job requirements. Trying to "woo back" the employee in withdrawal is usually an unsatisfactory management response. This attempt shifts power to the employee, for he now can choose whether or not to accede to the request implied by the manager's approach. This form of appeal to the employee mistakes the withdrawal for a passive move; actually withdrawal is an active confrontation move.

In the psychological, dyadic interpretation, power results when one person is dependent on another for goals mediated by that other, such as salaries, promotions, praise, or approval. The degree of power held by the power user is proportional to the power recipient's desire for achieving those goals and his lack of other sources for achieving them. The degree of power also depends on the cost to the power user of influencing the power recipient.

Power also is viewed as a social phenomenon. From this perspective, French and Raven list five sources of power[4]:

1. Legitimate power. Held as a result of social or organizational position.
2. Referent power. In which the holder is followed because of who he is. Charismatic power is included here.
3. Reward power. Includes its opposite: punishment power. In the organizational setting, promotions, raises, or firings would be typical examples.
4. Coercive power. Actual force.
5. Expert power. Based on knowledge or skills held by the power user and needed by the power recipient.

Legitimate power and reward power are inherent in the nurse executive role and together are often called *formal* power, as contrasted with *functional* power, or referent power. Obviously the nurse executive who combines both formal and functional power is both a manager and a leader. Where these powers combine in the same person, the degree of power possessed is great. Some nurse executives are able to convert functional power to formal power, using their charisma to convince others to invest more formal power in their positional role.

All too often the nurse executive faces an inequitable distribution of power in her organization. Often the nurse executive has to struggle for title and power commensurate with her responsibility as head of the largest division of the institution. The historical and social reasons for such power inequities in nursing are well known. Nursing has made strides in correcting these inequities. In many instances the formal goals have been achieved: the nursing service executive reports to her institution's director and holds title as assistant or associate administrator or vice president.

The remaining battles for equitable power are even more difficult, for they are psychological struggles. For example, the nurse executive with an appropriate administrative title needs to examine the informal structure of her organization. What is her status in the informal circle where the problems of the institution are identified and formulated? Many nurse executives have satisfactory titles and attend all the official high-level meetings, yet have no entrée to the informal power structure.

The nurse executive needs to ask, Does the chief administrator regularly consult with a particular group of executives? If she is not included in the informal group her executive role is still titular. She must be sensitive to informal lines of communication, for the philosophy and direction of an organization originate in informal power groups rather than in discussions at formal meetings. Formal meetings serve to crystallize and authorize thoughts and plans that are generated in the informal structure.

The nurse executive who lacks access to the informal power groups is in a weak position. Entrance can be difficult because entrée depends upon invitation. Failure to receive access to an informal power group is not always the fault of the nurse executive. Often, she can counter by extending her own invitations for informal occasions to the important individuals. If she is skilled at it, entertaining may be the backdoor entry to the power group or groups. Even here, there is no assurance that the groups will necessarily include her in their work-related informal sessions.

The nurse executive should set acceptance into power groups as a primary goal. She must not let herself be misled as to the nature of her power simply because she has an appropriate title and attends high-level meetings. She also needs to be part of the major informal power groups that determine organizational direction. At the very least, those power groups include the group surrounding the institution's chief administrative officer and the power formations among trustees.

Related to this aspect of power acquisition and politics is the need to build colleague relationships with physicians holding equivalent positions in the organization. Establishment of colleagueship does not simply happen. Often the nurse has to reeducate the physician to a new concept of nursing, insisting upon colleagueship not only by her method of interaction but also by exhibiting that she is every bit as professional in her domain as he is in his area of expertise.

Another power issue is in the continuing trend toward putting a non-nurse in the nurse executive's place. Often this is done under the guise of creating two positions: clinical nursing director and non-nurse manager of the nursing division. This division is promoted as a way to keep the nurse expert in the clinician role, leaving the "extraneous management features" to a person with special education in management. This proposal is dangerous and is likely to rob nursing of the power it has struggled to gain. Whether one likes it or not, purse strings and decision-making power go together, and ultimately, what the clinical nurse director is able to do will depend on the distribution of finances and regulation of policies by the non-nurse manager of the division. If the clinical nursing director gives up management of the division, control of nurs-

ing practice will soon follow. The clinical nursing director's "copartner" will soon be her boss. The nurse executive must be especially wary of such attempts to divest her of her division in the present era when schools of health care administration are turning out an excessive number of graduates—all looking for some high-level health administrative job. The nursing division, usually the largest one in an institution, appears to be a ripe plum to such job seekers. Furthermore, though this is not true in all cases, some hospital administrators would be more comfortable dealing with someone whose educational experience (and possibly sex) are the same as their own.

A related mechanism for divesting the nurse executive of organizational power is that developed in the name of "decentralization." Many nurse executives have discovered too late that where decentralization occurs, consolidated power of the nursing division may disappear. Shortly after decentralization nursing chiefs often find themselves reporting to a medical director rather than to the chief nurse executive, whose role has become totally titular.

Clearly, the nurse executive must attend to preservation and expansion of both her formal and functional power. If she neglects either aspect, her position is in jeopardy, and her effectiveness as a leader and manager is threatened.

Status. Just as it is difficult to separate the concepts of power and politics, it also is difficult to separate power and status. Power often is reflected in high social status. Conversely, high social status itself is a source of power. Viguers identifies five status systems that occur in the hospital[5]:

1. Scalar status. Attributable to place on the organization chart. This is positional authority.
2. Functional status. Attributable to one's functions in the hospital and their demand. At the top is the physician's function.

3. Informal status. Gained through personal relationships.
4. Sociological status. Based on social traditions and the mores of the community.
5. Psychological status. Various patterns, but especially the physician's status over that of the patient by virtue of the patient's need and the physician's power.

States That Contribute to Power Cumulation. Numerous authors identify states that contribute to the cumulation of power. Claus and Bailey discuss this factor adequately[6]. Such states may include:

1. Broad human networks. The more networks and the more extensive, the more power.
2. Broad information networks. The more diverse types of information controlled, the more power.
3. Multiple leadership roles. Formal and informal.
4. Ability to assess accurately situations (especially unstructured ones) and to solve problems.
5. Authority over others and resources via legitimate work or organizational roles.
6. Vision into the future.
7. Ability to grant services to others which build "debts."
8. Expertise that is sought by others.

Politics

The process of influencing others in order to achieve one's own ends—politics—is viewed in relation to two discrete domains in the nursing literature: the domain of the nurse executive in her own organization and the broad domain of influencing the political process at local, state, and federal levels. While the domains differ, and the publics to be influenced differ, the political tactics are similar in these two settings. Common tactics include:

1. Opportunism. Moving when the time is right.
2. Use of trade-offs. Selling votes on one issue for votes on another.
3. Negotiation. Two sides each give up lesser values to achieve greater values.
4. Formation of coalitions. Two or more smaller powers band together to defeat a larger power.
5. Compromise. Each side settles for a partial win, part of what it hoped to achieve.
6. Lobbying. Attempting to build collectible "debts" with persons who may exercise influence (or votes) in one's favor. This may also include trying to win favor with rightness, fairness, or nobility of one's cause.

Political moves are possible because people may agree on ends and means. Alternatively, people may agree upon actions (means) because the same action may be seen as contributing to different ends. Hence politics deals with both means and ends.

Power and Politics Applied to Nursing

Politics and power may be difficult themes for some nurse executives. Until recently, it may not have been considered right for a female nurse manager to admit that she sought to gain or use either one. Some nurses still decry these methods because they tend to seek to manipulate others covertly rather than openly trying to win others to their respective causes. Politics escapes that all-or-none mentality still held by some nurses for politics is the art of the gray—of the possible, not the ideal. The nurse executive who refuses to negotiate because her "cause" is not negotiable because it is right might do well to remember the adage, "The best is the enemy of the good." Politics and power both clearly attempt to manipulate others—even if in a good cause.

There are some applications of power and politics that apply within the nurse executive's own organization. We are just coming out of an era when a nurse had to "apologize" if she held a role away from the patient's bedside. Obviously, the nurse manager who casts herself in an apologist's role is an easy target for her enemies. The nurse manager must recognize the significance of nursing management; she must recognize that clinical nursing depends upon her own skill in creating an environment where vanguard practice and research can take place. Without powerful nursing management, clinical nursing cannot advance.

Control by physicians is still a power issue in health care organizations. Physicians will not voluntarily give power to nursing (power is seldom voluntarily shared in any circumstance), but nurses may learn from those groups of health care workers who did develop power enough to "free" themselves from the dominance of physicians. When one examines the paths of dentists, opticians, and podiatrists, for example, one sees that they managed to define their work domain as exclusive from medicine. There is no reason why nursing should not try the same tactic. Surely it is possible to differentiate nursing from medicine, whether one does that by the caring versus curing discrimination or by some other model.

With physicians and with others, nurse executives must learn to negotiate wisely. They must learn when to negotiate, and when *not* to negotiate. The nurse executive must be sure of her own authority, and she must not negotiate it away. Often this happens to a nurse executive who, because of her nursing background, prefers a cooperative mode and therefore fails to recognize that she is in a competitive mode until it is too late. One director of nursing allowed another institutional division to "help her" find her problems, until the representatives from that other division had totally taken over the power centers in the nursing division. She was "cooperated to death" because she failed to see a power move when it was hidden behind "good intentions."

The nurse executive must learn to recognize power plays when they are made, be they positive or negative in their outcome. Power plays proceed either by extension of a power network or by formation of a coali-tion. Extension of a power network is an equalizing power move that may occur in the organizational structure (when a manager seeks more employees or more sections to manage) or it may take place on the informal level (when a particular leader is sought out by more and more people). The nurse executive may choose to block or to encourage this power mechanism.

Some of the best contributions to any organization are made by industrious and capable individuals in the midst of expansion moves. The nurse executive who is secure in her own authority may allow the organization to benefit from challenges of this sort. For example, if a clinical specialist is trying to extend her informal power by making her skills available to more nursing personnel, the organization is likely to benefit if the nurse executive encourages the personal expansion. Similarly, if a capable supervisor is trying to increase her power by absorbing duties or functions ignored by others, the nurse executive might be wise to legitimate these added functions by a corresponding change in the supervisor's official position.

Coalition formation is the other equalizing power move. This move transfers separate individual powers into a single, greater collective power. Since coalition requires the cooperation of individuals normally competitive with or indifferent to each other, the administrator must accept this as a threat to her position and a critique of her management. Growth of a coalition does not indicate that the nurse executive necessarily is a poor manager. Coalitions are likely to form also in response to unpopular but needed management changes.

In any case, the formation of a coalition should be cause for the nurse executive to sit down and examine her course of management. How the nurse executive handles such power moves depends upon how she estimates the costs to herself and to her organization. At least the executive should be able to recognize such moves when they are developing, so that both actions and reactions can be analyzed effectively.

The nurse executive needs to evaluate both

the organization's managers and its informal leaders. The forward-looking nurse executive will want to consider the best people in both groups as a potential pool for future organizational leadership positions. She will plan ahead for the future management needs of her division by providing these individuals with work experiences and educational opportunities designed to enhance their developing abilities.

Sometimes a nurse executive holds back the careers of those individuals whose abilities are seen as potential threats to her own position. In such an instance she places less capable persons in the important management positions. The very fact of their inferior skills assures the nurse executive of their loyalty; they must depend upon her beneficence rather than on their own abilities in order to maintain their positions. This practice may protect the nurse executive, but it spells disaster for the nursing division. Capable individuals, perceiving that they cannot advance in the division, soon leave in search of better opportunities. Gradually the nursing division loses its talented people and sinks into a state of mediocrity, where maintaining the status quo is the highest goal of which it is capable.

The nurse executive who uses this strategy is incapable of being both a leader and a manager. The responsible leader-manager builds on strengths, not on weaknesses. She encourages the development of strong leaders in the organization. She thinks of such strength as an asset to the organization, not as a personal threat. Indeed, the executive who is effective in her job seldom feels threatened, for she is likely to be continuously developing her own abilities as well as those of her promising staff members.

The nurse executive also must be aware of symbols in the power game. One symbol of power is the physical environment of the executive. Where is the nurse executive's office located? Close to the president or chief executive officer? Or is it the only executive suite on the third floor? Or, worse yet, in the basement? Does the nurse executive have equal space and equivalent furnishings to that given to other officers of her positional status? Or is hers the only office which is not carpeted? I know of one case where the director of nursing was the only officer without air conditioning. This director bragged that she had told her boss that "her" air conditioning should be given to a patient's room; that any patient needed air conditioning more than she did. While she was proud of her dedication to patient service, her office gave an unspoken message to every visitor about her importance in the institution. The nurse executive must recognize that her environment speaks not just of her personal power, but of the power and significance of the nursing division in the institution.

The nurse executive should be careful what titles she gives to managerial personnel. Do the titles convey to outsiders the notion of power? Many nurse executives have given up as old fashioned titles like supervisor, head nurse, director, often replacing them with "soft" words like coordinator or facilitator. Words such as these indicate to those educated in a managerial tradition, staff positions rather than powerful line positions. Connotations are important, and the nurse executive should be aware of the subtleties conveyed by her choice of titles.

Finally, the nurse executive should be looking for ways to make the function (and necessity) of her division evident to others. The present move to cost out nursing services is one such attempt; it defines what nursing services can be had for what cost. Attempts to make the nursing division more visible are important in establishing power. If the nurse executive fails to grasp the power inherent in her role, someone else will be there waiting to take over—power abhors a vacuum.

In relation to legislative politics, particularly national, other issues pertain. Here one must look at nursing as a profession rather than specifically at the nurse executive. It is evident that this is a time when nursing could make a significant advancement in its status for this is a time when the country is not willing to put ever-increasing portions of the gross national product into health care. One way to decrease health costs for the nation is to use nurses for those tasks and domains for which they already are qualified—if seldom allowed to practice at the peak of their education and abilities. Were nursing ready for this challenge—if it had a strong and representative organization that could speak for all of nursing—it could advance significantly now. Unfortunately, lack of experience with politics and power are evident in the collective action, or lack of action, of nurses.

Were nursing in a position for collective, strong action, it would be making moves to take over well care, chronic maintenance care, convalescent care, and the nursing home industry, among areas of health concern that could be better handled on a nursing model than on a medical model. But it would take powerful moves to gain this control.

Nurses' naiveté in politics also is evident in our collective approach to federal policy. Inevitably, the nursing profession does not become involved until an act has already been passed and is perceived to be detrimental to nursing. The Professional Standards Review Organization (PSRO) act is a case in point. Nurses should have seen the disenfranchisement of nurse power before, not after, the act was passed. To work at changing laws after they are passed is much less beneficial than to work to change them before they become law. Nursing needs to develop a proactive rather than a reactive response to legislature.

Where should nursing go from here? What moves would have the potential to increase nursing's political clout and power? Several tactics suggest themselves for consideration. First, movement into mainstream university education is a power move. It is foolish to think that nursing can improve its influence without increasing its educational status, given the values of this society. Next, nursing may choose between two modes of "advancing" its practice, either continuing

to take over more specialized tasks from physicians as they advance to newer, more complicated technology, or increasing the science of nursing as a separate domain of practice from medicine. (These two options are not incompatible should nursing decide to move on both fronts.) Also, nursing might aim to take over control of health care settings. Certainly this should already have happened in the nursing home setting, but has not. Nursing is the logical body of health care workers to control the practice setting—if it is to be controlled by a professional group. (Of course, we are preparing too few nurse executives to make this route feasible in the near future.) Finally, one may view unionization as a mode to power, but one must be aware of the nature of that power: it is financial, not intellectual or professional. Obviously, the first step in *any* power-based, political-based move is to create a unity among nurses on goals to be achieved; nursing is a long way from achieving unity today.

SUMMARY

Continuity, change, and modes of creating change are subjects of serious concern for the nurse executive. She needs to be able to place all the recommendations concerning change and its achievement in an appropriate context. She needs to be able to determine when change is needed, how it is to be achieved, and when it is not to be desired. In understanding change, she may be benefited by many bodies of knowledge: change theory, conflict theory, political theory, and theories of power, to name a few. In relation to change, the nurse executive must be cautious not to accept without analysis, the fads and themes which come and go with regularity. Change in itself is merely a process to achieve another end. The nurse executive must not forget that the end in view determines the efficacy and appropriateness of change.

REFERENCES

1. Hart, B.H. *Strategy.* New York: Frederick A. Praeger, 1967, pp. 348–349.
2. Schmidt, W.H. Conflict: a powerful process for (good or bad) change. *Management Rev.,* 63(12):5–10, 1974.
3. Jacobson, W.D. *Power and Interpersonal Relations.* Belmont, Calif.: Wadsworth, 1972, p. 2.
4. French, J.R.P., Jr., and Raven, B. The bases of social power. In Cartwright, D. (Ed.) *Studies in Social Power.* Ann Arbor: University of Michigan, Institute for Social Research, 1959, pp. 150–167.
5. Viguers, R.T. Who's on top? Who knows? In Rakich, J.S. (Ed.) *Hospital Organization and Management.* St Louis: The Catholic Hospital Association, 1972, pp. 13–20.
6. Claus, K.E., and Bailey, J.T. *Power and Influence in Health Care: A New Approach to Leaders.* St. Louis: C.V. Mosby, 1977.

BIBLIOGRAPHY

Belanger, C. Do you confront the boss? *Supervisor Nurse,* 9(12):36, 1978.
Bell, D.V. *Power, Influence, and Authority.* New York: Oxford University Press, 1975.
Bernal, H. Power and interorganizational health care projects. *Nursing Outlook,* 24(7):418, 1976.
Cain, C., and Luchsinger, V. Management by objectives: applications to nursing. *J.O.N.A.,* 8(1):35, 1978.
Clark, C.C. Assertiveness issues for nursing administrators and managers. *J.O.N.A.,* 9(7):20, 1979.
Cleland, V. Implementation of change in health care systems. *J.O.N.A.,* 2(6):64, 1972.
Colls, J. Future shock invades nursing. *J.O.N.A.,* 5(3):27, 1975.
Cotton, C.C. Measurement of power-balancing styles and some of their correlates. *Am. Sci. Quart.,* 21(2):307, 1976.
Courtade, S. The role of the head nurse: power and practice. *Supervisor Nurse,* 9(12):16, 1978.
Deal, J. The timing of change. *Supervisor Nurse,* 8(9):73, 1977.
Dicken, A. Prescription for role conflict. *Supervisor Nurse,* 5(11):143, 1974.
Diers, D. A different kind of energy—nurse-power. *Nursing Outlook,* 26(1):51, 1978.
Doona, M.E. A nursing unit as a political system. *J.O.N.A.,* 7(1):28, 1977.
Froman, L.A., Jr. *The Congressional Process: Strategies, Rules and Procedures.* Boston: Little, Brown, 1967.
Henderson, H. Toward managing social conflict. *Harvard Business Rev.,* 69(3):82, 1971.
Kalisch, B.J. The promise of power. *Nursing Outlook,* 26(1):42, 1978.

Kalisch, B.J., and Kalisch, P.A. An analysis of the sources of physician-nurse conflict. *J.O.N.A.,* 7(1):50, 1977.
Kalisch, P.A., and Kalisch, B.J. The what, why, and how of the political dynamics of nursing. In Marriner, A. (Ed.) *Current Perspectives in Nursing Management.* St. Louis: C.V. Mosby, 1979.
Kanter, R.M. Power failure in management circuits. *Harvard Business Rev.,* 57(4):65, 1979.
Kotter, J.P., and Schlesinger, L.A. Choosing strategies for change. *Harvard Business Rev.,* 57(2):106, 1979.
Kramer, M., and Schmalenberg, C.E. Conflict: the cutting edge of growth. *J.O.N.A.,* 7(8):19, 1976.
Levenstein, A. Effecting change requires change agent. *J.O.N.A.,* 9(6):12, 1979.
Lewis, J.H. Conflict management. *J.O.N.A.,* 6(10):18, 1976.
Longest, B.B., Jr. Institutional politics. *J.O.N.A.,* 5(3):38, 1975.
Lourenço, S.V., and Glidewell, J.C. A dialectical analysis of organizational conflict. *Admin. Sci. Quart.,* 20(4):489, 1975.
McClelland, D.C., and Burnham, D.H. Power is the great motivator. *Harvard Business Rev.,* 54(2):100, 1976.
McDonald, A. Conflict at the summit: a deadly game. *Harvard Business Rev.,* 50(2):59, 1972.
McFarland, D.E., and Shiflett, N. *Power in Nursing.* Wakefield, Mass.: Nursing Resources, 1979.
McMurry, R.N. Power and the ambitious executive. *Harvard Business Rev.,* 51(6):140, 1973.
Manez, J. The untraditional nurse manager: agent of change and change agent. *Hospitals,* 52(1):62, 1978.
Marriner, A. Conflict theory. *Supervisor Nurse,* 10(4):12, 1979.
Marriner, A. Conflict resolution. *Supervisor Nurse,* 10(5):46, 1979.
Mullane, M.K. Nursing care and the political arena. *Nursing Outlook,* 23(11):699, 1975.
Nash, A. Conflict relations between nursing supervisors, practical nurses, and attendants. *J.O.N.A.,* 7(6):9, 1977.
Nehls, D., et al. Planned change: a quest for nursing autonomy. *J.O.N.A.,* 4(1):23, 1974.
Peterson, G.G. Power: a perspective for the nursing administrator. *J.O.N.A.,* 9(7):7, 1979.
Shiflett, N, and McFarland, D.E. Power and the nursing administrator. *J.O.N.A.,* 8(3):19, 1978.
Thurkettle, M.A., and Jones, S.L. Conflict as a systems process: theory and management. *J.O.N.A.,* 8(1):39, 1978.
Veninga, R. The management of conflict. *J.O.N.A.,* 3(4):12, 1973.
Wolff, K.G. Change: implementation of primary nursing through ad hocracy. *J.O.N.A.,* 7(10):24, 1977.
Zand, D.E. and Sorenson, R.E. Theory of change and the effective use of management. *Am. Sci. Quart.,* 20(4):532, 1975.

Chapter 14   The Role of the Nurse Executive

In examining role theory as it relates to the position of the nurse executive, it is useful to look first at the diverse approaches that have been taken historically to studying the process of management itself. Management literature reflects a basic division between a focus on people and a focus on tasks. Some researchers and authors approach management through examination of tasks; others view management by observing those involved in the work process. Even authors who take a broad view of management tend to do it by viewing *both* tasks and people, rather than by developing other categories. Figure 14-1 identifies the categories under which most research and writing on management may be placed.

Notice that the concept of role breaks down the traditional dichotomy between task and person. The chapter will examine the concept of role and its utility in nursing management after reviewing briefly the major management literature relevant to the categories denoted in Figure 14-1.

THE "PEOPLE" ELEMENT OF MANAGEMENT

Managers

Literature that focuses on the manager himself or herself tends to look at *traits,* personality factors, or at *leadership styles,* modes of approaching the task of the leader. Early management studies often sought to decide what constellation of personality traits best characterizes a leader. Supposedly, if one could recognize a leader, one could put recognized leaders in the managerial positions. Notice that this in-

terest shifted study away from management to leadership. Managers are persons who hold positions where they are responsible for other workers; leaders are persons who, for one reason or another, have a followership. Obviously there may be people in managerial positions with little or no leadership ability; conversely there may be leaders with no formal position. The early literature often ignored this difference, blurring the use of the terms, manager and leader.

The studies which sought to identify leadership traits often were disappointing because they generally revealed that leaders have many and diverse traits of personality. The Ohio State University studies improved on this negative finding by switching from traits to leader behaviors[1]. The leader of a group was found to be the person who 1) defined the roles of self and others in relation to goal achievement, 2) structured and interpreted the situation to the group, and 3) showed respect and consideration for the ideas of other group members.

Of the studies that concentrated on style rather than personality traits, perhaps the best known is one that classified managers according to their tendencies to be autocratic, democratic, or laissez faire[2]. Although the study calls these three tendencies leadership styles rather than managerial styles, the term leadership styles is a misnomer since one may have a laissez faire manager but a laissez faire leader, by definition, does not exist.

A more useful set of managerial "styles" is that one which discriminates among idiocratic, democratic, technocratic, and bureaucratic tendencies[3]. An idiocratic supervisor is one who tends to relate to her staff as individuals, in a one-to-one manner.

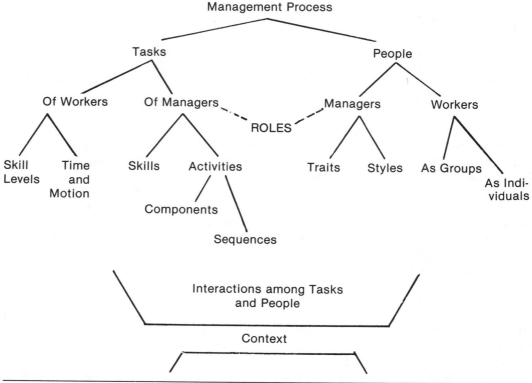

Figure 14-1.   Domains of Inquiry in Management Literature

In contrast a democratic supervisor is likely to relate to her staff as a group. Note that in both these styles, the "people," not the "task," component is dominant. The technocratic supervisor perceives herself as the "super technologist"—in the case of nursing, this might be a supervisor who sees her role primarily as a clinical consultant. The bureaucratic supervisor is one who perceives her role to be enforcement of the policies and procedures of the institution. The latter two styles relate to the work or tasks rather than to the workers directly. Hence even this perception of styles reflects the traditional division between people and tasks.

For a manager, the mere identification of instinctive styles of management is a meaningless exercise. One must go beyond identifying natural styles and examine them to decide which are good and which are bad and then proceed to convert a "natural style" into a learned behavior. In examining the four styles—idiocratic, democratic, technocratic, and bureaucratic—for example, one can make several judgments. First it would be useful for an individual to know which style (or what combination of styles) she uses in her own management. It also makes sense to select a style rather than to assume one unthinkingly. Mere knowledge of the options may assist the nurse executive in broadening her perspective of management.

Combining the styles is the contextual, situational approach to management, an approach sometimes called contingency management, whereby different styles are utilized as needed in different management situations. (This is the approach I prefer.) Note that the "context" is included as a base for management in Figure 14-1. For evaluating and improving performance of staff members, an idiocratic approach might work best for the nurse executive, for example. At her level, it is likely that her staff would have highly discrete functions, so individual management might succeed in relation to specific job performance. In contrast, for the general work of the nursing division, she probably will meet with top management staff nurses as a body, using the democratic style of management. Alternatively, when meeting with a group of clinical specialists in cardiovascular nursing, perhaps to plan nursing services for a new unit, she is likely to use the technocratic style. Finally, in the legal day in which we live, the nurse executive must function on a bureaucratic model in relation to many aspects of her work. For example, if she is administering a labor contract, she is not free to deviate from its contractual agreements. Ideally, then, the nurse executive becomes aware of her own instinctive style of management, learns other styles that are not instinctive, and learns to decide when to apply each style, making sure the style fits the situation.

An important work that borders on the style-oriented approach is that of McGregor[4]. McGregor defines two different perspectives, two managerial beliefs about workers. While these perspectives do not actually equate with given styles, each perspective encourages a different style of treating workers. McGregor's theory X describes a manager with the following beliefs about workers:

1. People dislike and avoid work if possible.
2. Direction, coercion, and control are needed to obtain performance from workers.
3. People inevitably try to avoid responsibility.
4. Personal goals inherently conflict with company goals.
5. It is not reasonable to have high expectations of people.

The manager with a theory Y perspective holds contrary beliefs about workers:

1. Work is natural, and people generally like to work.

2. People are capable of self-direction and self-control.
3. People seek and enjoy responsibility.
4. Personal goals can be achieved through company goals.
5. It is reasonable to have high expectations for people.

Obviously, a manager who holds McGregor's theory X will be likely to be a task master; he will focus on high control of workers, and his attention will be riveted on task completion. The manager who holds to theory Y, in contrast, is likely to be people-oriented. He will focus on providing an environment where human potential will develop and be productive. (Here again one can see a task-orientation versus a people-orientation.)

Workers

Some of the "people-oriented" management literature focuses on the worker rather than on the manager. When the workers are viewed as a group instead of as individuals, then two approaches are evident: a structural one and a psychological one. In nursing, one structural approach advocates participative management (sometimes even to the extent of recommending that groups elect their own managers). Another group structure recommends management by committees. Committees become the line structure. Although it has been successful in some academic settings, it is difficult to apply management by committees to a situation like nursing service, which calls for many rapid decisions.

Team nursing and the health team concept also may be seen as arising out of the structural approach to management via consideration of the worker, not the manager. Peer evaluation mechanisms also fall into this grouping.

Psychological approaches to the work group include attempts to analyze the roles of group members. Further psychological techniques such as transactional analysis and sensitivity training often have been imposed on the work setting. Group dynamics has also been studied in relation to the work group.

Workers are viewed as individuals as well as members of groups. Several major managerial movements have sprung from this consideration: the job enrichment movement, the clinical ladder, and the coaching notion of management, for example. Nursing's focus on employee self-development reflects this perspective.

Some of the best-known work on the individual employee is that of Herzberg[5], who studied work motivation and discovered that the things that cause job satisfaction or dissatisfaction are not opposites but separate entities. He found, for example, that the satisfying factors in a job relate to work tasks whereas dissatisfaction is related to the job environment. Poor salaries, short lunch periods, or cramped office space can create dissatisfaction; Herzberg calls these hygiene factors. Good salaries, long lunch periods, and spacious offices, on the other hand, do not provide contentment. What gives people satisfaction are factors such as ability to manifest talent, a sense of having turned out a good piece of work, or recognition of work achievement; Herzberg calls these motivation factors. Herzberg's findings have been the basis for many subsequent studies, including some that arrived at contradictory conclusions.

THE "TASK" ELEMENT OF MANAGEMENT

Workers

Most studies of the tasks of workers have primarily examined time and motion. Many health care institutions have had nursing activity studies done in order to find out how long various nursing procedures normally take. These time norms often have been used as a basis for patient classification systems and as a basis for calculating staffing needs. In industry, time and motion studies typically are used as one mechanism for improving efficiency. There has been little use of this sort made of the time and motion studies in nursing; there have been few instances when a particular nursing procedure or practice has been reviewed in order to revise it and streamline its motions and time. Most time and motion studies are done by "outsiders" who may not wish to presume to tell the professionals how to do a specific technical procedure.

Time and motion studies often are used as a basis for dividing workers according to skill levels. For example, if a given skill is classfied as belonging on the aide level, it is considered poor management to have that task done by a higher-level worker. The problems with this simplistic skill-level concept were discussed in Chapter 9.

Managers

Managers' tasks are discussed in two different ways: in terms of the manager's skills required to complete the tasks, and in terms of the specific tasks themselves. Katz illustrates the former pattern by differentiating three managerial skills: the technical, the human skills, and the conceptual[6]. He breaks with the task versus people dichotomy, adding the conceptual skill that is necessary to see an enterprise as a whole and to relate it appropriately to its environment.

When managers' specific activities are examined, two approaches are used. In one, the managerial tasks are seen as occurring simultaneously; in the other, managerial acts are seen as following an invariant sequence. Among definitions of management following the former pattern is the old standby, POSDCORB, an acronym standing for planning-organizing-staffing-directing-coordinating (or communicating)-rating (or reporting)-budgeting.

The sequential models include management by objectives, which sequences activities starting with goal definition; the management cycle—planning, organizing, directing, controlling; or the systems model which is the equivalent of the management cycle—problem definition, systems design, programming, operating, feedback, and evaluation.

As Figure 14-1 indicates, some authors combine both the "task" and the "people" side of management. Blake and Mouton[7] do this very well, noting that it is not necessary to take an either-or view in management. In contrast to McGregor's manager, who has one perspective or the other, Blake and Mouton's effective manager has a high concern for both production and for people involved in production.

Blake and Mouton have devised a grid in which the two factors, concern for work output and the human orientation, are placed on a scale with ratings from 1 to 9. A manager with a score of one on the work output scale would have low concern for work output of his staff; a manager with a score of 9 would have high concern for work output. Similarly, a score of 1 on the scale of orientation toward people indicates low concern for staff members, and a score of 9 indicates optimal concern for people. The 1-9 manager sees production as merely incidental to lack of conflict and good fellowship; from his perspective, the manager's job is to create a pleasant work environment and to see that employees are happy. The 9-1 manager has the opposite view; he sees workers as objects to be used to get out the work. The 9-9 manager has high concern for production and for people; he sees the manager's job as one of integrating task and human requirements. The 5-5 manager has a modicum of concern for both people and production.

Finally, some authors look at both people and tasks elements as they relate to the work context, as does Fiedler[8]. Although Fiedler takes an either-or approach to the task versus people orientation, the orientation is not an instinctive perception or a personal preference as in McGregor; instead it is a selected strategy. The manager selects either the task orientation or the human orientation on the basis of three variables rated high to low:

1. How well the leader is accepted by the group
2. How structured the group's task is
3. How strong leader's formal position power is

Where these variables fall to either extreme, Fiedler suggests a task-controlling style be elected; where the variables fall within a middle range, he suggests a permissive, human-relations approach.

ROLE THEORY AND THE NURSE EXECUTIVE

Role theory breaks down the division between people and task orientations because the concept of role involves a set of expectations concerning how a person will enact a given societal position. Both the person and the acts are included in the concept of role. There are at least two opposing views of how a person interacts with his or her roles. The first views the role, much like a stage role—something to be put on at appropriate times and taken off at others. In this conception, the role and the person are separate; the person "plays" or enacts a role, and then leaves it off when he moves, temporarily, out of that particular role. An existentialist would disagree with this concept of the person as separate from the roles he plays. An existentialist would say that the person is nothing more or less than the roles he dons: a person's essence is in the roles he elects and how he plays them; he is nothing separate from the roles. One can equate this with Sartre's old tale of the person looking for the "essence" of the onion by removing layer after layer—only to finish with nothing left.

Whether the person is separate from or part of his roles, it is clear that the role has both a psychological component and a sociological one. The person is highly involved with the roles he plays and he plays them in light of (or conscious of) social expectations for the roles.

There are two kinds of roles which people play: ascribed roles, for which one has no choice, e.g., white female, and achieved roles, e.g. nurse executive. Of course, one may argue that there are some roles which bridge these categories; for example, a person may have elected motherhood, but she may not have realized that it would cast her in the role of "Laurie's mother" for all the small fry of the neighborhood.

We are concerned in this book with an achieved role—that of nurse executive. This is a peculiar type of role, a highly prescribed occupational position. A role of this sort comprises three major components:

1. The sociological. What others in the society expect from a person in this position.
2. The rationalized. The specifics of job function and responsibility as detailed in the job description.
3. The personal. How the role incumbent chooses to enact this job based upon his or her unique being.

Much of the nursing literature encourages role making instead of role taking for the nurse executive, in keeping with the executive's need for an active instead of a merely contemplative role as manager. It is important that the nurse executive decide in advance what sort of role she wishes to play as administrator. She can then construct her behaviors purposefully to convey that notion of her role to others. The reason it is possible to change the content of a role is that each role has elasticity, leeway in the social component, the job description fulfillment, and in the personal component. Considerable elasticity is allowed in role performance in most cases; usually it takes severe deviancy before the role incumbent is questioned as to fitness for the role. The nurse executive can use this elasticity to create the role image she desires.

It is easier for a nurse executive to "make" a role when beginning a new position than after she has held a position for some time; if she has been in a position for a while, staff come to expect a given pattern of behavior from her. Suppose that a nurse executive has taken a new position and wished to play the executive role in a more powerful way than her predecessor. If she knows her predecessor was weak in decision making and control on the executive level, she will deliberately act so that others see her from the start as decisive and in control. One nurse executive in a new position recently had the following experience. During her first month in the new job, she announced a policy that no nursing personnel could add vacation time to their Christmas holiday. When the personnel manager saw the announcement, he immediately called her to say she could not do this. The nurse executive told him not to worry, that she certainly could. He then informed her that he could not allow her to go ahead with the policy. She then—politely but firmly—called his attention to the fact that she was a vice president of the institution whereas he was only a department head, and that he was in no position to countermand an order of hers. In this case, the nurse executive had to firmly enforce the obvious: that she had the power to make the decision. The previous nurse executive, who also had been a vice president, had established the social expectation that the nurse executive would act as if she reported to the personnel manager—even though the job description indicated the opposite. Though the personnel manager may not have consciously thought about it, his unquestioned expectation was that the new nurse executive would fill the role as it had been filled in the past. The new nurse executive, using role elasticity, had systematically set about changing his expectations of that role.

Even if a nurse executive has been in a position for a long period, she can change others' expectations of her role though the task is more difficult since social staff members' expectations for her behavior have probably jelled. There is an informal adage that the nurse executive should begin a job in an authoritarian style and as a firm disciplinarian. It is simpler to ease up from stern disciplinarianism to a democratic, informal position with friendlier, closer staff relationships, than it is to go the opposite direction.

Role Models

Observing executives at work, Mintzberg has identified ten major roles executives play[9]. These might be viewed as subroles within the executive role. Mintzberg's roles include:

1. Figurehead. Functioning as symbolic, formal head of the division, filling ceremonial functions.
2. Leader. Directing subordinates to goal achievement, motivating and working with staff.
3. Liaison. Building a communications network; establishing contacts outside the vertical chain of command.
4. Monitor. Scanning the environment for information pertinent to the job; keeping abreast of changes in the power structure or the organization direction.
5. Disseminator. Sharing and distributing information with staff; determining what goes to whom, when, where, why.
6. Spokesman. Speaking for the division, addressing key external and internal publics.
7. Entrepreneur. Looking for improvement opportunities, taking the initiative in new projects and developments.
8. Disturbance handler. Mediating and resolving disputes and disruptions among work groups.
9. Resource allocator. Determining how the division's resources are to be distributed.
10. Negotiator. Managing formalized and informal bargaining with both internal and external groups.

It may be useful for the nurse executive to consider the significance of each of these roles. Different nurse executives may spend different amounts of time on each, but it is difficult to imagine an effective nurse executive ignoring any one of them.

Katz offers a different perspective on executive roles, identifying just three[10]:

1. The remedial role. The director acts by correcting deficiencies and past inefficiencies of a division.
2. The maintaining role. The director acts by preserving a steady balance within a division.
3. The innovative role. The director seeks to start new projects in new directions.

Unlike Mintzberg's roles, Katz's are mutually exclusive rather than complementary. Note also that these roles are defined in close relation to the organization (or division). In a contextual model, the nurse executive would elect one of these roles, depending on the situation.

Katz relates his roles to his set of identified executive skills, asserting that the remedial role requires conceptual and technical skills; the maintaining role needs primarily human skills, and the innovative role demands both conceptual and human skills[11]. Whether or not one accepts the relations Katz asserts between skills and roles, the notion of relating role to organizational status and to executive abilities is useful.

The categories Katz terms "roles" are reminiscent of what Mintzberg terms "strategies"[12]:

1. Entrepreneurial. An active search for new opportunities; proactive, dramatic leaps forward in the face of uncertainty.
2. Adaptive. Reactive decisions, remedial, reducing conflict; negotiating with the environment; incremental decision making.
3. Planning. Anticipatory decision making; reliance on rationality and scientific techniques; goal setting with systematic plans for goal achievement.

Although there is not a one-to-one correspondence between Katz's roles and Mintzberg's strategies, there are resemblances and the components seem derived from a similar categorization. Perhaps the difference has to do with the flexibility and duration: a strategy may be seen as an approach selected for a single problem or project, and where a strategy is used consistently for all projects and problems, it may be logical to use the term, role.

As indicated earlier, Katz's roles clearly tie the executive to the organization by describing executive roles specifically in relation to the nature of the executive management. These roles—remediation, maintenance, and innovation—may reflect the state of the organization as much as the role of the nurse (or other) executive. Greiner[13] has categories that he calls organization stages, roles for the organization rather than the executive. He claims that organizations are organic, that they grow and evolve, going through the following sequence of states:

1. Organization. Entrepreneurial and technological orientation; informal and frequent communications; direct interaction with the market.
2. Direction. Formal systems introduced; accounting, purchasing, work standards, inventories; communication formalized; functional specialists and managers differentiated.
3. Delegation. Characterized by decentralization; direct control by top executive lost; powers distributed.
4. Coordination. Decentralized units are merged; companywide programs of control established; certain specialized functions centralized.
5. Collaboration. Greater spontaneity in management teams, problem-solving teams across functional areas, matrix organization.

Combining the notion that organizations have specific stages or roles at given times with the idea that executive roles may be defined in relation to the managerial approach, I have identified the following role categories demonstrated among nurse executives:

1. Innovator. Focusing on starting new programs, new methods, new ideas, her role is characterized by creativity and new expression.
2. Expander. Is interested in growth and expansion, she increases the size and scope of her division. Her moves are primarily political.
3. Refiner. Acting by tidying up the division, she cleans up loose ends, formalizes policies and practices, completes needed documents and systems, and provides a rationale for what the division does.
4. Stabilizer. Maintains harmony and equilibrium of the division, she balances the various interests and group demands and provides for smooth continuity of operations.
5. Revolutionary. Aiming to tear down outmoded structures and practices, she institutes methods, policies, and practices radically different from those in existence when she assumed the position.

Testing these categories with over 100 directors of nursing revealed that most were able to classify themselves, to recognize themselves in one and sometimes two of these dominant role patterns. I postulate that each has a particular skill associated with it, as follows:

1. Goal setting. The innovator is creative because she is visionary, not tied to the past. She looks to new ideas and new methods because she envisions new goals.
2. Bridging. The expander is good at building bridges—making the personal and political linkages which will advance her division, building the communication networks which will open doors for her.
3. Analyzing. The refiner puts the pieces together in logical patterns. She makes the "fine strokes" that give a division

that intellectual glue which makes it "all fit together."

4. Problem solving. The stabilizer excels in handling issues and resolving problems which threaten to upset the balance of her well-running machine.

5. Negating. The revolutionary excels in nest cleaning. She gets rid of unnecessary red tape, outmoded practices, and any other unnecessary baggage.

It is my hypothesis that organizations have stages of growth and development that correspond to the executive roles: innovation, expansion, refinement, stabilization, and revolution. Directors of nursing tested under this model were able to identify stages both for their respective organizations and for their divisions. Unlike Greiner's model, this one does not state that organizations necessarily go through the stages in an unvarying sequence, only that the organization is likely to be in one of the five states listed at any one time.

I hypothesized further that the success of the nurse executive might be a reflection of the match or mismatch of her state to the organization's state. To date, testing has only involved executives' self-reporting, but several interesting findings have been reported. First, executives confirmed that a successful pattern in one situation often was a disastrous pattern in another situation. (Many directors added long written illustrations to the questionnaire. This was interesting in that the questionnaire did not request further explanatory material. It may be that the model provided the nurse executives with the first intellectual explanation for their success/failure pattern, thus stimulating the spontaneous additions to the questionnaires.)

Other nurse executives noted that they only stayed in an institution so long as the need and the role function matched. A typical response (again, spontaneous) might be, "I only stay until I have a place straightened up. Once it is running well, I start looking for a new job with a challenge." A person who made such a comment inevitably marked herself an innovator, revolutionary, or both.

Other nurse executives reported having been able to change roles to match their institutions' needs though they could identify a stage which they most enjoyed, a role which was their preferred behavior. Peculiarly, the only "write-in" question in the questionnaire, which gave the nurse executive a chance to identify her role in her own terms if none of the five named roles fit, was seldom filled in; in those few instances when some answer was offered, it dealt with a category other than role definition. Apparently the nurse executives tested either were comfortable with the five role distinctions or were unable to formulate alternatives if not content.

In looking at this and other role classifications, it is important to note that several relations may be explored: 1) roles may be related to skills and abilities of the role incumbents, 2) roles may be associated with the state of the organization in which the role incumbent serves, 3) roles may be related to the strategies which the role incumbent selects in addressing specific issues and problems, and 4) roles may be related to subroles selected for emphasis in the role performance.

THE NURSE EXECUTIVE'S PERCEPTION OF HER ROLE

The roles discussed in this chapter are highly rationalized ones and would be unlikely to enter into the nurse executive's concept of her own role unless she were a scholar of role theory. It is useful, therefore, to consider also some role images and thoughts concerning role performance which might be likely to occur to the nurse executive. Since nurse executive's perception of her role greatly influences the character of her organization, it is important that she analyze this perception and its underlying assumptions. Typically, she perceives her role as related to her special talents. It is not surprising that she, like most people, prefers to work at the things she does best.

If a nurse executive has great ability in interpersonal relations, for example, she is likely to see her role as one of coordination. If a nurse executive is an exceptional practitioner, she is likely to view her role as that of chief clinician. On the whole, an organization is apt to receive optimal benefit when the executive acts out her role on the basis of her strengths. When a mismatch does occur and the strengths of the nurse executive and the needs of the nursing division are quite dissimilar, it is essential that the nurse executive recognize the dissimilarity and change her role focus.

Suppose, for example, that a given nurse executive sees her role as chief liaison person with other organizations and community groups. Such a focus could be defended in some nursing divisions but would be detrimental in a nursing division whose greatest need is for revision of deficient internal nursing practices. Hence it is important that the nurse executive be aware of her own role interpretation and that she analyze the interpretation critically in light of the needs of her organization.

Typically nurse executives perceive themselves as the expert clinician, the manager, the educator, or the human relations expert. Many nurse executives focus on human relations and are frequently involved in one-to-one relationships with staff members on all levels. The nurse executive with this focus probably is more concerned with personal growth and development of nurses than with analysis of the delivery modes for care, and she is likely to spend considerable effort in establishing the kind of social atmosphere conducive to interpersonal and interprofessional exchange of communications.

The nurse executive who perceives of herself as educator acts out her role with different stresses. She may focus on staff education, patient education, or on clinical nursing research. She is likely to be interested in such things as job enlargement programs or clinical ladders to recognize and reward clinical practice at different levels of skill and knowledge. Thus the role content represents the nurse executive's major self-concept in relation to her job. It is the self-image from which she acts, whether or not she is able to verbalize that image. The four examples mentioned here (clinician, manager, educator, and human relations expert) are not the only possible images; they are, however, common ones among nurse executives.

SUMMARY

It is vital that the nurse executive critically examine her role conception and her role performance. She should take an activist's position in regard to her role, making it the sort of role it should be rather than merely filling the role as others expect or anticipate. Every role has much elasticity in it, and this enables the nurse executive to manipulate and alter the role if she tries. She also should learn to be sensitive to attempts to cast her in lesser roles than that which accords with her position in the organization. Role is an excellent concept by which to consider and link such various elements of management as managerial skills and abilities, managerial functions, organizational status, and strategies for management.

REFERENCES

1. Korman, A.K. Consideration, initiating structure, and organizational criteria—a review. In Sorensen, P.F., Jr., and Baum, B.H. (Eds.) *Perspectives on Organizational Behavior*. Champaign, Ill.: Stipes, 1973, pp. 134–135.
2. Stogdill, R.M. *Handbook of Leadership: A Survey of Theory and Research*. New York: Free Press, 1974, pp. 365–370.
3. Nelson, C.W. *The Leadership Inventory*. (rev. ed.) Chicago: Industrial Relations Center, University of Chicago, 1957, pp. 6–7.
4. McGregor, D. *The Human Side of Enterprise*. New York: McGraw-Hill, 1960, pp. 33–57.
5. Herzberg, F., et al. *Job Attitudes: Review of Research and Opinion*. Pittsburgh: Psychological Services of Pittsburgh, 1957.
6. Katz, R.L. Skills of an effective administrator. *Harvard Business Rev.*, 52(5):91–92, 1974.
7. Blake, R.R., and Mouton, J.S. *Corporate Excellence through Grid Organization Development*. Houston, Texas: Gulf, 1968, p. 15.
8. Fiedler, F.E. A contingency model of leadership effectiveness. In Berkowitz, L. (Ed.) *Advances in Experimental Social Psychology*, vol. I. New York: Academic Press, 1964, pp. 150–190.
9. Mintzberg, H. The manager's job: folklore and fact. *Harvard Business Rev.*, 53(4):49–61, 1975.
10. Katz, R.L., 1974, p. 102.
11. Katz, R.L., 1974, p. 102.
12. Mintzberg, H. Strategy-making in three modes. *Calif. Management Rev.*, 16(2):44–53, 1973.
13. Greiner, L.E. Evolution and revolution as organizations grow. *Harvard Business Rev.*, 50(4):37–46, 1972.

BIBLIOGRAPHY

Conway, M.E. Management effectiveness and the role making process. *J.O.N.A.* 4(6):25, 1974.

Douglass, L.M., and Bevis, E.O. *Nursing Management and Leadership in Action*. (3rd. ed.) St. Louis: C.V. Mosby, 1979.

Etzioni, A. *Modern Organizations*. Englewood Cliffs, N.J.: Prentice-Hall, 1964.

Georgopoulos, B.S. *Hospital Organizations Research: Review and Source Book*. Philadelphia: W.B. Saunders, 1975.

Heimann, C.G. Four theories of leadership. *J.O.N.A.*, 6(5):18, 1976.

Kast, F.E., and Rosenzweig, J.E. *Organization and Management: A Systems Approach*. New York: McGraw-Hill, 1972.

Knable, J., and Petre, G. Resistance to role implementation. *Supervisor Nurse*, 10(2):31, 1979.

Koontz, H., and O'Donnell, C. *Principles of Management: An Analysis of Managerial Functions*. (5th ed.) New York: McGraw-Hill, 1972.

Leininger, M. The leadership crisis in nursing: a critical problem. *J.O.N.A.*, 4(2):28, 1974.

Levitt, T. The managerial merry-go-round. *Harvard Business Rev.*, 52(4):120, 1974.

Likert, R. *The Human Organization: Its Management and Values*. New York: McGraw-Hill, 1967.

Massie, J.L., and Douglas, J. *Managing: A Contemporary Introduction*. (2nd ed.) Englewood Cliffs, N.J.: Prentice-Hall, 1977.

Mintzberg, H. Planning on the left side and managing on the right. *Harvard Business Rev.*, 54(4):49, 1976.

Moloney, M.M. *Leadership in Nursing: Theory, Strategies, Action*. St. Louis: C.V. Mosby, 1979.

Newman, W.H., and Warren, E.K. *The Process of Management: Concepts, Behavior, and Practice*. (4th ed.) Englewood Cliffs, N.J.: Prentice-Hall, 1977.

Szilagyi, A.D., Sims, H.P., Jr., and Terril, R.C. The relationship of leadership style to employee job satisfaction. *Hospital Health Services Admin.*, 22(1):8, 1977.

Chapter 15   Nursing's Middle Management

"Middle management" is a term that covers many and varied roles in nursing. A middle manager is one who has responsibility for lower-level managers rather than direct responsibility for staff, but who is not in top management, that is, not part of the team with the view of the whole institution. Even this definition is only a rough guide, for nurses fill diverse positions and cross levels in the modern institution. The following criteria may be used to outline a middle management position:

1. Territory (geography). A supervisor/ middle manager may have her job defined by the nursing care units assigned to her; she is responsible for a delegated number of care units linked typically by their geographic proximity.
2. Patient condition. A middle manager may be assigned to cover all areas which deal with a specific type of patient; she may be supervisor of spinal cord injury units and clinics, supervisor of obstetrics. Often the patient condition criterion and territory criterion join since all patients of a single type tend to be geographically grouped.
3. Specialized function. Middle managers may be assigned by function rather than by territory, e.g., inservice education, staffing/scheduling, home care.
4. Time of work. Evening and night middle managers fall into this category, typically assuming responsibility for larger units than is the case for day managers. Their "units" typically incorporate numerous types of patients and/or various functions.

Where one of the foregoing criteria is extended, another may be limited. For example, if a supervisor has 24-hour responsibility, she usually maintains that responsibility for a smaller number of units than does the supervisor with 8-hour responsibility. Similarly, a night supervisor may have an extensive number of units, but she is not expected to carry the weight of long-term planning as is her day counterpart with fewer units. An inservice middle manager has a similar situation. She may be responsible for education on a large number of units—but her function is limited to education, not direct patient care.

FUNCTIONS OF MIDDLE MANAGEMENT

What are the major functions of middle management? How do they differ from those of first-line and top management? The critical function of middle management is to serve as the link pin between the other two layers. Middle management serves as an active conduit of messages throughout the nursing managerial structure; it carries goals, policies, purposes downward to first-line managers and monitoring information (state of the units) up to executive management.

It is useful to examine the link pin function in relation to goals. The linkage is not so simplistic as it might first appear. Middle management is not merely a conduit; it must not only convey the executives' goals to first-line managers, but it must explain, support, and sell those goals. The middle manager must broaden the understanding of the first-line managers so that they are able to attend to goals that advance beyond the day-to-day operations. Furthermore, the middle manager must serve as an authority and consultant concerning means by which first-line managers may reach executive-determined ends.

In addition, the middle manager will evolve her own goals specific to her own area of managerial responsibility. She also will help the first-line manager set goals for that manager's domain. This mutual goal-setting effort requires skill on the part of the middle manager. Typically, her first-line managers are far less experienced than the middle manager, and she may be tempted to dictate all goals to them. Here another function of the middle manager must be brought into play: the middle manager is the chief developer (educator) for upcoming managers. Hence she must be careful not to substitute her own judgment and ideas for those of the first-line managers. She must give the first-line manager the freedom and managerial responsibility that manager needs to develop her managerial skills. This means that the middle manager often serves in a consultant function, helping the first-line manager to analyze issues and problems, suggesting resources, but not providing the decisions for her.

A second link pin function comes into importance: the middle manager knows a wider world than does the typical first-line manager. She has knowledge of the institutional systems beyond just those of the nursing division. She also knows what people in what departments may be useful to the first-line manager for a given problem. The linkages of the middle manager extend beyond the base institution; she knows how to use community resources. Indeed, one of her major teaching functions is to introduce her first-line managers to the wider picture, a greater expanse of resources than those of the unit, the nursing division, or the home institution. She teaches the first-line managers, not only what the resources are, but how to manipulate the systems, to make

them work effectively in delivering care to patients.

The middle manager may or may not also function as a clinical expert. Some supervisors, for example, become both expert clinicians and expert managers. In other systems, the middle manager primarily becomes a manager, focusing on making the system work. Even here, however, the manager is capable of recognizing and responding to clinical emergencies. Indeed, if she lacks this good basic clinical expertise, she will not know what systems, what resources, to invoke at what times.

Since she is indoctrinating new managers, inexperienced managers in most cases, the middle manager also has a heavy responsibility for monitoring and evaluation; she must know whether or not the first-line managers are safe and effective in the positions of responsibility they hold. Here again, she must be careful to use her evaluations thoughtfully; she must not substitute her own activities for first-line inefficiencies; she must use those examples of inefficiency as a teaching mechanism, as a way to improve first-line performance. If she is unable to bring a first-line manager up to desired performance level, then she must replace her rather than continue to substitute for her, tolerating poor managerial performance.

This is not to say that the middle manager has no direct responsibility for management and managerial decision making herself. What is important is that she limit decision making to those issues which fall specifically to her advanced level of management; she should not make head nurse level decisions in lieu of the head nurse. The middle manager serves as advice giver to first-line managers, especially when they must make decisions in unprogrammed areas, when they must deal with new or unique problems.

The primary domain for middle management decisions lies with the nursing systems and nursing managers rather than with patients or staff directly. Every middle manager should be her own systems analyst, seeing that the supply lines, communication systems, and systems of care delivery function at peak performance. She must facilitate getting the work done by providing the environment where that is possible. The logistic questions in a complex institution are difficult and require more than incident-by-incident, patchwork attention. The middle manager is ideally equipped to deal with systems problems since she has a good overview of the functioning of the total organization or at least of a good portion of it.

In her relations with first-line managers, then, the middle manager serves as "horizon-lifter," helping the first-line manager to develop a wider conception of the managerial role. She also serves as troubleshooter, educator, and consultant.

The next major responsibility of the middle manager is upward, to the top nurse executive (or her superordinate). Middle management is responsible for conveying the state of the department to the division level. This assessment must be accurate for effective planning by top management. Inaccuracy occurs through two possible routes: 1) the supervisor/middle manager may wish to mask her own inefficiencies in running her department, or 2) the middle manager may have gotten a false image of what is going on from her own subordinate managers. The nurse executive simply cannot tolerate a middle manager who, for whatever reason, fails to see or reflect the state of the department.

Just as middle management is responsible for development of first-line management, so executive management is responsible for further development of those middle managers who have potential for executive management. Often this potential is recognized and developed by allowing middle management (all of it or selected members) to participate in or observe executive management decision making and goal setting.

In addition to some degree of participation in or observation of top management, middle management is responsible for maintaining the equilibrium of that unit which constitutes a department. Hence the middle manager is responsible for solving problems which involve more than one patient unit

and for setting goals for groups of patient units. If the middle manager has a functional instead of unit assignment, then these problem-solving and goal-setting activities relate to that function.

Additionally, some middle managers may serve as administrative officers for the division, for example on nights or evenings. While this appears to cross lines and enter top management, the responsibility is limited to immediate performance.

PROBLEMS IN MIDDLE MANAGEMENT

In some ways, the middle manager's position is the most difficult in the nursing hierarchy. This is primarily because middle management roles are seldom clearly defined. This section will look at the problems inherent in the regular nursing supervisor's job, since she is the most common middle manager in the health care institution. Problems of content and of definition of role will be reviewed. The role of the nursing supervisor, whatever the official title, is often the most ill-defined role in the hospital hierarchy. Inability to clarify the role has led many organizations to eliminate the position and to give the head nurse more authority. Unfortunately this solution is not always practical in large institutions.

Basic management principles for span of control indicate that in most situations, no more than six to eight persons should report directly to one boss. The director of nursing who tries to have 20 head nurses report directly to her will quickly confirm the validity of this rule. Unless she has an exceptionally experienced, capable, and self-directed group of head nurses, middle management becomes a necessity. Where middle management is needed, identifying a clear role for the nursing supervisor is a problem of first priority.

In most organizations the nursing supervisor has from two to eight head nurses (or key areas) under her supervision. This range satisfies the management principle concerning span of control and the director's need to limit contacts. Creation of a middle management layer merely to satisfy span of control, however, may create more problems than it solves.

Granted, occasionally a remarkably adept and clever person comes along and makes a significant contribution to the supervisory role. Unfortunately, the remarkable individual is rare. More commonly, the nursing supervisor is a competent, industrious, intelligent, normal human being with problem-solving ability within the frame of the policies of the given institution. The nursing supervisor who has all these attributes, however, is still likely to do a mediocre job because of obstacles built into the supervisory role.

The Territoriality of the Head Nurse

The head nurse has strategic advantages over the supervisor. The first advantage is quite simple: the head nurse knows where she works. She can physically "mark off" her territory, her patients, her staff. There is no question about what is hers. Consequently, when the supervisor appears, the head nurse may react as though a "foreigner" had invaded her territory. She is immediately on the defensive. In spite of her knowledge of organization charts, job descriptions, or lines of authority, the head nurse responds with a feeling that the unit she heads is *hers*.

The supervisor, on the other hand, often comes to feel that her only real territory consists of elevator shafts, back stairways, and halls between wards. She can periodically retreat to her office, of course, provided it is not in proximity to the office of the director. The director reasonably expects her to be on the patient units.

The head nurse's second advantage is that she, unlike the supervisor, really knows what her job is. If she never gives her role a thought or never defines one work objective, she still can come to work, let the events of her ward direct her activity, and go home feeling that she has accomplished something.

The supervisor, however, is usually forced to ask herself, "What is my role, and how do I go about fulfilling it?" The answer to this question is difficult, for the role of the supervisor is often one of her own making. Her job is limited or productive, depending on her ability to use creativity, insight, and to influence others. She "proves" her value by altering (interfering with) the domain of the head nurse. Even if the supervisor has good ideas, it is very difficult for a head nurse to accept these ideas from a person she regards as competition.

Most of the recent attempts to alter the supervisor's role have been designed to soften the competitive response to this position. The title has been changed to that of coordinator, and job descriptions have been altered to define the nursing supervisor as a "resource person." Nevertheless, attempts to change the image of the supervisor have minimal effect if the position retains line authority over the head nurse. Such alterations in image do not change the essential problem inherent in the supervisor's role. The problem, simply defined, is that the commonly assigned supervisory tasks are merely extensions of the head nurse's responsibilities rather than discrete, separate functions. For example, the supervisor might be expected to be more expert in patient care decisions or in planning for staffing, but these tasks can be handled by the head nurse. Thus the supervisor is expected to do the same job as the head nurse, only "bigger and better." The difference in jobs is simply quantitative; essentially the supervisor and head nurse have the same job. The supervisor has a greater number of patients, but not different patients; she has greater knowledge, but she uses it to make the same kinds of decisions.

The lack of a clear job differentiation is demonstrated in the manner in which the average supervisor deals with head nurses reporting to her. She usually relates to each head nurse separately, and whatever she does with the head nurse is only an extension of what is happening on that particular head nurse's ward. Thus the supervisor has neither a synthetic nor a distinct function; her functional unit, similar to that of the head nurse, is the individual ward. This basic failure in role differentiation undoubtedly is the reason so many supervisors spend excessive time in checking employee time cards, transferring employees from one ward to another, or in other trivial duties they have managed to usurp as their own prerogative.

Middle Management as Obstruction

Middle management may be the source of both upward and downward communication problems. In the first instance, the nursing supervisor may have the human tendency to minimize problems in her wards in order to prevent stressful relations with the nursing director. This tendency causes considerable frustration for the head nurse, as she must cope with the concrete work problems while awaiting higher-level decisions. A nurse executive may face similar communication obstacles in trying to make changes at the patient care level. Theoretically the director should transmit objectives and plans through the defined lines of authority, i.e., she should communicate with the supervisory level. The supervisor, to support her position of authority, should be the person to interpret objectives and plans at the head nurse level.

Even if the supervisor tries to translate the director's intentions and plans, the head nurse, as previously noted, may have a vested interest in complying only so far as necessary, and then reasserting her own ideas (protecting her territorial rights). Frequently the director, in her need to produce results, is tempted to bypass the supervisors, either by holding meetings directly with the head nurses or by placing both supervisors and head nurses in a common group for meetings she conducts herself. Either of these methods errs by confirming what the head nurse already suspects—the infirmity of the supervisory role.

STRUCTURING MIDDLE MANAGEMENT

What then can be done to strengthen the supervisor's role when the director elects to maintain a middle management level? There is no single or simple answer. One guideline for the director is that the supervisory level must have a job function that is different from that of an extended head nurse.

One possibility for restructuring the supervisor's role is to analyze the nursing management components and to assign each supervisor to the management of a specific component. For example, suppose a hospital has 15 units (15 head nurses) and three supervisors. The director might decide, on the basis of their number, to divide tasks into the following areas: evaluation and improvement of patient care; staffing and regulation of personnel; and administrative processes and nursing systems. Each supervisor then would be responsible for guiding and directing her assigned specialty in each of the 15 units. With this chance to specialize, it is likely that each supervisor could become expert in her particular field.

The head nurse in this restructuring would be responsible to the appropriate supervisor for each area of function on her ward. For example, her ongoing patient care would be evaluated in consultation with supervisor A, while her staffing would be done in consultation with supervisor B.

The psychological advantage to this scheme merits examination. The head nurse is less likely to react negatively to the supervisor who has only a partial interest in her "territory," thereby making it easier for her to accept each supervisor in the "expert" role and to take advantage of the guidance offered.

The system of divided function must be carefully structured for it infringes on the time-worn principle that each person should have to report to only one boss. Actually, this principle is broken every day without major incident. For example, the nurse director is not responsible only to her immediate boss; she also is responsible to the personnel director for upholding certain contracts and policies of his division. This division of authority causes no problems. The nurse director is quite capable of differentiating what is "owed" to the personnel director and what is not within the scope of his authority. Clearly the head nurse cannot be responsible to three supervisors who may give incompatible orders, but she can be responsible to each supervisor within a clearly defined and delimited scope of activities.

This system can work well if each supervisor has a clear understanding of her function and insists that problems outside her range be referred to the proper supervisor.

In addition to giving each supervisor a job unlike that of the head nurse, the proposed system offers the director other advantages. Since the job division requires close coordination, the director has a real purpose for her staff meetings with supervisors. Too often meetings between the director and supervisors evolve into meaningless recitals of patient admissions, discharges, and deaths. With the proposed system, immediate inhouse patient data is not the only focus, and proper attention can be given to relating patient data to delivery systems and policies. Thus staff meetings can become dynamic problem-solving, decision-making sessions rather than simply informational reports.

A Second Alternative

The previously described supervisory pattern is only one possible application of the basic principle of giving the supervisor a job different in nature from that of the head nurse. As a second alternative, it would be possible to create a functional unit larger than the patient ward. For example, suppose a supervisor manages three wards and a common basis for action can be identified in spite of the differentiated functions of the wards. Possibly all wards serve surgical patients, or perhaps they serve geriatric patients. If a unifying factor can be identified, it can guide the establishment of common goals and needs of the wards. The unity could be of a broad nature and still serve the purpose.

The supervisor might then begin to weld her separate wards into a single functional team. She could hold staff meetings with her head nurses to set common goals or to try common projects. Any transferring of personnel to meet daily variations in patient numbers and needs among these wards could be managed cooperatively rather than reaching outside the new functional unit. Indeed, the head nurses could plan a methodical interchange of personnel so that each employee is properly oriented to the other two wards and to their special equipment and patient care needs. Necessary staff relocations then would not cause the usual employee protest and resistance, since workers would be prepared for such interchange.

If an assistant head nurse role does not exist in the institution, the head nurses could also orient themselves to their related wards in order to be available as resource persons during their coworkers' days off.

With this proposed structure, the job of the supervisor is clearly differentiated from that of the head nurse. She has a territory of her own, the larger (combined) unit. She functions within the larger unit as a whole rather than interfering in the everyday function of the head nurse. She helps the unit evolve group goals and long-range objectives and no longer attempts to usurp the day-to-day head nurse functions. She maintains a broader objective and serves to coordinate the activities of the new functional unit. She now meets head nurse needs through the staff meetings more often than in individual conferences.

Consider the difference in response to the following situations: 1) the supervisor informs a head nurse that she is weak in interviewing techniques and makes learning suggestions; 2) the supervisor, in a staff meeting with the head nurses, proposes that the group work on building expertise in interviewing skills and proposes a study program. In the second situation the threat to the individual head nurse is removed. What would have appeared to be criticism now can be accepted as a group goal for increasing head nurse expertise. The head nurse no longer sees the supervisor as a competitor; the supervisor now has a role that is validly larger and more complex than that of the head nurse. The head nurse now can respond to the supervisor without being on the defensive, without taking each suggestion as a criticism of her performance.

In addition to the two described, many other alternatives can be identified which could give the supervisor a credible role. The answer for any one organization depends on its individual needs and capabilities. In all cases, however, it seems logical that if the director of nursing needs a middle management, then she should recognize it is both unfair and unwise to lose the contributions of the best head nurses in an organization by placing them in ill-defined supervisory jobs with built-in obstacles that will surely reduce them to mediocrity.

SUMMARY

The middle management role is one of the most difficult to enact in the nursing hierarchy. Often this is due to blurring of role responsibility because of poor job descriptions and position practices. The middle management position is becoming even more complex under new matrix management and 24-hour responsibility plans. As an increasing number of nurse specialists enter organizational practice, the supervisor/middle manager may be threatened further for her role functions often are blurred with functions of persons in other categories (see Chapter 17 for illustration). The nurse executive must have a clear understanding of what she expects from her middle managers, and she must convey that message to them. Just as first-line managers need support in their position, middle managers need support and counseling from the executive. Since middle management includes so many and varied roles, it is not possible to generalize further on this level of management.

BIBLIOGRAPHY

American Management Association. *Supervisory Management Course for Hospital Supervisors: Part I, Management Principles.* New York: AMA Publishers, pp. 3-11.

Amundson, N.E. Caught in the middle: nursing supervisors. *J.O.N.A.,* 5(5):15, 1975.

Consolvo, C.A., and Schmidt, P. Clipboard supervision—not reasonable in 1977. *Supervisor Nurse,* 8(6):29, 1977.

Falls, E.B. The supervisor—is she necessary for good patient care? *Supervisor Nurse,* 1(2):14, 1970.

Hersey, P., Blanchard, K.H., and LaMonica, E.L. A situational approach to supervision: leadership theory and the supervising nurse. *Supervisor Nurse,* 7(5):17, 1976.

Parker, J.K. Job description of nursing supervisor. *Supervisor Nurse,* 9(4):15, 1978.

Stagnitto, M.R.E.B. Nursing supervision: leadership or police work? *Supervisor Nurse,* 10(1):17, 1979.

Stetler, C., and Downs, C. The supervisor/consultant: a difficult role. *J.O.N.A.,* 4(4):50, 1974.

Uyterhoeven, H.E.R. General managers in the middle. *Harvard Business Rev.,* 50(2):75, 1972.

White, H.C. Perceptions of leadership styles by nurses in supervisory positions. *J.O.N.A.,* 1(2):44, 1971.

Chapter 16   First-Line Nursing Management

The title "first-line manager" indicates a management position that is one step above the workers. "Foreman" or "leadman" are industrial terms that indicate first-line management positions. In the military, the sergeant or noncommissioned officer holds a first-line management position. In nursing, first-line management positions may be filled by head nurses, charge nurses, team leaders, and module leaders. While the degree and duration of responsibility may vary with these positions, all involve managerial responsibility for staff workers, that is, for nonmanagerial personnel.

In addition to this responsibility for non-managerial personnel, the first-line manager is concerned with the materials necessary for completion of the work and the systems that regulate and turn out the work. The foreman on a production assembly line, for example, is responsible for the flow of materials to and from the workers. Similarly, the first-line nurse manager is responsible for the provision of equipment and supplies and for the systems that delegate and control the work.

The primary responsibility of the first-line manager is the production of the desired product. On an assembly line, the product will be some physical object; not all products are physical objects, however. In nursing the products are desired patient health outcomes and desired patient states during the course of illness, injury, or health-related adjustment.

The first-line manager works close to the actual steps of production, being responsible for turning out the desired product through effective use of personnel, materials, and systems. In nursing the first-line manager is responsible for producing desired patient states and health outcomes through use of nursing staff, equipment and supplies, and systems that organize the work to be done.

The first-line manager has three important characteristics. She works "where the action is," that is, at the juncture between administration and creation of the desired product. She knows which products are desired. She discovers the means appropriate for production of the desired product.

WHERE THE ACTION IS

First-line management is the critical juncture in the nursing organization; if it fails, all higher-level planning becomes meaningless. If the nursing division's objectives never filter down to the patient care level, then the planning is futile. The first-line manager works at the juncture where administrative plans are converted into action. This is what makes the role so exciting. Indeed, many head nurses refuse upward promotions for just this reason; they prefer to stay "where the action is."

Much of the satisfaction derived from a first-line management position arises from closeness with the finished product. The head nurse or team leader has the satisfaction of seeing the direct effects of her management in patient outcomes, whereas the director of nursing and the supervisor cannot see the effects of their work in this same exciting way.

The challenge of first-line management is to convert planning into action. Because her plans are immediately concretized in action, the first-line manager deals with the realities of nursing care delivery. There is no way she can escape the reality of nursing action and its results by flight into nonrealistic planning for the plans of the first-line manager are tied to the everyday results, and these results provide loud and clear feedback.

The danger in first-line management tends to be an overinvolvement in immediate problems and a relegation of planning to the backburner. Working in the midst of many people and events, the first-line manager may easily spend all of her time responding to the here and now. The greatest trap facing first-line management is action without a plan.

Planning requires a definition of goals and imposition of one's plans upon the environment. Because nursing takes place in a very complex environment, inflexible plans have little chance of realization, for the environment may well require some alteration of goals and plans. Unanticipated events will occur on the patient unit, the team, or the module. Courses of illness and recovery can be anticipated but never entirely predicted. Working in a coordinated system, the first-line manager cannot regiment the behavior of others. For example, most physicians on a given patient unit may make rounds between 7:00 and 10:00 A.M., but some of them may diverge from this pattern on any given day. Thus, planning must be flexible and open to revision as circumstances may require.

The nature of planning will depend upon the responsibility of the first-line manager and the capabilities of the person filling the position. For example, the head nurse's planning will involve long-term projects, while the planning of an inexperienced team leader may include nothing more than completion of all designated nursing care programs and therapies for her group of patients. In either case, the manager must know what objectives are to be accomplished by the end of the shift so that she may organize and reorganize the shift toward that accomplishment. Sometimes objectives for the shift must be revised. One of the important tricks of first-line management is knowing when a plan must be altered or even scrapped in favor of an alternative one. Changing a plan, however, is not the same as operating without one.

KNOWING DESIRED PRODUCTS

All planning rests on the assumption that the first-line manager has a clear idea of the goals to be achieved, or the products to be created. The head nurse is likely to have a set of long-term objectives for her unit, formulated according to the types of patients for which she is responsible and the unique characteristics of her particular environment, in addition to objectives imposed from above by top and middle management. These objectives dominate her activities although they are mixed with interim and immediate objectives, formulated on the basis of the day-to-day situation. Thus, for an eight-hour shift a head nurse may plan a mix of activities, some directed toward formalized unit and division objectives, and others directed toward immediate and interim objectives arising out of the particular state of the unit and its occupants at a given time. The first-line manager subordinate to the head nurse is more likely to set intermediate or interim objectives than long-term ones, although she may contribute to the achievement of long-term objectives set by others.

Whether the ends are long-term objectives that require a series of activities for their achievement, or short-term objectives that might be accomplished on a single shift, managers have different ways of perceiving objectives and goals. Not only are perceptions different, but ways of formulating objectives are quite different when they are presented as informal guides rather than as formalized documents. The first-line manager does not need to formulate her day-to-day objectives in terms understandable to others, for these objectives serve primarily as her own internal gyroscope.

Compare, for example, the objectives for Team Leader A and Team Leader B on a day that is experiencing a critical shortage of staff.

Team Leader A's Objectives
1. To get all the ordered treatments and medications done

2. To leave nothing hanging over for the evening shift to finish
3. To skip rounds with doctors in order to save time
4. To get nursing care plans up to date only if there should be any time left

Team Leader B's Objectives
1. To set care priorities based on immediate patient needs
2. To give clear orders to staff about action priorities for the day
3. To let no patient go home without understanding his follow-up care
4. To achieve the best possible patient states with the short-handed staff

Although these objectives are not articulated in the same manner as official ones and may not even be consciously formulated, it is quite likely that they could direct the actions of the respective team leader for the day. Team Leader A generally sees nursing actions as ends in themselves, while Team Leader B sees patient states as the ends. Team Leader A identified two tasks to be dropped in the short-staffed day—rounds with physicians and completion of nursing care plans. Team Leader B identified a criterion for determining what would be dropped, i.e., patient needs.

Clearly, Team Leader B's perspective seems more attuned to the patient, for his needs direct the actions and serve as the criterion by which the "success" of this particular day will be measured. Team Leader A, on the other hand, has no measure for success other than the total number of tasks she can manage to squeeze out of her reduced staff.

Formal objectives also show two approaches to nursing. For example, most standards for practice set by the ANA or its divisions focus upon the nursing process itself. For example, the Division of Orthopedic Nursing Practice formulated such standards as Standard II, whereby nursing diagnosis is derived from health status data, and Standard VI, whereby the plan for nursing care is evaluated[1]. Such standards (or

objectives) tell the nurse what to do, not what happens as a result of that activity. Many head nurses identify unit objectives in this manner.

Other head nurses prefer to state unit objectives in terms of patient outcomes. A long-term care unit, for example, might have the following objectives for its bedridden patients: skin surfaces remain intact, and joint mobility is maintained.

MEANS AND ENDS

In truth, the first-line manager must consider *both* nursing actions and patient outcomes. It is critical, however, that she see these in an appropriate means to ends relationship. Otherwise many nursing actions (means) mistakenly become formalized into patterns of invariate behavior (traditions) which take on unwarranted significance apart from their effectiveness in the production of desired patient health outcomes (ends). If the first-line manager judges nursing actions by their ability to produce desired patient outcomes, detrimental tradition and meaningless "standard operating procedures" will not prevail.

Such a view of the means-to-ends relationship requires the first-line manager to give more attention and credence to nursing research. Only through research are nursing practices or traditions proved to be useful, meaningless, or detrimental to patient health states. Where research indicates that traditional care patterns are detrimental, it is up to first-line managers to program new patterns of nursing behavior that are in keeping with research findings. Nursing has too few resources to invest them in nontherapeutic procedures and actions. The first-line manager's job is to relate nursing actions to patient health outcomes in a manner that judges the effectiveness of the former by the improvements in the latter.

But effectiveness of a nursing action is not the only criterion for choosing it. The first-line manager also must consider efficiency and economy. If a given set of actions can produce the desired outcome more quickly, more cheaply, and with less staff, it is to be preferred over another set of actions that produces the same outcome. Sometimes nurses are uncomfortable with considerations of efficiency and economy, for the nursing profession has taught them the ethos that human health is priceless and that every patient deserves the best possible care. Some nurses feel that nursing values are debased with the introduction of managerial criteria such as efficiency or economy.

Nurses must realize, however, that everything, including nursing, has a price tag. Someone must pay the price for the personnel, supplies, equipment, and support systems that make nursing possible. Nurses tend to be very concerned when they know that a patient is financially affected by his illness and they typically do all they can to lighten the financial load. This attitude disappears, however, when the payer is a third-party insurer or the government. Nurses must realize that sooner or later the consumer pays for health services, whether it be directly, through insurance premiums, or through taxes. In a world of limited resources, the money that goes into health care does not go into other valuable activities—education, recreation, cultural pleasures. The first-line manager has a responsibility to develop a pragmatic approach to the financial facts of nursing. Economy and efficiency cannot be overlooked in the provision of nursing care.

CONTINUUMS OF FIRST-LINE MANAGEMENT

The first-line manager may perceive of her work as taking place along two special continuums: the real to the ideal and the programmed to the unprogrammed. Each of these continuums will be explored, and the two poles of each continuum will be contrasted in order to make explicit the major dangers in first-line management. In real practice, the manager seldom will deal with polarized alternatives. Instead, she will ask herself to what degree her thinking is dominated by the real or the ideal, to what extent a problem is dominated by programmed or unprogrammed knowledge.

The Real versus the Ideal

One of the most important tools of the first-line manager is her direct and personal knowledge of each patient and each staff member. This knowledge enables her to temper general management principles according to the realities of the situation. This knowledge enables her to utilize the unique talents and abilities of each staff member and to match these talents and abilities to the unique needs of patients.

The inexperienced first-line manager often has trouble reconciling her picture of the ideal employee with the reality of the workers on her patient unit, team, or module. According to the textbooks, every employee cheerfully gives his all, does every assigned task, and generally is a paragon of virtue; the task of the first-line manager simply is to provide proper guidance. The new manager usually is surprised to learn that she is not skillful enough to provide such guidance and that even if she is a skilled leader, some employees will not turn in star performances.

The first-line manager soon learns that while she aims to build an ideal work team, her plans had better be based on the average, not the exceptional, employee. In management, one must plan around what are—not what ought to be—the capabilities of staff members. Management realism may clash with nursing idealism, but the effective first-line manager starts with her staff members as they are, not as they should be.

For the inexperienced first-line manager, personal knowledge of staff members may be a problem. For example, if staff members are her friends and peers, she may have difficulty giving them orders. It is not unusual to find a new manager doing too many tasks herself simply because she is ill at ease in delegating tasks to others. The first-line manager must recognize that her job requires delegation of tasks. No matter how efficient she may be at doing the tasks herself, she cannot compensate for the care time lost when her staff is underemployed.

Inexperienced first-line managers may rely too heavily upon a few unusually talented workers. This may cause resentment from all workers, for some may see it as favoritism while the "favored" ones may feel over-burdened by the increased work load. Not only should the first-line manager be careful not to penalize the unusually talented or willing worker with too much work, but also she should not deny to the less capable worker the opportunity to acquire further skills through practice.

The first-line manager may find that not only her employees but also her environment and its resources are far from ideal. If the manager acts as if she were in an ideal setting when in fact she is not, she will set unrealistic goals, frustrating her staff and accomplishing little. If, instead, she regards the environment and its resources realistically, then she will set achievable goals and reasonable priorities.

The real versus the ideal also may influence the first-line manager's relationship with patients. Some first-line managers act upon an unspoken assumption that the patient will respond ideally and achieve all the goals formulated by the nurse. But in cases where the nurse's goals, however well-intentioned, are beyond the present capabilities of the patient, the patient is likely to feel the nurse's expectations as an additional burden upon his already diminished capacity for self-care and autonomy.

The Programmed versus the Unprogrammed

The first-line manager deals with both pro-grammed and unprogrammed nursing knowledge and application. Some nursing knowledge is programmed, that is, well accepted by the nursing community and supported by nursing research. Other nursing knowledge is unprogrammed; it is in the early stages of investigation and is not yet validated by research or generally accepted by the nursing community.

Similarly, the application of nursing knowledge may be programmed or unprogrammed. For example, a nursing unit may have a routine teaching program for obese patients. Yet that program may not be adequate for the needs of an obese patient with a language problem. Hence, the nursing knowledge must be applied to such a patient in an innovative, unprogrammed manner.

Clearly, the greater the amount of pro-grammed knowledge and programmed application, the simpler the job of the first-line manager. However, the manager has a particular responsibility when an unprogrammed situation arises. It is her responsibility to chart a course of action, to solve problems. This does not mean that the first-line manager will make all unprogrammed nursing care decisions herself. Indeed, the wise first-line manager will use her best resource people for this purpose; resource people may include her supervisor, clinical specialists, experienced nurse team members, or nurses from other units or institutions who have special expertise. Although it is not up to the first-line manager to make all decisions, it is her responsibility to be creative and effective in finding the best resources for each unprogrammed situation.

Many inexperienced first-line managers make staff assignments purely on the basis of the difficulty or simplicity of each patient's care needs. In making assignments, it is suggested that the manager also consider what aspects of that care are programmed or unprogrammed. For example, the care of a given patient may be complex but relatively well programmed; in such a case, a competent LPN may be able to offer care just as satisfactorily as could an RN. The RN might be assigned to a simpler case that requires some thinking, planning, and searching for new ways and means.

It is the responsibility of the first-line manager to document new approaches and new theories of care as they are tested in the clinical area. Where satisfactory results are obtained from a new course of therapy, it is important that the findings be preserved and shared with other nurses. Results obtained in any given case are shared in order that a similar plan of care may be tested again in a similar case. In this way programmed nursing knowledge grows and is verified.

First-line management is an exciting role because it offers the ideal synthesis of management and nursing. It offers the nurse a chance to observe the effects of her direction and it enables her to accomplish more than she could do alone, through the careful use of her staff. All first-line positions share this potential. The most important first-line position, however, is the permanent one, the position of head nurse. This position will be examined in more detail.

HEAD NURSE MANAGER

The head nurse fills one of the most critical first-line roles in the administration of nursing services. The majority of objectives for any nursing service relate to what happens to the patient, and the head nurse is the administrative channel through which these objectives ultimately are implemented or fail to be implemented. The nursing director has planned in vain for these objectives if the head nurse is unable to translate these plans into concrete action.

Role Analysis

The head nurse is in the pivotal position linking nursing management to nursing care. This conversion of plans and concepts into action is one of the most difficult parts of management. It may be easier, for example, to derive a set of rules by which to make assignments of patients than it is to use these rules in actually assigning a given set of patients to a given staff. Typically it is the function of the head nurse to apply the policies, practices, procedures, objectives, concepts, and goals to the concrete situation on a given patient unit. Such application de-

mands clear perception of the concrete situation and good judgment as to which concepts apply and how they apply in each instance. To be successful, the head nurse must be able to both conceptualize and concretize.

Because the head nurse has one foot in the work and the other in administration, she needs a wider scope of abilities than is required in most positions. First, she must be a clinical nursing expert in order to direct and teach her staff and to maintain their respect in her as a leader. In addition to nursing expertise, she also needs management skill to direct the work of others effectively.

One reason management can be difficult for the head nurse is inexperience. Typically the head nurse role is the first management position in the individual's nursing career. High turnover in the nursing profession, unfortunately, is also evident in head nurse positions, thus contributing to the problem of inexperience. The practice of promoting to head nurse positions nurses without preparatory education further compounds the problem.

Another complexity specific to the head nurse role is that of interaction with multiple divisions and departments. The head nurse is the primary manager to interact with physicians. Since part of her job is to implement physicians' orders, it is not surprising that some physicians try to impose their own authority on the head nurse. Whatever the situation, it is necessary that the head nurse work out acceptable role relations with physicians. Head nurses achieve these relationships by using every means from submission and colleagueship to intimidation. In any case, some resolution must be made to facilitate the accomplishment of the goals of both nursing and medicine, and the head nurse is the person who must accomplish this resolution.

Another ongoing interaction is that between the head nurse and the unit management or secretarial staff. Most institutions today attempt to relieve the head nurse of some non-nursing tasks. Plans range from providing simple clerical assistance to providing a coequal manager to handle all non-nursing elements of the unit. While such assistance is usually welcome, the problems of coordinating and adapting role relations increase in proportion to the power and authority of the non-nurse manager. As "services performed" increase, the need for interaction and role resolution also increases.

In addition to working with physicians and unit managers, the head nurse must maintain smooth coordination with all other divisions and departments concerned with direct patient services or nursing supportive services. It is essential that this coordination be smooth because when there are break-downs the problems revert to the head nurse as custodian of the patient. Thus, because of the high number of interactions, the head nurse role is subjected to more sources of potential frustration than are most management roles.

Seen in its full scope, the head nurse role is that vital management position through which the patient-related objectives of the nursing division are concretized by firsthand direction of nursing activities. The head nurse's role is also the management position with greatest responsibility for day-to-day coordination with all other departments and divisions that relate directly or indirectly to the patient.

Management Issues

It is important that the head nurse see herself as a manager, otherwise she is likely to be directed by her environment rather than directing it. The head nurse is particularly vulnerable to this management defect because of the nature of her environment, which is usually bustling; there are always things that need to be done. It is very easy for a head nurse to put in an eight-hour day without ever organizing the events that occur on her unit.

In order to avert this tendency toward immersion in the immediate events, the head nurse needs to have a framework by which to interpret, plan, and evaluate the ongoing activities of her unit. Concepts of management and nursing theories will be required for an adequate framework.

Even before building a conceptual framework, however, the head nurse must internalize her concept of herself as a manager. Unfortunately the usual institutional system for selecting and employing head nurses presents some obstacles to development of their self-image as manager. Typically, selection of a head nurse is by promotion upward of a staff member rather than the hiring of an individual experienced in the head nurse role. Thus the first obstacle is the earlier peer relationship of the head nurse with the staff. This established pattern of interaction complicates the internalization of the management role.

A second obstacle concerns selection of the individual for the head nurse position. One criterion is clinical excellence. The nurse selected on this basis is likely to have justifiable pride in her capacities as a clinician. A nurse with a strong commitment to the clinical self-concept may have difficulty in assimilating the management role. Indeed, she may have great difficulty in reconciling the two roles, and her resolution may be to minimize the importance of the management role. Even when the clinician nurse satisfactorily internalizes the management self-concept, there is no reason to assume that excellence in individual clinical practice predicates excellence in management of the work of others. Indeed, the personality traits that lead one into a profession that stresses nurturing and caring for others may be inconsistent with the personality traits required of a manager. While most nurses would believe that it is possible to combine clinical talents with management talents, there is no assurance that this will be the case for any particular nurse.

The second common criterion for selection of a head nurse is that of observed leadership ability. Natural leadership ability is usually conducive to internalizing of the management role, and it may be a better predictor of success in a head nurse role than is the criterion of clinical excellence. Leadership ability, however, is only one component of good management, and by itself it is only an indicator of potential management success.

Promotion of a staff nurse to a head nurse position does not in itself assure that the nurse will internalize a concept of herself as a manager. Indeed, some nursing divisions encourage the head nurse to undervalue her management role by using her as a fill-in worker. Where a nursing division chronically uses its head nurse to fill in for missing team leaders or bedside nurses, it is clear that the division sees management as an epiphenomenon—something unessential, to be done when there is lots of help. This type of attitude from higher management certainly does not encourage the head nurse to see the significance of her management role; nor does it encourage her subordinates to look on her as a manager.

A nursing division with a clear appreciation of what good management can do will know that a manager is needed on an understaffed day more than at any other time. Appropriate head nurse management will assure the institution of optimal output from each employee.

Not only the institution but the head nurse herself may need to adjust to the concept that her time away from the patient's bedside contributes just as much to the patient's welfare as does her direct care. Once the head nurse has developed administrative skills, she will be able to see the impact that good management has on patient care.

Management Framework

The head nurse role is more complex than the staff role in both its responsibilities and its resources for action. The head nurse may share the same concept of good nursing as the staff nurse, but she has more variables at hand for implementing that concept. The staff nurse has essentially one resource for accomplishing her job: the use of self. The systems she will use and the assignment she will fill are set. The judgments the staff nurse makes concern use of self in that predetermined environment and within the prescribed systems and practices.

The head nurse has a larger number of resources at her command; she has at least three potential variables: use of self, use of staff, and use of delivery systems. The head nurse has the right to determine the most valuable use of her own time. She decides how and in what ways she will relate to her staff and her patients. She also has the freedom to use her staff in any way that is most appropriate to producing the kind of nursing that is her objective. She can determine methods of staff assignment, set criteria for performance, and educate and indoctrinate her staff to her concept of nursing. In addition, she has the right to determine and regulate those systems that control the day-to-day delivery of nursing care on the unit. She can determine the nature and timing for such routine events as hygiene, bathing, and temperature checks. She can decide on the systems for implementing physician's orders, and, most important, she can establish systems for evolving and implementing nursing care orders.

In addition to the larger number of resources for action, the head nurse also has a larger scope of responsibility for patient care, staff management, and administration of nursing division policies; thus a basic head nurse management framework can be developed by identifying both her key responsibilities and her key resources for action. (See Figure 16-1.)

If the parts of this model are seen as pivoting around a central point, it becomes clear that there are nine possible combinations in the framework. Every resource can be brought to bear upon every responsibility. Obviously, not every resource will be of equal importance in meeting each responsibility, but it is important that the head nurse not limit her effectiveness by failure to consider all possible options. Not all of these combinations of responsibilities and resources will be discussed, but several critical ones will be examined.

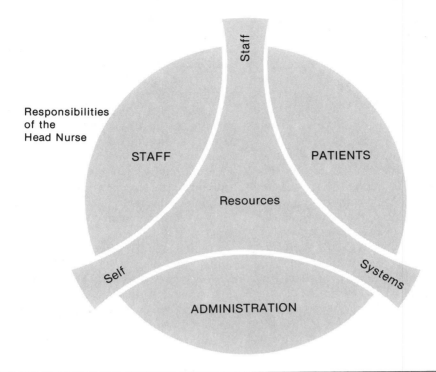

Figure 16-1. Responsibilities and Resources of the Head Nurse

In her management of staff, the inexperienced head nurse often fails to make optimal use of self. It is easy for her to rely on management systems such as assignments and periodic evaluations to manage the staff. If she is fortunate, she can also rely on the staff to provide their own management through self-motivation and internalized professional standards.

In what ways, then, can the head nurse consciously use self in the management of staff? Three major staff management functions (directing, teaching, and controlling) can be improved by planned use of self.

For directing staff, it seems absurdly simple to suggest that the head nurse tell her staff what she expects of them. Obvious as this sounds, it is a step often neglected. The head nurse may assume that her staff will want the same goals she does. This assumption, unfortunately, is often faulty. Even if all staff members are highly motivated to give "good patient care," there is no reason to assume that they all mean the same thing

by this phrase. Therefore the head nurse has an obligation to make clear to her staff the kind of performance she wants.

Telling the staff what is expected is an obvious answer to the communications problem, but telling alone is seldom adequate. The head nurse should reinforce the telling with the appropriate use of incidental questions during the work day. Consider the following questions directed to two staff nurses by two different head nurses. Assume that both head nurses have told their respective staffs that they want to focus upon patient assessment and care planning.

Head Nurse A:
   "Are your baths done?"
   "How are you doing?"
   "Can you get done in time for an early lunch hour?"

Head Nurse B:
   "What is your assessment of Mr. X's progress in use of his left arm?"

"How can you modify Mrs. B's care to clear up that reddened area I saw during rounds this morning?"

Clearly, Head Nurse B is reinforcing her directive, whereas Head Nurse A is telling her staff nurse that other things are far more important than patient assessment and care planning.

Staff members have a healthy sense of self-preservation, so they soon learn the real interests of the head nurse. If her professed interests do not coincide with the rest of her behavior, particularly the questions addressed to staff, she should not be surprised if those interests are ignored by her staff. It is an interesting exercise for a head nurse to keep a log of all her questions to the staff for a day. This will give her a clear idea of what things the staff see as important to her.

Head nurse's use of self in teaching staff members is especially important. If she fails to see teaching as an integral part of her role, it is likely that staff may develop the same attitude and neglect patient teaching. The head nurse is the individual best able to identify the teaching needs of her staff, both as a group and as individuals. She therefore needs to be alert to situations that provide an opportunity for meeting educational needs.

It is important that the head nurse do some teaching herself, for this establishes her competence in nursing in the minds of her staff. Overreliance on an inservice education department robs the head nurse of this valuable means for relating to staff.

One of the best ways for a head nurse to teach is by demonstration. Since the head nurse's time for giving individual patient care is limited, she should use her direct care occasions as teaching episodes. She should be selective as to what direct patient care she does so that in her care she will be teaching as a role model.

Control of staff members is another primary obligation of the head nurse, and control will be poor if it is left to the formalized system of personnel evaluations and disciplinary notices. The head nurse can make clear to staff what behavior is acceptable, what is required, and what is unacceptable by simple verbal communication. She must make her expectations explicit and not assume that the staff will intuit her standards and limits for behavior.

The same resources for action (self, staff, and systems) can be examined as they apply to the responsibility for patients. The conscious use of care delivery systems is often underutilized by head nurses. It is easy for a head nurse to continue with her institution's traditional delivery systems without ever really evaluating them or seeing that they exist.

The first step therefore in meeting responsibility for patients is to identify what delivery systems exist. The assignment of staff is the most obvious delivery system. It is also one in which the head nurse has great latitude. Even if she is in an institution committed to a specific assignment method such as team care or primary care, there is still great variation possible in the interpretation and application of the selected method.

Some other delivery systems are not so immediately obvious as the assignment method. The system of communicating new orders is one such example. This system, like many others, usually was evolved by circumstance and passed on by tradition rather than being the result of a considered decision. Bath times and routines as well as temperature times and routines are other such examples. There are systems for reporting on and off duty and for transmission of information regarding patients, as well as for interacting with physicians visiting patients on the unit, for coordinating with various practicing students, and for permitting exchange of shifts.

All these systems and others like them have impact upon patient care. They determine how staff will spend their time, they regulate many of the safety and comfort factors of the environment, and they channel relevant information to, from, and about the patient. It is important therefore that the head nurse identify the systems in effect in her unit and subject them to rational scrutiny. Are the existing systems appropriate for attaining her patient care objectives? Should some systems be eliminated as serving no valuable purpose?

In looking at the delivery systems as they relate to her patient goals, the head nurse can streamline and secure the activities of her staff. When such systems are subjected to scrutiny one will not find such absurdities as nurses passing morning basins to up-and-about patients when they do not have enough time to do the teaching these patients need or nurse assistants spending hours taking unnecessary temperatures on afebrile patients who could better have had the time spent in skin care. Nor would patients who need optimal rest be awakened at an early hour for a bath they do not need. Most of the well-publicized absurdities of institutional nursing care are defects in the delivery systems rather than acts of individual incompetence.

The last major responsibility of the head nurse is administration of nursing division policies. Here use of self is the most important resource. The head nurse must recognize that she is part of the administrative sector and that interpretation of the nursing administrative decisions to staff members is a crucial part of her job. It is her obligation to communicate nursing division goals and to translate those goals into actions; the head nurse is the major implementer of nursing policy and policy decisions. She also must remember that as an administrative representative, all her decisions bear the weight of precedent-setting judgments. She cannot afford to make a hasty decision that gives an employee an advantage that would not be offered to another employee under similar circumstance. She has to recognize that all her decisions and actions must be consistent with general administrative rules and policies. The new head nurse should be assisted to develop this sensitivity to the administrative role by her supervisor.

As an important member of nursing administration, the head nurse should accept responsibility for input into, and participation in, administrative decisions. Included in this is not only responsibility for committee participation but for the conscientious feedback to her supervisor of any information or opinion important to administrative decision making.

In accepting the administrative role, the head nurse also accepts the obligation to learn the new craft of management. Some institutions are able to offer the new head nurse a management course, others are not. When not, the head nurse should assume the responsibility for basic management reading so as to equip herself for her new function. The supervisor or director of nursing should be able to provide an appropriate reading list.

The head nurse will need to know basic management principles and how they apply to nursing. Thus she should learn basic concepts underlying all common forms of assignment of staff—functional, team, modular, and primary systems. She should learn concepts of staffing and relevant issues such as cyclical plans and irregular-hour shift concepts. She should study systems of assessing quality of patient care and systems of estimating patient work load and patient classification. These and other nursing-related management concepts will need to be accommodated to the head nurse's idea of the nursing process.

In summary, it is important that the head nurse understand the scope of her role. Since her education seldom prepares her for the management aspects of that role, the head nurse needs assistance in developing management skills. The nursing division should assume some responsibility for management development by providing educational programs or resources and by making clear its expectations for managers. Adjustment to the head nurse role is facilitated if the head nurse can use a role-descriptive framework by which to identify and order her functions. The head nurse needs to recognize the unique nature of her role at the juncture of administration and staff; that unique factor is the responsibility for translating concepts and goals into concrete activities.

SUMMARY

The nurse executive must be very sensitive to the needs of her first-line managers. These needs are strong because first-line management is the first administrative position and is often filled by inexperienced managers and because first-line management occurs at the critical point of patient care delivery. While the nurse executive needs to develop good channels for communication with head nurses (and other first-line managers), she needs to do so in a way that does not undermine the authority of her supervisory staff. The nurse executive also will want to develop mechanisms whereby she or her supervisory staff can discover which staff nurses have managerial potential. Often this potential can be developed in the informal first-line positions, as in charge experience or team leading. The wise executive is planning well ahead by identifying today the potential leaders and managers of tomorrow for the institution and for the profession.

REFERENCES

1. Orthopedic Nurses' Association and American Nurses' Association. *Standards of Orthopedic Nursing Practice.* Kansas City, Mo.: ANA, 1975.

BIBLIOGRAPHY

Alexander, E.L. *Nursing Administration in the Hospital Health Care System.* (2nd ed.) St. Louis: C.V. Mosby, 1978.

Beyers, M., and Phillips, C. *Nursing Management for Patient Care.* Boston: Little, Brown, 1971.

Clark, C.C., and Shea, C.A. *Management in Nursing: A Vital Link in the Health Care System.* New York: McGraw-Hill, 1979.

Ganong, J., and Ganong, W. Are head nurses obsolete? *J.O.N.A.,* 5(7):16, 1975.

Holloman, C.R. The nurse enters management. *Supervisor Nurse,* 2(4):54, 1971.

Joy, P.M. Maintaining continuity of care during shift change. *J.O.N.A.,* 5(9):28, 1975.

Kron, T. *The Management of Patient Care—Putting Leadership Skills to Work.* Philadelphia: W.B. Saunders, 1971.

O'Donovan, T.R. Leadership Dynamics. *J.O.N.A.,* 5(7):32, 1975.

Plachy, R.J. Head nurses: less griping, more action. *J.O.N.A.,* 6(1):39, 1976.

Chapter 17

The Clinical Specialist and Nursing Management

The clinical specialist now has an accepted nursing role in most health institutions, and resistance to her role that existed initially no longer exists. Accountability of the clinical specialist remains a perennial issue, however. The major difficulty is that the clinical specialist's role, as envisioned by educators, was not designed to fit into the bureaucratic, hierarchical management system typical of health care institutions. The role is an administrative anomaly, grafted to a system in which it does not comfortably fit. Clinical specialism cannot be faulted; no other movement in nursing has contributed so much, so rapidly, to the professionalization of nursing. Nevertheless, the fact remains that clinical specialism is structurally ill adapted to the typical bureaucratic management system.

It is unrealistic to assume that this system of management will be replaced on a large scale in the near future. For all its flaws, a bureaucratic system still enables an average group of people to do a credible job of providing services. One suspects that some of the newer management trends, such as matrix organizations and use of design groups for management, require a concentration of better-than-average managers for effective organizational management. Since neither clinical specialism nor bureaucracy are likely to vanish, it is necessary to establish a livable relationship between them. Methods of determining the accountability of the clinical specialist spring from this relationship.

In order to determine accountability, the clinical specialist's authority and the place it reserves for her inside the institution must be discussed. There is a direct relation between authority and accountability; it is illogical

for a manager to hold anyone accountable for activities or events over which she has no authority or control.

Authority can be defined in two ways. First, it is the power or right to give commands, to enforce obedience, to take action, or to make final decisions. This kind of authority is vested in the holder by virtue of organizational position. To have such authority requires that one serve in a line position, having responsibility for the actions and management of other employees. Such authority really is granted to a position rather than to a particular individual, for it goes with the role, regardless of who fills it. In this discussion this power will be called *administrative authority*.

Secondly, authority can be defined as power or influence resulting from knowledge and expertise. A clinical specialist achieves such authority among her peers through their respect for her expertise. This authority is granted to the person by choice, not to the position by fiat; this authority will be called *professional authority*. Professional authority applies to every competent and respected clinical specialist, while administrative authority depends upon her job description and her place in the organization.

PROFESSIONAL AUTHORITY

Appropriate accountability for the clinical specialist depends upon the authority she holds. When she has only professional authority, her accountability is necessarily limited. Professional authority is granted to the clinical specialist by others when they perceive that her expertise is superior to their own, but there is no assurance that they will seek her services voluntarily. If she is perceived as a threat or as competition, her expertise may not be sought even when it is needed. Utilization of the clinical specialist depends upon several factors: the staff's understanding of her role and functions, their personal reactions to her, and their perceptions of patient needs.

Because use of the clinical specialist by staff is dependent upon their perception of her, it is hardly fair to hold her accountable for her impact on staff behavior. Nor is it fair to hold the clinical specialist accountable for the general quality of patient care if her access to patients is determined by the perception of others. Therefore, when the clinical specialist is given professional authority alone, the nurse executive should only hold her accountable for the direct patient care she renders. Of course, the executive has a right to expect from the clinical specialist a higher level of patient care, in terms of better patient outcomes, than that expected from the general nurse practitioner. The clinical specialist has claimed to be an expert and is accountable for providing expertise.

Since no one (including the nurse executive) is likely to have sufficient expertise with which to assess the nursing process of the clinical specialist, she must be held accountable on the basis of patient outcomes. Improved outcomes are expected for patients receiving the specialist's care, and judgment of the clinical specialist's performance is based on the total numbers of cases handled and their cumulative outcomes. Some individual failures are expected, even for the clinical specialist, since no plan of care is foolproof.

Unfortunately, nurse executives often overlook the logic of holding the clinical specialist accountable only for her independent practice. Although she is limited to professional authority, in a staff position the clinical specialist is expected to work with line managers and staff, select her own case load, serve as a consultant for nursing care problems, and function as an educator and role model for staff members. Clearly, these activities require the specialist's clinical knowledge, but they also require other unrelated abilities of an interpersonal nature. The acquisition of these interpersonal skills may or may not have been part of the clinical specialist's education. All too often the clinical specialist's graduate education gives her no notion of how to interact effectively in an organization or with people. Indeed, the clinical specialist often naively cannot understand why others fail to follow her recommendations when they are obviously clinically sound. Usually the answer lies in her inability to influence people within the organizational setting.

When unstated job requirements exist for performance through others (without line authority over them), the clinical specialist's effectiveness depends not only on her skill with interpersonal and intraorganizational processes, but also on the nature of the work environment. The attitudes of staff members with whom she interacts are a critical element of that environment. Environments may range from those that welcome and accept the clinical specialist to those in which hostility, suspiciousness, and resentment predominate. The clinical specialist must be sensitive to the fact that her positional autonomy may be a source of envy to the staff nurse. Indeed, many a staff nurse has said "If I could pick my own case load, doing only as many patients as I determined I could manage, then I could give the same kind of care the clinical specialist does." Although such a statement may be false, it reveals the source of envy—the specialist's ability to pick and choose and to determine the quantity of work to be done.

Because of such problems the clinical specialist role is fraught with sources of discord, but this does not mean that clinical specialists can never be expected to be responsible for achieving better care through others. If a clinical specialist is expected to perform in this manner, however, the interpersonal and intraorganizational skills she will need should be identified as part of the job requirement in the position contract. When these skills have been agreed upon as part of the job, then both employer and employee understand what is expected from the start. The clinical specialist who takes a job that specifies these skills would be wise to seek education to develop them.

Given the realities of a staff role, the clinical specialist will want to make a good assessment of both the work environment and her own skills before agreeing to take a position which includes responsibility for changing the behaviors of others not directly under one's authority. Similarly, the nurse executive must assess these factors in order to be sure that she is not contracting for an impossible task. The difficulty for both parties lies in their ability to assess each other. If the clinical specialist has not had previous contact with the institution, she will find it difficult to assess the work environment accurately. If the nurse executive has not worked with the clinical specialist before, she will have difficulty assessing the specialist's interpersonal and intraorganizational effectiveness. It is almost impossible to predict the mutual compatibility of an individual clinical specialist and a particular work environment.

From an administrative viewpoint, it is risky to hire a clinical specialist for a staff rather than line position in which she must change staff behaviors. A position's likelihood for success should be built into the design of the job; it should not depend on the chance factor of the incumbent's personality and how that personality "fits" or is responded to by others in the environment. This risk factor is the reason that directors hesitate to hire clinical specialists for staff positions. The salary of a clinical specialist is usually a major investment of scarce resources, and the director has to justify such a high risk investment in a staff position. Further, if the staff clinical specialist position is justified only on the individual care the clinician gives, it is difficult for the nurse executive to justify the position. How, for example, can the nurse executive justify giving a small selected group of patients more expert care than other patients of the same sort? This is especially dif-

ficult when all patients are paying the same fees for nursing care. In an era of heavy emphasis on cost containment, it is difficult to say that general staff care is acceptable for all patients of one kind but that some will be picked out for better care than that which already has been judged as acceptable.

Given these conditions, many nurse executives do not feel that they can hire a clinical specialist unless that specialist is able to exponentially extend her impact on patient care through others. For staff positions how can this be done? One way is to hold the clinical specialist responsible for the behavior of others even without authority to modify their behaviors. Although this is risky for both director and specialist, some may choose this route in any case. Aydelotte suggests an alternate staff use of clinicians[1]. She suggests that most nurses be expected to follow protocols of patient care, to apply the known nursing knowledge to care. She suggests that clinical specialists be cast in the research role, investigating care regimens for those nursing problems yet to be solved. When a clinical specialist has worked with patients demonstrating a given care problem and has solved—or partially solved—that problem, then she would devise a protocol to be used by the nursing staff. In this model, the clinical specialist is the person who researches and turns the unknown into the prescribed; she takes previously unprogrammed nursing problems, studies them through individual care of selected patients, and programs a plan of care to be shared with other nurses.

An alternate staff position for the clinical specialist would be that of teacher-role model. In this instance, her direct patient care would take place only as role modeling, and her primary responsibility would be for staff education. In either this model or Aydelotte's model, the nurse exponentially extends her capabilities for care by increasing the quality of care given by the staff; both allow her to do this through a staff position. An alternate model for exponentially extending expert care is the line position for specialists.

ADMINISTRATIVE AUTHORITY

What about the clinical specialist who assumes line responsibility? In accepting such administrative authority, the clinical specialist assumes the same accountability for management as any other line manager. She has no right to use her clinical interest as an excuse for second-class management. Typically, the clinical specialist is given line management for a limited number of patient units, preferably only those served by her speciality. The objective here is to have the best of both worlds: if she has limited administrative scope, then she should have time to use her skills as a specialist. In this way her administrative authority enables the clinical specialist to implement her clinical expertise fully: she has the authority to issue orders to staff

For what should the clinical specialist in a line position be held accountable? Management tasks? Improved clinical outcomes? Typically the nurse executive expects her to accomplish both. However, unless the clinical specialist's management scope is limited, this is an unrealistic expectation. A clinical specialist cannot carry the same scope of administrative responsibility as other managers and still have special impact on bedside care; this discounts the reality of administrative demands. Moreover, a clinical specialist is not prepared by her education for the management role. When she assumes line authority, she will need additional education for this function. In most cases her clinical graduate degree will not have prepared her for management.

Use of the line position for clinical specialists has become more popular in an era of economic cutbacks. Additionally, many clinical specialists have sought line positions after being frustrated in trying to change a care delivery system from a staff position. Unfortunately, few graduate programs presently prepare the clinical specialist for line positions in management. Few programs allow the clinical specialist time for more than a cursory review of basic management.

ROLE AMBIGUITY

Given that some problems attach to almost every organizational position for the clinical specialist, it is important that the nurse executive and the clinical specialist agree on the job responsibilities before such a job is accepted. It is particularly illogical for a nurse executive to mislead the clinical specialist by inviting her to come and "do her own thing." No environment is this pliable and responsive to the whims of a single employee. Indeed, the offer to "write your own job description" should be viewed with suspicion by the clinical specialist. Every nurse executive has expectations for the clinical specialist—otherwise she wouldn't be hiring her. Every nurse executive is going to hold the clinical specialist accountable for meeting those expectations. Sooner or later the clinical specialist will be made aware of how she measured up.

Given the realities of life within an organization, the clinical specialist has nothing to lose and everything to gain by getting a clear idea of her boss's expectations. Unstated expectations do not increase the clinical specialist's autonomy; they merely force her to work in the dark, providing no external criteria by which to assess her performance. Autonomy is not anomie; it is freedom to select one's own means for reaching accepted goals.

REFERENCES

1. Aydelotte, M.K. Organizational Climate and Measurement of Clinical Specialist Effectiveness. Speech given at University of Illinois, Chicago, October 14, 1975.

BIBLIOGRAPHY

Anders, R.L. Matrix organization: an alternative for clinical specialists. *J.O.N.A.,* 5(5):11, 1975.

Blake, P. The clinical specialist as nurse consultant. *J.O.N.A.,* 7(10):33, 1977.

Castronovo, F. The effective use of the clinical specialist. *Supervisor Nurse,* 6(5):48, 1975.

Disch, J.M. The clinical nurse specialist in a large peer group. *J.O.N.A.,* 8(12):17, 1978.

Donovan, H.M. The clinical specialist—where does she fit? *Supervisor Nurse,* 1(2):35, 1970.

Feutz, S., and Jackson, B.S. Justifying clinical nursing specialists. *Supervisor Nurse,* 10(6):28, 1979.

Kirkman, R.H., and Miller, M.E. The clinical specialist in a community hospital. *J.O.N.A.,* 7(1):30, 1972.

Parkis, E.W. The management role of the clinical specialist—part I. *Supervisor Nurse,* 5(9):44, 1974.

Parkis, E.W. The management role of the clinical specialist—part II. *Supervisor Nurse,* 5(10):24, 1974.

Passos, J.Y. Accountability: myth or mandate? *J.O.N.A.,* 3(3):17, 1973.

Shaefer, J.A. The satisfied clinician: administrative support makes the difference *J.O.N.A.,* 3(4):17, 1973.

Smith, M.L. The clinical specialist: her role in staff development. *J.O.N.A.,* 1(1):33, 1971.

Part IV

Resources of Nursing Management

Part IV of this book examines some of the resources of nursing management, specifically, financial resources (Chapter 18), space and materiel (Chapter 19), and legal resources, especially those relating to personnel and management interaction (Chapter 20). This part of the book is limited, not because resources are limited, but because many of the resources available to the nurse executive were already discussed when the structures and processes of nursing management were considered. Some of the most important resources for the nurse executive consist in manpower, discussed under staffing, and her own intellectual capabilities, discussed under thought processes. Indeed, all the structures and processes of nursing management are, in a sense, the resources used by the nurse executive.

Resources will be considered from two perspectives: what they contribute and what they limit. Resources may be conceived as limitations to the extent that they curtail executive action; legal constraints exemplify this perspective.

All nursing management takes place in a situation of scarce resources; that is what makes management the pursuit of the possible, not the pursuit of the ideal. The function of the nurse executive is to achieve the greatest result with the resources available. It also is her function to know when resources are simply too scarce to deliver safe nursing care. In this case, she cannot conscientiously continue to participate in such a situation. She either must acquire additional resources or withdraw, making the danger known.

Chapter 18

Institutional Finance and Nursing Management

In order to be an effective administrator, the nurse executive must have a good grasp of the financial side of management in her institution. This chapter will review several important aspects of health care finance including institutional finance and budgeting, cost containment, nursing division budgeting, costing out of nursing services, and mechanisms of cost accounting which can be used for accountability and divisional decision making.

INSTITUTIONAL FINANCE

The financial system of the health care organization is headed by the chief financial officer, sometimes called director of finance; sometimes this function is performed by the controller. Whatever title, the chief financial officer usually oversees the following functions and/or departments.

1. Financial planning and auditing is the function that prepares and administers the institutional budget and audits funds. The department charged with this function should provide services to the nurse executive unless she has her own financial manager, in which case, the nursing financial officer will closely coordinate with the department of the budget.
2. Accounting services control payroll, accounts payable, cash control, and taxes. This function is primarily mechanical with activities designed to follow prescribed protocols, or decision rules set by others.
3. Reimbursement and fiscal projects deal with external regulatory impacts on finance, for example providing admin-

istration of Medicare, Medicaid, and interactions with other third party payers such as Blue Cross, Blue Shield, and major medical coverage plans and handling the cost reports required by such external agencies so as to assure reimbursement.
4. Data processing collects data which affect finance, such as census, patient days, admissions and discharges, visits to various clinics. What data are collected depends upon executive decisions and the capabilities of the collection systems used.
5. Patient financial services handle patient billing, credit and collection of fees, and the cashier function. This is another mechanized system, following decision rules made by others. The complexity of this function may be reflected in the fact that the average hospital has 20 to 30 independent revenue centers and approximately 2,000 billable items. This number is growing as many institutions attempt to more closely associate actual costs and fees.

The major policy issues and problems of financial management in a health care institution include establishing rates and charges, funding unprofitable departments, adjusting financial policies to the demands of the medical staff, managing cash flow, and developing a strategy for depreciation.

Establishing a rate structure and charges is a difficult balancing act. The rate is set so as to achieve financing which is above the break-even line, even in institutions which are not for profit. This is to offset loss on uncollected debts and Medicare, which pays the lowest—the charge or the cost. The rate structure is set so that the unprofitable departments are carried by the profitable departments. Departments where charges typically do not cover costs include obstetric units, emergency rooms, and small specialty units such as pediatrics. Obviously when third-party payers reimburse charges rather than real costs in the unprofitable departments, costs must be carried by other departments. Similarly, when the profitable departments only are reimbursed according to the real costs, they can no longer compensate for unprofitable departments. Hence the basic rate structure must be high enough to compensate for reimbursement plans which work to the detriment of the institution.

On the other hand there are pressures to keep the basic rate structure as low as possible. One such pressure is created by local competition. If the rate is such that potential customers elect another institution, low occupancy will cause a loss of funds. Further, approximately half of the states in the United States have rate review boards which must approve any increase in rates. Since these boards are designed to hold down health care costs, increases require justification before they are approved. It is to be expected that the number of rate review mechanisms in the states will continue to increase.

Funding of departments that operate at a deficit is a real problem for health care finance. One solution, where there are several small hospitals in a community, is for each one to "specialize" in offering a potentially unprofitable department. Hence, three hospitals in a given town might agree that only one would offer emergency services, only one an obstetric department, and only one a pediatric unit. In this way, these specialized services might each have a large enough population to increase economies of scale. Further, each would have only one potential deficit department instead of three.

Such a solution is not possible in an institution which serves a population in a geographically isolated district with no other health institutions close enough to "share services." Further, even where a sharing plan is possible, some communities have made a political issue out of the closing of a local emergency or obstetric department, claiming that the extra time to reach the alternate institution endangers lives. The health care institution is forced to draw the line between good community relations and cost effectiveness.

Adjustment of financial outlay to physicians' demands is another problem for the financial officer and for the chief executive officer. Understandably, physicians desire that the institution where they work have all the latest equipment. Where advanced equipment improves the health care outcomes, it is to be expected that physicians will apply heavy pressures for the purchase of such equipment. That pressure may include the economic threat to "take one's patients and go to another institution." This problem is accelerated in an era of rapid technological advancement, where equipment is technically obsolete before it is either old or fully depreciated.

This is an interesting area in which to compare the political clout of nursing and medicine. Nursing, comparatively, is powerless to make its demands for nursing equipment (or manpower) heard; unlike medicine, nursing cannot threaten to take its patients elsewhere. This fact of life explains why nurses so often are denied a financial investment that would help numerous patients in order that physicians may have some piece of equipment that can help only a few. Decisions are often based on power rather than upon logic or an assessment to total health care outcomes of clients.

Management of cash flow is another financial problem for the health care institution. Cash flow becomes a problem because the health care institution is slow to collect on its accounts receivable (patient bills). Private insurers and government payers both delay payment. Even where a patient is paying independently, he is likely to arrange timed payments. Hence, money is slow to come in, but employees still want to be paid on time and suppliers are not happy to wait for their payments.

Another problem for the financial officer is to determine a depreciation strategy that will be financially advantageous to the institution. Straight-line depreciation allows for the same amount of depreciation every year until an item has been fully depreciated. Accelerated depreciation allows for a larger deduction in the first years. Depending upon the third-party payment arrangements, one plan may be preferable over the other. A typical solution is to arrive at a mixed strategy which reflects the types of coverage held by the average patient population. For example, what is allowable under a Medicaid or Medicare plan may be different from what is allowable under private third-party payment. The depreciation strategy would reflect the type of payment used by the institution's clients.

While the nurse executive is seldom involved in finances beyond the budgeting of her division, it is important that she have an appreciation of the overall financial structure and problems of the health care institution. For greater detail concerning hospital finance, see the bibliography of this chapter.

COST CONTAINMENT

Cost containment is a major concern of all health care institutions today. The expense of health care in the nation has risen to a level that is unacceptable to everyone. Indeed, the cost containment effort may be seen as running counter to a highly esteemed value in nursing: optimal nursing care for everyone. Such optimal nursing care or total health care has a high price tag, and nursing as a profession must reconcile its ideal with the reality of the world in which it practices. The average nurse must be educated to consider health as one value among many. Since present nursing education systems so often function from the perspective of ideal care, it is up to the nurse executive to educate her staff as to the place of health (and nursing care) as one value among many, competing for scarce national resources.

In the past, there was little incentive to control cost in the health care system. Health care was and still is illness-based, costing far more than a prevention-based system. Until recently, third-party payers usually would pay the bills without questioning the cost or source of the rate setting. Finally, public service institutions accumulated power in relation to the size of their budgets. Hence the organization that spent more became more powerful. The same was true intraorganizationally: the department which spent more money received more money to spend the next year.

All of this has changed in our present economy. Third-party payers, especially the government, have begun placing ceilings on what they will pay. Fear of a federal takeover increases the voluntary efforts at cost containment, and external monitoring—in effect or impending—is on the rise. Cost containment efforts have followed the ever-increasing, exponentially-rising costs of health care. What are the reasons for the increasing costs?

Among the many conditions blamed for the increased costs of health care, are increasing wages for health workers, often due to unionization; increasing cost of equipment and supplies, with inflationary costs of the society passed on to the health care institution in its purchases; and increasingly expensive and complex technology, with lifesaving but very complex equipment requiring more highly skilled, and better paid, technologists. Other causes of increased costs include a steady increase in patient acuity. Institutionalized patients are sicker than the patients who populated institutions even ten years ago. Sicker people are surviving longer because of advanced technological measures. Further, utilization review systems dismiss patients from institutions earlier, leaving the institutionalized clientele cumulatively more acutely ill.

Ironically, the increased attention to

utilization of beds has produced some increases in cost by emptying out beds—sending patients home sooner. When this occurs in an institution or community which provided too many beds, these beds are not filled. Instead, the beds stand empty, even though a full complement of staff may be paid to tend to the unit. Ironically, then, in an "overbedded" community, utilization review may cost rather than save money —and it is a fact that many hospitals in this nation presently have a surplus of beds.

Increased administrative costs also spiral health costs upward. Some of the increased cost here is due to the expense of meeting reporting requirements of regulatory bodies. Complaints concerning the "cost of compliance" are rampant in health care institutions; requirements, especially federal ones, may be contradictory and confusing as well as requiring similar data to be collected and formulated in diverse (time-expending) ways—an expensive requirement.

When an institution attempts to control costs, nursing inevitably will be involved. Since the nursing division may constitute 60 to 80 percent of an institution's budget, it will necessarily be one place where the chief executive officer of the organization will seek to make cuts. Also, since the major part of a nursing budget is salaries, it is likely that cuts will involve staffing patterns. Some nurse executives assume that they have been singled out for financial cuts because they direct a "female" division. In truth, in this instance, nursing may be the only division large enough to contribute substantially to cost savings on a large scale, and this is probably the reason the nursing division is selected for serious cutbacks.

It is ironic that the present era of cost containment occurs simultaneously with a demand for improved quality control. While there is some truth that nurses can "practice smarter" in the same length of time, it also is true that smaller and smaller nursing staffs cannot continue to give better and better care. Sooner or later, staff cutbacks are reflected in the quality of care given. For this reason, it is important that nurse executives identify the levels of care that can be given for given resources (manpower and other) in order to relate quality logically to cost. This subject matter will be addressed later in this chapter.

What are some of the ways in which an institution and a nursing division may contain costs? Several suggestions at the institutional level already have been given: where possible eliminate unprofitable departments, share expensive equipment such as CAT scanners between institutions, and plan realistic levels of care rather than idealistic ones. Steps should be taken to ensure that beds remain filled; often this may involve converting excess beds to other types of care, such as nursing home, convalescent care. Managerial control systems should be improved. At one time, it was suspected that inefficient management was a great source of excessive cost, but ironically, when the specialists came in to dictate "good management" to those already in the hospital industry, costs often increased rather than decreased. One managerial tactic that is effective is the conversion to a multi-institution corporation; when a number of health care institutions join together, they achieve economies of scale by common purchasing, standardization of operating procedures, and sharing of equipment, facilities, and even personnel.

Cost Containment and Nursing Personnel

Within the nursing division, many personnel factors should be reviewed for cost containment. One is staff education. Whereas staff development directly related to job performance can be justified as a valid investment, it is difficult to justify an institution paying for education that is not related to the employee's present job but instead prepares the employee to advance to a higher level of functioning and a higher salary. The nursing division must question whether the patient and the health care institution can afford to assume the burden of cost of a nurse's education when she will be the direct beneficiary reaping personal benefits from that advanced education.

Nursing divisions also must streamline their evaluation and control systems. If a patient classification system which takes four minutes of the head nurse's time daily gives information almost as complete as a system which requires 20 minutes, it may be reasonable to settle for a little less information at a lot less cost. Outmoded "routines" also should be streamlined; they must be justified if they are to be retained.

Nursing management must be careful to maintain its managerial flexibility in negotiating labor contracts. If a nurse executive gives up the right to move nurses from one unit to another, she is necessarily increasing her personnel costs. Expensive management practices such as shift differentials, extra money for critical care, and use of agency nurses will have to be examined also. Obviously, where institutions compete with each other for nurses, these practices cannot be controlled unless all the nurse executives of an area mutually agree to modify practices in their respective institutions.

Major savings in the nursing division can result from improved staffing practices. It often "takes money to save money"; an adequate and well-supervised orientation period for personnel costs more than does a hasty orientation, for example, but the higher investment is usually recovered in higher retention of personnel. It is no secret that inadequate orientation followed by too much responsibility too soon is a major cause of premature resignation. And turnover and recruitment costs are a major expense in nursing. When staffing is too short, another false economy occurs. When staff are unable to "cover" normal deviations in the workload because they have been pared too thin, then the cost of overtime and agency replacement staff is far greater than the amount "saved" by inadequate staffing. And, of course, such staffing also leads to resignations and increased recruitment and orientation costs.

Poor management is always expensive. Keeping employees who do not give a full day's work for a day's pay increases costs because more staff are needed. It is also wasteful to pay for credentials rather than performance; in a cost-conscious environment, there is little justification for paying a baccalaureate nurse more than a diploma nurse *if* her performance is evaluated to be identical.

Careful examination of the policies on illness and tardiness can produce cost savings. Are the policies intelligent? Are they enforced? Or is a lot of work time abused by employees? Time is money in the nursing division. Meetings also can be a source of great expense. Are 20 people put on a committee when five could do the job adequately? Hours of time sitting in committees cost money, especially when the committee members are professionals receiving high salaries.

Unfortunately, most of the measures of cost containment suggested thus far are not those which produce easily visible results. Especially where nursing services are included in room rate, savings on staff elements may not be "visible." It is up to the nurse executive to illustrate the savings made by good personnel management. Though it may take a lot of work, she must be able to show how good orientation, adequate staffing, and firm enforcement of policies save money.

Savings on personnel costs can easily be greater than savings on materiel since the greater part of the nursing budget is spent in salaries. Unfortunately it is easier to identify savings on equipment and supplies and easier to attach a specific dollar amount to them.

Cost Containment in Nursing Materiel

Although savings may not be so great on materiel (equipment and supplies) as on personnel, there is still enough potential to merit the concern of the nurse executive.

One major source of loss is theft by staff—nursing, medical, or other. The nurse executive, therefore, will want to investigate her systems for management of equipment and supplies. Is accountability built in? Is it possible to determine who has missing equipment? What accounting systems monitor supplies? Do these systems function so as to protect supplies without frustrating staff who must deal with the systems in getting the needed supplies?

Often it is useful to facilitate discount purchase by staff, through the institution, of those items which might otherwise be stolen. Scissors, stethoscopes, and sphygmomanometers may head the list. Each institution has a good idea of its primary theft items. The systems which guard against theft should focus on development of fail-safe systems for management of these supplies. Even here, common sense must reign. The reader will not want to follow the example of the nurse executive who instituted such tight procedures that nothing was stolen, but under whose theft-prevention system hundreds of hours of staff time went into filling out vouchers and reports on equipment and supplies. One must always be sure that the costs of administering such a system actually are less than the loss that could be incurred by thefts if the systems did not exist.

It is also worthwhile not to mistake pettiness over trivial expenses for economy or frugality. If staff perceive that changes have more to do with "cheapness" than frugality, they are more than capable of finding ways to subvert the purported savings. Consider the following sad example of petty economy. The chief executive officer of a city hospital was making rounds one night and observed policemen drinking coffee in the emergency room. He inquired about the practice and was told that the nurses "keep a pot on" for the police in the late evening and early morning hours. He calculated that this practice was costing the institution several hundreds of dollars yearly, and insisted that it be stopped immediately. The policemen, who

had enjoyed this "stop" on their rounds, ceased to patronize the emergency room. Indeed, they heard of the executive decision and were so insulted they took police-related emergencies to another hospital thereafter. Not only did this cut down on emergency room cases, but word soon got out that emergency room nurses were on "alone" at the night hours. Two assaults occurred on emergency room nurses, followed by two resignations and two requests for immediate change of assignment. The administrator, then, was forced to hire two private guards to cover the night hours. In this case he "saved" a few hundred dollars on coffee and ended up paying two full-time salaries for two new employees—guards. The nursing division also had the expense of replacing the two nurses who resigned before the guards were hired.

In summary, the nursing division can save money on personnel and materiel by some careful review of its systems. It may be useful to hire a systems analyst if no one on the staff is adroit at systems analysis. The logistic systems of the divisions may be examined for streamlining and standardizing where economies of scale may be gained. The nurse executive should not be overconcerned with every minor divisional system; she should concentrate her inquiry on the big systems, those where there is potential for significant savings. No system is really fail-safe, but many systems can be improved with a little work. Sometimes employees are good analysts of systems, and most institutions find that a small bounty for cost-saving ideas is worth the effort.

The nurse executive also must relate cost savings carefully to budgeting. If the frugal department is "punished" by having its next year's budget lowered by the amount saved, while the wastrel department is "rewarded" by continuing to receive a high budget, all motivation for cost containment will soon be lost.

The nurse executive will want to examine the budgetary system of the institution to see if the procedures encourage or discourage cost saving. For example, a nurse executive may be buying some equipment (perhaps bedside tables) in small numbers, month by month, because she can slip them into her operational budget in this manner. However, if the budgetary system would allow her to make one major purchase in a year, she might be able to get a big discount on the tables, a discount that is unavailable if she purchases them a few at a time. Similarly, the nurse executive may find that she is "waiting" to purchase an expensive item in a particular budget period. This, again, is wasteful if an increase in price is to be expected and the money for the item has already been budgeted.

The nurse executive must use sense in selecting equipment and supplies. Many people advocate looking outside of the usual hospital suppliers for items such as furniture because of the significant savings that can be made this way. The nurse executive will need to be very careful in going outside of the usual suppliers, however, for many items simply are not made for the hard wear equipment and furnishings receive in a hospital setting. It is important to learn to specify exactly what is needed in supplies so that a purchasing department, in its own attempts to save, does not buy an inferior product for the nursing division or one that does not do the task for which the item is being purchased. The nursing division and the purchasing department cooperate for both cost saving and appropriate purchases.

NURSING DIVISION BUDGETING

Budgeting will be examined first as it concerns the nursing division alone, then as it concerns the total health care division, and finally, as it related to other fiscal activities of the organization.

Generating and controlling a divisional budget is a major responsibility of the nurse executive. The budget is a major operating document of the nursing division. It can best be thought of as a third-level statement of the division's activities. The first level is the statement of basic objectives of the nursing division and the elaboration of those objectives into departmental and unit objectives. The second-level statement is the translation of those objectives into specific, identified activities that will accomplish the objectives. The third-level statement, the budget, is the financial description of those activities.

To predict budget expenses for any anticipated period of time, the nurse executive needs to identify clearly the present activities of her division, the activities she plans to institute during the projected financial period, and those activities she plans to delete during the projected period. The planned activities may be partly dependent upon events occasioned by others: the opening of a new patient unit, a new surgical physicians' group in the community, or a medical research project that will require extra nursing hours. As a starting point the nurse executive will require the financial records from prior financial periods as a basis for planning. Budget planning can only be as good as the institution's accounting system permits.

The nurse executive needs to identify her cost centers. A cost center is the smallest functional unit for which cost control and accountability can be assigned under the existing accounting system. Ideally each separate functional unit in the nursing division should have its separate account for expenses. For example, a nursing service budget should make it possible to charge each separate patient floor for the actual supplies used on that single unit. Logically, a head nurse cannot be held responsible for costs on her unit unless they are identified and separated from costs accrued by other nursing units.

Some institutions put out financial statements in which they allot costs by formula rather than by fact. They may buy supplies in bulk quantity and distribute the cost of these items among nursing units based upon bed count or patient occupancy figures. Such distribution of costs by formula does not reflect the actual use of such supplies on the units. Thus, financial statements showing nursing units as cost centers do not necessarily indicate that the nursing unit is in fact the cost center.

Accounting objectives and nursing objectives often conflict on establishment of cost centers. For example, an accounting department may be very willing to make a ten-crib nursery a separate cost center (because its supplies are different from those of other cost centers); the same accounting department may resist separating accounts for several 30-bed medical units that use similar supplies. On items such as this, the needs of the nurse executive for appropriate management have to be weighed against the actual capacities of the institution's accounting department.

The problem of traditionally established cost centers failing to coincide with management centers makes financial management of a large division extremely difficult. To match accounting cost centers to management centers is usually a prime objective of a nurse executive. Where such matching requires a change in accounting systems, the nurse executive must be aware that the change requires increased manpower hours on the part of the accounting department and may require the keeping of double books until the new system is firmly established. Such a change is a long-term project. Where cost centers have been made to coincide with management centers, however, fiscal responsibility can be more easily shared with lower nursing management levels.

Divisional Income and Expenses

Most nursing budgets are simply expense budgets. Such budgets reflect only what the nursing division spends; they fail to indicate the income resulting from that department. This is because most nursing income is undifferentiated from other income and is "hidden" in the so-called room rate. The psychology of this form of budgeting is disastrous because other managers and often nursing managers themselves come to think of the nursing division as non-income pro-

ducing—in contrast to the X ray department or pharmacy, or other departments where patient fees are evident. Suggestions to put nursing on the income, as well as the expenditure budget, will be made later in this chapter.

The nursing budget usually is a line item budget, with items budgeted according to specific departments or units. Another form of budgeting—planned program budgeting—to be discussed later in this chapter, allocates expenses per activity or project rather than by department or division. In determining the content of a nursing budget, it is not feasible to rely merely on a review of items that seem to belong to the nursing budget. All items that are in fact presently charged to the division must be identified. Since most accounting departments group like expenditures in their financial statements, the nurse executive needs to learn what individual items are included in each grouping. There often is no clear-cut logic as to which items are charged against nursing accounts and which are charged against other departments, so this step of identifying each separate charge item is unavoidable. Much equipment, for example, is shared by nursing and medicine, but usually only one of these departments bears purchase and upkeep expenses.

Clear explanation of all line-by-line content items also makes the nurse executive aware of expenses that she may not have anticipated, such as depreciation costs, service contracts, and in-house service charges. Once she has a clear understanding of those items charged to her budget, the nurse executive can plan for reallocation of expenses to other divisions if needed. At least she will be able to budget adequate funds to meet the demands upon her division.

The Manpower Budget

In generating a budget, most institutions project costs of activities in three categories: manpower costs, operational costs, and capital expenses. As mentioned earlier, the manpower, or personnel, budget is usually the largest single expense in a nursing budget. Planning this budget requires determining the number of persons needed in each job category for the planned fiscal period.

A baseline for this prediction can be established by first determining if the present manpower is adequate for the current divisional activities. The first step in this process is to attain an exact accounting of employees on the nursing payroll. Only persons directly responsible to the nursing division should be on this account. If necessary, once the nurse executive knows which employees are charged to her division, she can adjust this figure on the basis of the planned alterations in divisional activities for the proposed fiscal period.

Adjustments in personnel may include changes in the manpower mix (number of persons in each job category) as well as absolute changes in the total number of hired persons. For control of staffing during the proposed fiscal period, the nurse executive will need to know if she is to work by position control or by budgeted expense control. In the first instance, the positions identified in the budget serve as the criterion for hiring of new personnel. In the second instance, the nurse executive is free to change positions if she desires, but she is restricted to the original budgeted total salary figure.

Indicators for needed adjustment in manpower in nursing service would include such items as increasing or decreasing rate of patient occupancy, change in general complexity of patient cases handled, functional changes in role expectations, or addition of new departments and functions.

The nurse executive who is new to budget-making is cautioned to allot extra manpower hours for vacations, illness, education time, and overtime. It is a good idea to review the overtime of the prior financial period. If it is a large expense, then overtime cost may need to be weighed against the cost of creating some new positions. Usually three types of staffing need funding: regular staffing, anticipated replacement staffing, and emergen-

cy situation replacement or incrementing of staffing. (See Chapter 8.)

Besides actual salary expenses, what employee fringe benefits are charged to the division? In most institutions a formula using a set percentage of the gross salary is used to calculate fringe benefits. Anticipated increments in wages also must be calculated for the proposed financial period. The personnel department usually can supply the nurse executive with estimates for both fringe benefit costs and anticipated raises.

Employee turnover must be considered in estimating manpower costs. Recruitment costs such as advertising and agency fees often are charged to the division seeking to hire new personnel. Orientation costs also should be calculated, including sufficient funds to allow for the new employee to be hired and inducted into the position before the employee he or she is replacing leaves. Where such "overlap" funds are not available, the new employee suffers. Eliminating overlap funds usually is a false economy because poor orientation and rushed assumption of new duties are the primary source of premature withdrawal of the new employee. To lose an employee shortly after investing both recruitment and orientation costs in his hiring is poor management.

Some nursing divisions depend heavily upon graduating classes of new nurses for position replacements. Here again, there may be a need for "overlap" funds, for it may be necessary to hire nurses at the time of their graduation in order to have them available later, to replace staff lost for various reasons. If the nurse executive has no leeway and cannot hire these nurses when they graduate, it is likely that they will not be available later in the year, when she needs replacements.

Often the nurse executive builds flexibility into her personnel budget by requesting funds that she would need to cover all positions in her staffing plan. If some periods then occur when some positions actually are vacant, this will build in additional funds that may be used for overlap. When, instead, she is on a tight position control system, she may lose funds that were allotted to positions that were unfilled. When possible, the nurse executive will want to control these monies. Some institutions decrease the nursing manpower budget by the percentage of funds not spent the previous year because positions were unfilled. If the nurse executive budgets this way, there is no way that she will be able to fill all positions were that to become possible.

The nurse executive should inquire as to where funds for unemployment compensation are charged: the nursing division may have to pay these costs if an employee is discharged rather than resigning.

In planning a manpower budget, it is useful to work with estimates for each class of worker. Except in a very small institution, the time spent in calculating raises specifically for each employee presently at the institution is unnecessary work. Such exact calculation for the coming year is fruitless because there will be unexpected resignations and changes within the staff. A budget requires only a gross estimate. It is important, however, to know the turnover rate for each class of employee. One projects the turnover for the coming year because newly hired personnel are likely to be hired at a lower pay rate than received by the longer-tenured staff whom they replace.

The Operational Budget

The operational budget finances the ongoing needs for equipment and supplies to complete the divisional activities. Most institutions have a financial cut-off point above which purchases of equipment and supplies are termed *capital* instead of operational expenditures. The nurse executive will need to know which budget, the operational or the capital, should be used when bulk purchase of like items presents a total cost over the cut-off point on items that would not individually be capital expenditures. For example, if the nurse executive plans to buy ten dressing carts at $100 each, she will need to know whether to consider them ten items for the operational budget or one $1,000 item for the capital budget.

The starting point for operational budget planning is review of the cost of the division's activities during its last fiscal period. Next, projected increases, decreases, or alterations in divisional activities are calculated. In addition to actual changes in the specific activities, the influence of technological or methodological changes on the use of operational supplies and equipment is reviewed.

Planned changes in manpower will affect the need for selected supplies and equipment as well as changes in the anticipated number of patients. It is a good idea for the nurse executive to review the major grants and contracts in effect in the institution for the upcoming budget period. Often physicians (and sometimes nurses) write and receive funding for grants which have failed to take into account their effect on nursing division costs. It is not atypical for a physician to fail to calculate in his grant proposal the expenses of additional nursing equipment or nursing hours that will be needed to carry out the work to be funded by the grant. If the institution is one with major grant or contract funding, it is a good idea for the nursing division to have the right of review on all grants to prevent just such miscalculations concerning the impact of projects on nursing costs.

In addition to reviewing the cost of operations during the last financial period, it is important that the nurse executive identify each operational item in her past accounts to preclude mistakes of omission or commission in future planning. There is usually no way to predict logically which charges are made directly to the patient and which to the nursing unit. Similarly, nursing support equipment may be charged either to the nursing division or to the supplying division. The nurse executive must find out what is, and what is not, charged to her division.

Among the many problems in budgeting is coordination with the medical staff. Do new equipment requests from medicine come out of the nursing budget? Physicians often request purchases when new products or conveniences come on the market. Such items are frequently used by both the physician and nurse, so there must be a clear understanding of the budgetary procedures for such items. Unanticipated changes in physicians' modes of therapy also can tax the nursing budget and may affect the manpower budget as well as the operational budget.

Nursing not only interacts with medicine but with many other divisions and departments. Changes in management of equipment and supplies, for example, can affect operational and manpower budgets of nursing. Therefore, interdivisional discussion and comparison of objectives and projected activities for the planned financial period are essential.

Many unseen elements enter into the operational budget. Inflation is perhaps the most insidious. Anticipated price changes usually are available from the institution's purchasing agent or from product salesmen. Another unseen cost is depreciation. How is it handled in the institution? Also to be considered are repair and renovation costs, both those handled within the institution and those for services and contracts with outside agencies. Repair contracts for intensive care and coronary care equipment, for example, are major expenses. Are these items charged to the nursing division? The nurse executive must know.

Besides ongoing supply costs, there are such sporadic costs as recreation (Christmas parties, retirement teas), consultation and education fees, accreditation expenses, and travel expenses. Administrative overhead also should be added, including such indirect costs as plant maintenance, heat, light, housekeeping, and general administration. Many institutions add administrative overhead later to the total organizational budget, instead of calculating it by division. Again, the nurse executive will have to know if she is accountable for overhead in her budget.

Finally, even where equipment is donated or originally purchased by another division, there are costs of upkeep to consider. A simple "gift" piece of equipment may cost hundreds of dollars a year if it uses supplies and needs servicing.

The Capital Budget

The capital budget is the projection of costs for major purchases or projects. Each institution has its own definition of what qualifies as a capital expense. Two common criteria are that the item be above a certain baseline cost, and that the expected lifespan of the item be longer than a set time period. For example, an institution might decide that all items above $200 in cost with a lifespan of at least three years are capital expenses. Under that definition, a $300 purchase of admission kits expected to last one year would not be considered a capital purchase whereas a $250 resuscitation cart, with a seven-year life expectancy, would be considered a capital purchase. Capital items usually include major architectural renovations as well as discrete items.

One major problem the nurse executive has in preparing a capital budget for a technologically oriented environment is the inability to predict what new major equipment is coming on the market during the projected financial period. This problem may be averted somewhat if the nurse executive is allowed to budget for unspecified items or if items originally budgeted can be "traded off" for unanticipated technologically advanced equipment if it becomes available and is preferred over the original item budgeted.

Capital purchases can involve unseen costs. Operational and manpower budgets will require adjustment if planned capital purchases involve special upkeep, supplies or man hours. In addition, projected inflation must be considered when pricing items that will not be purchased for six months to a year. Either the accounting department or the purchasing department usually can advise what percent inflation to expect on individual capital items.

In preparing a capital budget, the nurse

executive is required to document the need for most major items. Where the purchase will partly pay for itself over a period of time (because it will mean decreased man hours or use of less supplies), the potential savings is calculated and included in documentation. For example, if the nurse executive wants "nurse server" cabinets in every patient room on a unit undergoing renovation, part of her supporting documentation should include an estimate of anticipated nursing hours saved by this convenience.

How purchase requests from physicians are handled affects both the capital budget and the operational budget. The chief problem here is that physicians are likely to request capital items during, rather than prior to, the planned fiscal period. It is sometimes difficult to get a large staff of entrepreneurial physicians to plan ahead as a body. The difficulty is accentuated when new items appear on the market at unexpected times.

Relating the Nursing and the Institutional Budgets

Typically, the health care institution has several types of budgets prepared simultaneously. These include the operating budget, the capital budget, the cash budget, the balance sheet, and the master budget. Nursing typically participates in the operating and capital budgets. The *operating budget* includes the revenue budget and the expense budget. The expense budget has two components: personnel (manpower) and operational (equipment and supplies). The nursing division usually completes both parts of the expense budget, but seldom submits a revenue budget.

The *cash budget* deals only with resources that are available or required in monies. It balances cash disbursements against cash receipts. The cash budget does not consider resources such as land, buildings, or other items which would have to undergo conversion into financial form. The *balance sheet*, however, includes all assets and all liabilities.

Here, assets include cash available, buildings and equipment owned, and portfolios of investment. Liabilities might include debt service, payroll owed, capital layouts, and outstanding debts. The master budget is the summary of all these budgets taken together—operating, capital, cash budgets, together with the balance sheet.

It is important that all divisions come together to discuss their proposed divisional budgets before a total budget is prepared, because actions in one division may have an effect on planned budgets of other divisions. The final summarized budget is taken to the trustees of the institution for approval.

Financial Control

Once a budget has been approved and implemented, it becomes a control system. Reports are distributed to each division periodically, usually monthly or four-weekly, comparing actual to budgeted figures. In this way the nurse executive can quickly determine if she is "on target," overspending, or not spending available funds. Where cost centers and managerial centers coincide, departmental or unit budget reports are shared with the subordinate managers responsible for these areas. These managers should be able to explain deviations from the expected expenditures. Not all overages are indices of poor management. For example, an increase in patient occupancy figures will increase expenditures. (Of course, this increase in patients is paying for itself in increased revenue.) Nevertheless, it is the responsibility of the nurse executive to track budget deviations and to have a clear explanation for these deviations.

In some instances, funds may be moved from one line item category to another to "cover" overexpenditures. The nurse executive needs to know what manipulations are allowable within her budget. The ideal budget is flexible enough to allow such movement of funds from one category to another. Since a budget is a prediction, it is not logical to expect absolute correspondence between the actual and the predicted expenditures.

An Alternate System: Planned Program Budgeting

Planned program budgeting is an alternative to the line item budget. With this method, every service program is viewed as a separate entity, with a separate budget cutting across traditional divisional lines. For example, an emergency room service would be one program, and its budget would include items previously charged to nursing, to medicine, to materials management, and to various other divisions.

The objective of a planned program budget is to put an accurate price tag on each program so that a realistic comparison of cost and income can be calculated. The institution can then accurately identify the true costs of any specific service program. A primary advantage of planned program budgeting is evident when funds are limited. In typical budget cutting of the traditional divisional budget, a nursing division (or any other division) simply is given less money with which to manage the division's proposed activities. The nurse executive, then, is forced to decide which activities to curtail. Her ability to make such decisions, however, is closely tied to the planned activities of other divisions. For example, how far can the nurse executive reduce the staffing in the operating rooms without impairing the activities of the surgical staff?

When heavy cuts are demanded in a divisional nursing budget, departments having minimal interaction with other divisions become necessary targets. Departments such as inservice education are hit hardest because their involvement in patient care is less direct. Typically, budget cuts reduce the quality of nursing service or nursing education.

The planned program budget avoids this sacrifice of quality. All programs offered by the institution are budgeted separately and given priorities. Then, if budget cuts are required, total programs of low priority are eliminated to assure adequate funding for the quality programs that remain.

Planned program budgeting is not without its faults. Computation of salaries of individuals who work in several "programs" is tedious. Calculating program costs is also difficult and often requires exacting care.

Whatever the budgeting and accounting systems of the institution, the nurse executive must recognize her responsibility for careful fiscal management. The nursing service executive usually manages the biggest division of her institution. In large institutions she may have accountants within the nursing division to help her in financial planning and control. In smaller institutions she may not have this advantage, but may still be responsible for managing millions of dollars. The nurse executive cannot use her professionally oriented education as an excuse for ignorance in financial management. Acceptance of an administrative position implies acceptance of the financial management responsibilities inherent in that role.

COSTING OUT NURSING SERVICE

When the nursing division cannot account for the monies earned by the provision of nursing services, as discussed earlier, the nurse executive lacks the power and influence which come with "paying one's own way." That nursing often is viewed as non-income producing is ironic since most patients are hospitalized either because their condition demands nursing or because their medical therapy will put them in a condition demanding nursing care. If nursing were not what they most need, most patients would be cared for in physician offices or in their homes rather than in hospitals. In fact, nursing is responsible for much institutional income; the problem is that nursing service is included with other services in the "room rate." Thus the nurse executive is at a distinct disadvantage, for she cannot identify specifically the income attributable to nursing services.

Several institutions and organizations are now working on differentiating the income earned by nursing services (and by other services such as the hotel function, housekeeping, dietary department). This movement not only will allow the contribution of nursing to become evident, but it also will enable the patient to pay for only those services extended to him. At present it is the case that the relatively well patient "pays" for the nursing services of his very ill roommate, for they both pay the same room rate. Costing out of nursing services would make possible separate billing for services received.

Several principles underlie the notion of separate billing. First is the idea that actual cost should be reflected in fees charged. This does not mean an identical cost or fee figure, but a proportional one. Legitimate management control of costs requires knowledge of real costs; once known, the real costs become the basis for fee setting. Another principle of separate billing is the notion that departments should be made self-supporting, that if patients pay according to costs of their care, then departments will be self-supporting. This principle, although overtly sound, will create some social problems. For example, the cost of the birth of a child, if the real costs of nursing services were completely itemized, would be prohibitive without insurance coverage. And eventually maternity care insurance might become prohibitively expensive were separate billing to become a reality. Such problems would pertain for other selected departments as well. Although such problems do not diminish the value of billing according to services rendered, they simply indicate that the whole financial structure of health care must be involved in a changing fee system.

Separate billing assumes that nursing care can be quantified in ways that connect care and cash. To date, there have been two major approaches to this task. In the first, specific billing is charged for each nursing act. This method encourages task-oriented nursing because the nurse constantly must identify her "tasks done for a patient" and record them for billing purposes. The accuracy of this system is great—if nurses actually do the required recording—but it presents a problem as an administrative system: billing per nursing task requires a mammoth amount of "bookwork" in keeping track of charges. Not only would billing per task be time consuming, but the record systems would be extensive and costly. For this reason, the second method of specific billing seeks to find a way to reflect the amount of nursing care given without specifically tracking and recording each nursing task. This seems to be a logical and feasible way to associate nursing costs with patient fees. Two distinct approaches have been devised to accomplish this task. The first, used by Holbrook at Montana Deaconess[1], utilizes a patient classification system in which average costs of nursing have been associated with each patient category. This represents a logical and simplified way to assess the costs of nursing services, especially in institutions which already have a patient classification system.

The original costs may be determined by a study of actual nursing tasks, relating those tasks back to nursing time and salary rates in the institution. A simpler system than timing and costing out actual tasks is a mathematical extrapolation from the comparative length and level of nursing care for each patient category. An accountant working with the nursing division will be able to figure out a system which takes present fees and redistributes them over patient categories.

A second method of associating costs with fees has been devised by Wood at Massachusetts Eye and Ear Infirmary[2]. In this system, costs are associated with diagnoses and expected trajectories of care required for each diagnosis. In this system it is possible to predict the added care needs of a first postoperative day as compared, for example, to a third postoperative day. This system differentiates all costs: ancillary services, dietary, laundry, medical supplies, nursing care and physician care. The professional services are calculated based on clinical care units of measurement. Wood uses the PETO unit for nursing services[3]. In this system the care trajectories are calculated, so that one can say that a patient typically uses so many PETO units on admission day, so many the day before cataract surgery, and so forth. In this way "case norms" have been worked out for every diagnosis seen at the Eye and Ear Infirmary.

Both the Holbrook and the Wood systems have advantages and disadvantages. In the Holbrook system or any other system relying on patient classification, the system is as fair as the classification is accurate. In such a system, one question to be answered is how often the patient is to be classified. Each shift? Each day? Obviously, a patient condition can change in one day or even during a single shift. The Holbrook system happens to use four patient categories and two classification times daily. The system derived in a given hospital would utilize the patient classification system extant there, and a hospital might decide to classify patients more or less frequently than the Holbrook system. A disadvantage of the system is the need for daily, or even more frequent, patient assessment. An advantage of the system is that it does not assume that a patient with a given diagnosis will be in a given state of health.

The Wood system has the advantage of avoiding the Holbrook system's frequent categorizations of all patients, but it has the difficulty of assigning costs for a patient whose illness does not follow a typical trajectory. It is easy to see that such a system might work well in the eye and ear infirmary setting where it is likely that most cataract surgery patients will follow similar patterns of entry, surgery, and recuperation. When the same principle is applied to the cases in a general hospital, it becomes more complex. Not all recuperating patients after a cholecystectomy, for example, have similar care needs nor similar convalescence trajec-

tories, thus a way is needed to vary daily PETO units based upon individual patient responses and needs. Also, the number of possible diagnoses, for which trajectories would need to be worked out, would increase greatly and many patients might combine one or more diagnoses. Nevertheless, the system still has great possibilities if a way can be found to insert differences into the fee structure.

The reader is advised to become familiar with both the Holbrook and Wood system as fee-setting protocols. Table 18-1 compares these and other potential methodologies for costing out nursing services.

Separate billing for nursing services has much to recommend it. First, it enables the nursing profession to identify in concrete financial terms its contribution to the total health institution enterprise. Being able to identify its contribution will enable nursing to justify further its claims on the resources produced by that contribution. Further, association of fees with costs will allow for a new level in nursing accountability. If a patient knows what nursing services he is paying for, he will hold the institution accountable for providing these services. This accountability also gives the nursing management the power to demand the resources it needs to deliver the promised care.

Association of fees and actual costs will force nursing management to be realistic about what levels of nursing care can be delivered at what cost. This realism can only work to the advantage of the nursing profession in an era when many expect nursing to keep delivering more and better nursing at ever-decreasing cost—an unrealistic expectation at best. Such a realistic assessment of the care delivery system may result in different levels of nursing care being derived. An institution might offer Plan A (basic, safe, no-frills nursing), Plan B (this might be defined in terms of number of hours per day or in terms of quality care, or both), and Plan C (which might include finest quality plus the "amenities" which make a hospital stay more comfortable). Ultimately, in-

Table 18-1.   Systems for Costing Out of Nursing Services

	Massachusetts Eye and Ear (Wood)	Montana Deaconess (Holbrook)	Other Possible Systems
Source of the new costs	Mathematical derivation from old costs	Mathematical derivation from old costs	Actual cost studies of nursing hours and equipment and supplies used
Basic assumptions	Nursing is reflected in time	Nursing is reflected in time	Nursing could be reflected in both time and level of personnel; intensity also could enter calculations.
Conversion system	1. PETO units cumulated into total nursing time per day in a trajectory for a given diagnosis 2. Patient charged by the "norm" of nursing units per the "day" of the trajectory in which he fits via his diagnosis and therapy	1. Four-level patient classification system used twice daily 2. Average nursing time associated with each level 3. Costs determined by multiplying level times average hours per level, cumulating per hospitalization	Any system could be devised to equate tasks or classes to time required for the tasks or classes.
Criterion	Medical diagnosis and/or medical/surgical therapy	Level of nursing care required	Nursing diagnosis as a third option; patient acuity as a fourth option
Relationship of criterion and conversion system	Daily nursing norms calculated for each medical/surgical entity based on average patient response trajectories	Nursing norms per patient classification calculated on a twice daily actual patient assessment	Could include billing per actual tasks, or could combine a classification system with "add-on" cost for particularly expensive or time-consuming tasks

dividuals might select their insurance plans according to the levels of nursing for which the plans will pay.

COST ACCOUNTING

The nurse executive often needs to know the basics of cost accounting, as when assigning costs for nursing services or assigning fees for an inservice offering. She may need cost accounting skills when arranging conventions or working on other mass-attended events in relation to her professional organization responsibilities as well as when arranging large events for her own institution. Grantsmanship also requires the ability to put a price tag on an event or series of events or projects.

Accurate cost accounting enables the nurse executive to associate costs with the purposes for which they are incurred. When the nurse executive has an accurate idea of the cost of a given project, she can determine whether the cost/benefit ratio is reasonable. She may determine if the cost per client served, in a proposed clinic for alcoholics for example, may be warranted in the expected benefit. Cost accounting will enable her to compare proposed programs when she does not have sufficient resources for all desired projects. Cost accounting might enable the director to compare the cost and benefits of the proposed alcoholic care clinic to cost and benefits of a proposed birth control clinic.

In business, the cost/benefit ratio is usually a financial one, with input costs identified and compared with expected profit. In nursing, it may not always be possible to state the ratio of cost to benefit in financial terms. Consider the accounting task of the nurse executive who is adding a human service for the community, a home visit program for patients discharged from hospitals after strokes. Here the financial benefits probably are not equal to the input costs; the real benefit may be in the number of senior citizens who are able to manage on their own without being placed in nursing homes. Of course, one might extrapolate a financial gain—in years lived independently versus years in a nursing home—if one could calculate the financial differences in lifestyle, and multiply those costs by life expectancies of persons in and not in the home program. In nursing, it often makes more sense to identify the benefit in human terms rather than in dollars and cents, since it is difficult to put a price tag on improved quality of life—on increased comfort, security, independence, or self-control. Nevertheless, it is useful for the executive to identify the costs and benefits of her programs and projects even if they must be stated in qualitative terms. If she can show that a clinic client typically has five more years of independent living than does a comparable patient who fails to utilize the clinic (at a cost of $500 to the clinic), then she has some facts upon which to base future judgments concerning the clinic.

In addition to calculating cost/benefit ratios for programs and projects, the nurse executive may calculate cost effectiveness ratios. In this construct, cost is related to the achievement of given, specified objectives. If, for example, the objective of a nurse executive is to prepare 10 staff nurses to give updated coronary care to patients in the coronary care unit, then she may compare the cost of two or more programs for reaching that goal. For example, she may calculate the cost of having her inservice education program offer a course versus the cost of sending the staff members to a program of similar education elsewhere.

In calculating such costs for program decisions, there are several terms with which the nurse executive should be familiar. A *sunk cost* is money already invested in some particular object or system which encourages further investment along a particular line. For example, if a nursing division or an institution has already invested in a given computer system on the patient care units, it is likely to invest in other programs which utilize this same system rather than investigating an alternate system. Sunk costs dictate future administrative decisions.

A *fixed cost* such as the salary of the head

nurse, is not related to volume of business, for a head nurse must be present no matter how small the patient load. A *proportional cost* does reflect volume of business: the use of 4x4's on a surgical unit reflects the number of patients on the unit or the number of surgeries performed. A *step cost* does not directly reflect volume of business as does a proportional cost; instead it increases or decreases at critical levels. For example, the staffing of an emergency room will not match the amount of patient traffic, but if traffic is accelerated for a sustained period, staff may be added, reflecting a higher "step" in activity. Both the proportional cost and the step cost are *variable* costs as opposed to fixed costs.

Besides knowing the nature of each cost, the nurse executive may want to differentiate controllable costs from real costs before making managerial decisions. The *real cost* of a project will include all the labor, materials, and administrative overhead required for the project's enactment. In contrast, the *controllable costs* are those which would not exist if the project were eliminated. Suppose, for example, that the nurse executive and the inservice director create a primary nursing education project. Suppose that the secretary for the inservice department devotes one-fifth of her working time to the project; also assume that one regular instructor is assigned for 50 percent of her time to the project. The project will include 10 hours of lecture by an "outside expert," and the distribution of materials on primary nursing to program attendees. It is anticipated that the program will be offered to 40 nurses on work hours, for a total of 30 hours per total course. In this example, real costs would include distributed materials, salaries (proportional) of the secretary and the inservice instructor, time of the inservice director, and the total time of the outside expert. Real costs also would include salaries of the employees for the hours that they are attending the program, administrative overhead (proportion of overhead charged to the inservice department), and depreciation on any audiovisual equipment used in the classroom. Charges also might be calculated for use of a classroom. Many of these costs would be eliminated if the executive only considers controllable costs. For example, if the instructor were a full-time employee, her salary would have been paid even if she were not involved in this project; the same is true for the secretary and the inservice director. Only the fees of the outside expert would be listed as controllable costs. Cost of materials are also controllable costs, but salaries of employees attending the course only would be counted if they actually were replaced on their units for the time of class learning. Similarly, if the classroom "belonged" to the inservice department and did not need to be rented from another source, then its cost would not be considered.

Obviously, it is important that the nurse executive have a good idea of both real and controllable costs for most major events that occur in her division. In some cases real costs and in other cases controllable costs will be dominant in her decison making. At other times she will wish to compare these costs. Some nurse executives repeatedly lose money on projects because when planning the projects they forget some real costs involved. For example, if a nurse contracts to run a new clinic on funds sufficient only for controllable costs she will be relying on institutional support for administrative overhead and other services; this may make a "funded project" a major expense to the organization in terms of real costs.

For some projects, it is important to have a *unit* cost as well as a *total* project cost. For example, the absolute cost of running a labor and delivery function may not tell the executive as much as would a figure that describes average cost per delivery. Similarly cost per clinic visit, and cost per employee hired may have more significance than the report of a total cost. A *unit cost* is one that is reported in terms of one unit of production, whether that unit be a patient, a surgical experience, a student, a visit, or any other item determined to be appropriate to the subject under consideration. It is particularly important to calculate unit costs if fees are to be associated with costs. In this way, it is possible to determine what to charge the clinic patient per visit, what to charge the student nurse for attending a continuing education course, or what to charge the patient for use of the surgical suite.

The nurse executive will discover that some unit costs vary depending upon the volume. It becomes expensive to staff an emergency room with two nurses if few patients wander in; costs of their salaries are covered if there is a high or normal volume of emergency room traffic. Costs for projects usually go down as volume increases, though the relation may not be exact. (Step or proportional costs may be involved.) There is often a critical volume at which costs invested in the project are recovered, and it is important that such volumes be determined by the nurse executive, especially for optional programs. For example, the fee for an inservice offering to "outsiders" may be determined based upon a certain volume of attendees. If that volume is not achieved, the program may lose money. Certainly the inservice director will need to learn how to calculate breakeven costs, as will any other nurse manager who is involved in fee setting where volume affects profit or loss.

SUMMARY

In budgeting or other financial matters, the nurse executive must have a good idea of accounting methods and of systems for accounting used in her own institution. If the nurse executive has a large division, she may have an accountant on her own staff. She should expect that employee to provide data and keep records—not to substitute his judgment for hers in major divisional decision making. Where the nurse executive does not have her own financial staff, she should learn to work with the financial officer of the institution. The nurse executive can neither ignore nor be intimidated by the financial aspects of management. A brief course in basic accounting may be a big help

to the nurse executive who is unsure in the financial side of management.

REFERENCES

1. Holbrook, F.K. Charging by level of nursing care. *Hospitals* 45(16):80, 1972.
2. Wood, C.T. Split-cost accounting: a more precise and equitable way to assign patient costs. *Health Services Manager* 9(9):8, 1976.
3. Clark, E.L., and Diggs, W.W. Quantifying patient care needs. *Hospitals* 45(18):96, 1971.

BIBLIOGRAPHY

Aden, G. Cost containment is principal purpose of rate review. *Hospitals* 50(14):69, 1976.

American Hospital Association. *Cost Finding and Rate Setting for Hospitals*. Chicago: AHA, 1968.

American Hospital Association. *Internal Control and Internal Auditing for Hospitals*. Chicago: AHA, 1969.

American Hospital Association. *Budgeting Procedures for Hospitals*. Chicago: AHA, 1971.

American Hospital Association. *Estimated Useful Lives of Depreciable Hospital Assets*. Chicago: AHA, 1973.

American Hospital Association. *Capital Financing for Hospitals*. Chicago: AHA, 1974.

American Hospital Association. *Chart of Accounts for Hospitals*. Chicago: AHA, 1976.

Anthony, R.N. *Management Accounting*. Homewood, Ill.: Learning Systems, Division of Richard D. Irwin, 1970.

Berki, S. *Hospital Economics*. Lexington, Mass.: D.C. Heath, 1972.

Berman, H.J., and Weeks, L.E. *The Financial Management of Hospitals*. Ann Arbor, Mich.: Health Administration Press, 1976.

Brown, M., Jr. An economic analysis of hospital operations. *Hospital Admin.* 15(2):60, 1970.

Cleverly, W.O. (Ed.) *Financial Management of Health Care Facilities*. Germantown, Md.: Aspen Systems, 1976.

Crabtree, M. Application of cost-benefit analysis to clinical nursing practice: a comparison of individual and group preoperative teaching. *J.O.N.A.* 8(12):11, 1978.

Curry, W. How hospitals are controlling costs. *Hospitals* 50(10):64, 1976.

Feldstein, P.J. Applying economic concepts of hospital care. *Hospital Admin.* 13(1):68, 1968.

Forsyth, G.C., and Thomas, D.G. Models for financially healthy hospitals. *Harvard Business Rev.* 49(4):106, 1971.

Fuller, M.E. The budget: Standard V. *J.O.N.A.* 6(4):36, 1976.

Glasser, M.R. What price health care? *Hospital Admin.* 20(4):7, 1975.

Helt, E.H. Economic determinism: a model of the political economy of medical care. *Int. J. Health Services* 3(3):475, 1973.

Herzlinger, R. Can we control health care costs? *Harvard Business Rev.* 56(2):102, 1978.

Klarman, H.E. Application of cost-benefit analysis to the health services and the special case of technologic innovation. *Int. J. Health Services* 4(2):325, 1974.

Kovner, A.R., and Lusk, E. Effective hospital budgeting. *Hospital Admin.* 18(4):44, 1973.

Lawlor, E. Hospital faces cost challenge with extensive, ongoing program. *Hospitals* 50(10):60, 1976.

Levey, S., and Loomba, N.P. *Health Care Administration: A Managerial Perspective.* Philadelphia: J.B. Lippincott, 1973.

Lille, K., and Danco, W. AHA recommends cost containment committees. *Hospitals* 50(10):69, 1976.

Lipson, S.H., and Hansel, M.D. *Hospital Manpower Budget Preparation Manual.* Ann Arbor, Mich.: Health Administration Press, 1975.

Macleod, R.K. Program budgeting works in non-profit institutions. *Harvard Business Rev.* 49(5):46, 1971.

Marram, G. The comparative costs of operating a team and primary nursing unit. *J.O.N.A.* 6(4):21, 1976.

Poland, M., et al. PETO: a system for assessing and meeting patient care needs. *Am. J. Nursing* 70(7):1479, 1970.

Rice, R.G. Analysis of the hospital as an economic organism. *Modern Hospitals* 151(4):87, 1966.

Sauer, J.E., Jr. Cost containment—and quality assurance, too—It can be done. *Hospitals* 46(21):78, 1972.

Schmied, E. (Ed.) *Maintaining Cost Effectiveness.* Wakefield, Mass: Nursing Resources, 1979.

Seawell, L.V. *Hospital Financial Accounting: Theory and Practice.* Chicago: Hospital Financial Management Association, 1975.

Sorkin, A.L. *Health Economics.* Lexington, Mass.: D.C. Heath, 1975.

Stevens, B.J. Cost accounting in inservice education. *Supervisor Nurse* 9(12):23, 1975.

Stevens, B.J. What is the executive's role in budgeting for her department? *Hospitals* 50(22):83, 1976.

Suver, J.D., and Brown, R.L. Where does zero-base budgeting work? *Harvard Business Rev.* 55(6):76, 1977.

Swansburg, R.C. The nursing budget. *Supervisor Nurse* 9(6):40, 1978.

Sweeney, A., and Wisner, J.N., Jr. *Budgeting Fundamentals for Nonfinancial Executives.* New York: American Management Association, 1975.

Thacker, R.J., and Smith, R.L. *Modern Management Accounting.* Reston, Va.: Reston Publishing, 1977.

Thueson, J. Hospitals' programs and progress in cost containment reported. *Hospitals* 51(18):131, 1977.

Weston, R.T. Adjusting your accounting for inflation. *Harvard Business Rev.* 75(1):22, 1975.

Chapter 19

Material Resources of Nursing Management

The material resources of nursing management include the supplies, equipment, and facilities of the division as they are distributed over space and time. This chapter will focus upon two major elements of this distribution: the design of facilities for patient care and the design of logistic systems to supply materiel within the health care facility.

DESIGN OF FACILITIES

Design of space for patient care involves both planning for new facilities and organizing the use of extant facilities. Focus here will be placed on the original design of facilities, because that element presents some unique problems. Whenever new facilities are planned for the health care institution, be they patient care units or other facilities, the nurse executive should be in on the planning. There are few departments which do not impact on nursing, so the executive will want to consider how any addition or renovation will affect her division. It is most important that the nurse executive be in on any facilities planning *from the start*. If she is not consulted until late in the process, it may be too late to make revisions in plans without incurring great expense. Often only late in the planning do others think to include the nurse executive; she should not wait for an invitation but should immediately request to participate the moment any building plans come to her attention.

Since facilities planning involves a special domain of knowledge, the nurse executive will want to become knowledgeable about this domain or else appoint a nurse specialist in this area to work on renovation and con-

struction projects. If a major building project, such as a new hospital, is involved, someone in the nursing division should work permanently on the planning, which should be that person's sole duty.

The Process of Building

There are several discrete stages in facilities building. The nurse executive will want to be involved at each phase. The first stage is the long-range planning. Here the goals and needs of the community and the organization itself are considered, and future needs are projected. This part of the planning involves both long-range goal setting and the gathering of much demographic and other data to support the legitimacy of those goals. Demographic data might identify the "service area" of the institution; projections of growth or decline in patient population from that service area; projections of subsidiary service areas expected to develop due to shifts in populations served; changes in health manpower capabilities of the community—physician, nurse, technician, other; and growth or decline of other health service agencies in the community. Data concerning financing for the planned new facilities also must be gathered. At the end of the planning phase the institution is ready to make a knowledgeable decision as to whether the construction is feasible and logical.

The next phase of building involves the development of a master site plan. This plan should take into account all foreseeable expansion, now and in the future. The site plan interrelates all lands owned by the institution, be they in geographic proximity or separated. Many institutions, with tunnel vision, have failed to acquire adequate land for expansion. In heavily built-up areas, it may be impossible to count on geographic expansion later, so that most planning will have to involve vertical, rather than horizontal extension. An institution often walks a fine line with a community: while the community may want medical facilities to expand, it may balk at such a project if it involves the displacement of community residents or businesses.

The third phase begins the actual design of facilities. First block schematics are drawn, simply to show how major areas to be built will relate to each other, both horizontally and vertically. Figure 19-1 is a simplified block drawing. In an actual block drawing, the scale would be indicated. When dealing with block schematics, the nurse executive must be careful to note the common pathways by which patients flow from one department to another. An ideal structure would allow all departments immediate access to all other departments; unfortunately the realities of space do not easily allow such construction and, therefore, the block design is a compromise, placing in close proximity those departments which most require it. For example, it makes sense if the recovery room is near the operating rooms, the nursery near postpartum, and so forth. In one institution that did not call in the nurse executive until late in the planning, and then only as a courtesy, for it was too late to redesign the plans, the woman immediately pointed out on the block diagram that the only way in which emergency room patients could be taken to the X-ray department was by moving them through the cafeteria or the front lobby (as in Figure 19-1).

In the next phase of planning, single-line sketches are composed for all areas to be constructed. Actual space constraints such as internal columns, elevators, and corridors are drawn to scale, and rooms are designed with beds and room equipment also drawn to scale. Entrances and exits are indicated in the single-line drawings. The finished single-line drawings reveal the configuration of each unit, the size and shape of planned

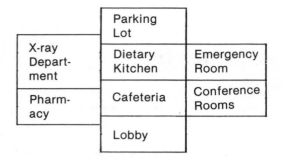

Figure 19-1.   Block Schematic for the First Floor of a Hospital

spaces, and the functional relationships (horizontal and vertical connections) between planned units.

Design development drawings are refinements of the single-line sketches. These drawings include such things as structural, mechanical, electrical systems, as well as any built-in equipment. By the time the architects reach this stage of development, they are very hesitant to make changes, and changes will cost significant amounts of money for the organization. The final planning stage is the development of blueprints—a refinement of the design development drawings.

Construction of facilities always is a compromise between what an institution wants and what it can afford. Few nurse executives have the privilege of having a building designed just as they desire. The nurse executive must beware of building "savings" that will cost money in the long run: a given architectural plan may be costly in terms of nursing hours, and if the institution will have to pay extra nursing salaries over the next 20 or more years, it will end up spending far more than was saved by some architectural shortcut. For example, if elevator service is limited because elevators were a major expense to install, thousands of nursing hours may be lost in waiting time. Similarly, if a work area is too small, nurses may have to wait until other nurses vacate the area to use it. If each patient room does not have an adjoining bathroom, thousands of nursing hours may be spent in accompanying unsteady patients to facilities at a distance.

Often nurse executives are successful in getting architectural plans changed by pointing out potential inefficiencies such as these.

It is amazing how often the managerial needs of a nursing unit are overlooked by planners if nurses are not adequately represented on the planning committees. Head nurses' offices and conference rooms certainly should be included on any modern design. The following tale was recently related by a director of nursing service. Her institution had attempted to "save money" by hiring a young and upcoming architectural firm, one that had never worked on hospital designs previously. In the single-line sketch stage, the director of nursing service asked where the nurses' bathrooms were to be located, only to find that the architects had given thorough attention to patients' bathrooms but totally forgotten that nurses might require such facilities. The architects argued in vain that the large nurses' bathroom in the basement locker facility would be adequate.

The nurse executive will need to be especially careful in the design of each patient unit. Many real life "horror stories" of major errors in these facilities are told by nurse executives. One director moved into a new facility only to discover that door proportions somehow had been changed, making it impossible to roll a bed directly into a room; thousands of nursing hours would be spent in unnecessary stretcher-to-bed transfers. Another new facility has bathrooms in which the patient had to be a healthy contortionist to use the bowl. Another has nurses' stations placed so that they are not in the line of vision of people walking patient halls but directly accessible from an elevator used by the public; hundreds of dollars worth of equipment—namely IBM typewriters— "walked off" before this nursing station was restructured.

While common sense will prevent some errors of this sort, more refinement of judgment is required to do a good planning job. The nurse in charge of planning should know such things as the legal requirements for space usage, the norms of space footage

for various facilities, and other "tricks" of facilities planning. If there is no one with such expertise in the nursing division, it may be wise to use a nurse consultant who is an expert in this area.

After blueprints receive final approval, the building phase is initiated. By then it usually is too late for any changes unless a catastrophic error is discovered. The nurse executive at this phase must try to carry on patient management in a noisy, interruptive environment with construction nearby. Where the nurse executive is fortunate enough to have the construction at a distance, she may face the problem of planning the logistics of the move of patients from one facility to another. This problem is no less complicated than the movement of troops in battle and will require long-term planning for each and every detail.

During the planning phases, then, the nurse executive will need to consider the proposed architecture as it relates to 1) flow patterns for patients, staff, and visitors, 2) security needs of the facility, 3) facilities' proximity needs, 4) movement of equipment and supplies, 5) placement of nursing offices and managerial space as they relate to the space of other key managers, and 6) patients' convenience in use of the facilities.

Basic Plans for Patient Units

A particular item of interest to a nurse executive in planning a new facility may be the design of patient care units. The oldest and least satisfactory design is the single corridor design, in which patient rooms as well as nurses' stations, treatment rooms, and other service areas all are rooms off the same long hall. Obviously, such a long-hall construction calls for many more man hours spent walking than needed with more compact designs. (See Figure 19-2 for illustration. Here and in subsequent design illustrations the dark areas indicate nurses' stations and other staff work areas.)

In the double corridor design (Figure 19-3), patient rooms branch off halls located

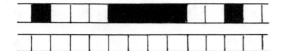

Figure 19-2.   Single-Corridor Patient Unit
(Dark areas indicate nurses'
stations and other staff work
areas.)

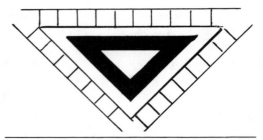

Figure 19-4.   Triangular Patient Unit

on both sides of a central core containing the
work areas of the unit. Advocates of this
design claim walking time is cut nearly by
half, compared to time required for a single
corridor with the same number of patient
rooms. Some nurses are uncomfortable with
the fact that this design cuts down visibility
of hall activities because only one-half of the
floor can be seen at any one time.

Each variation in unit design has both
advantages and limitations. The square,
triangle, and circle designs usually simplify
the nursing logistics but tend to waste space
by having more central work area than really
is necessary (see Figures 19-4–19-6). T-shaped
units attempt to solve this problem while still
shortening the length of any given corridor
(Figure 19-7). When a major decision such as
that concerning shape of nursing units is to be
made, the nurse executive will want to consult
with persons who actually have "lived with"
the designs under consideration. Some of the
newer designs of separate care pods, for example, may look attractive and efficient but
may decrease professional exchange by producing excessive spatial separation of staff
members; one cannot accurately anticipate
how it is to inhabit such a structure without
visiting one and asking those who have lived
there how they like it and whether it works.

As a general rule the builder will desire to
have large-census patient units because they

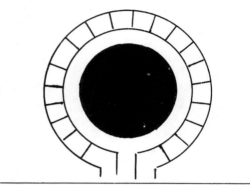

Figure 19-5.   Circular Patient Unit

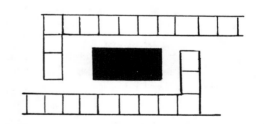

Figure 19-6.   Square Patient Unit

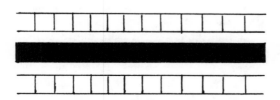

Figure 19-3.   Double-Corridor Patient Unit

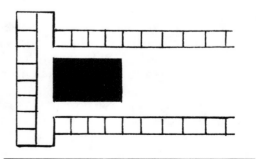

Figure 19-7.   T-shaped Patient Unit

are less expensive to construct than are small-census patient units. This is another area for negotiation. Obviously, the nursing systems of care delivery and staff assignment will be affected by the geographical distribution of patients and supplies. Typically the nurse executive prefers smaller units than does the architect or perhaps her boss, who is looking more for economy than for convenience and ease in the provision of nursing care. If the nurse executive is unable to get the size patient units she desires, however, it may be possible to negotiate for other architectural advantages that would lessen the problems of large patient units.

Interior design also may present problems. Typically the closet area in patients' rooms is inadequate. Another common fault is lack of counter space in bathrooms. Both of these faults arise out of attempts to save space, usually in order to increase the number of private over shared patient rooms. Another question in interior design is whether to go for "built-in" versus mobile equipment. Flexibility is maintained with mobile equipment, but such equipment typically needs more care and tending. Carpeting is another issue that is usually debated in relation to patient rooms. Arguments *for* carpeting include esthetic pleasure, noise prevention, fewer injuries in patient falls and psychological satisfaction. Arguments against carpeting are the difficulty of infection control, problems with moving stock such as stretchers and wheelchairs, and the problem of spills of various sorts. There is no single satisfactory answer, though the type of carpet used may make a radical difference in how satisfactory it is in patient rooms.

Interior design of the nurses' station deserves attention; typically these areas lack enough space to sit (probably a holdover from days when nurses were expected to "do" continually, not to "sit and think").

If the nurse executive, or one of her staff, has not had considerable experience in interior design, it is probably a good idea to hire a nurse consultant who specializes in this area. There are just too many possibilities of making mistakes that must be lived with for inordinately long times.

LOGISTIC SYSTEMS TO SUPPLY MATERIEL

There are two major types of supply systems in the health care institution, those that match supplies or services on a one-to-one basis with requests and those that supply items or services in accordance with usage norms. The dietary and pharmacy departments usually have the first type of supply system. Patient trays and drugs are supplied on the basis of specific requests. Some leeway may be established by maintaining stock and emergency drugs on a patient unit or by holding some stock food supplies on the unit.

On the whole, resource problems with departments, divisions, or sections that supply goods and services upon request turn out to be problems of timing or communication. Since the supplier and the user both are involved in the logistic system, it is useful to examine a defective system rather than to try to place blame for its failures. Many health institutions hire systems analysts or have a department of operations research just for the purpose of handling such problems. Where such a person or department exists, they should be used for analyzing resource supply failures.

When assistance is not available, the nurse executive or the nursing management staff involved in the systems breakdown may undertake an analysis of the system. A flowchart may reveal system defects and suggest solutions to the manager's problem. Consider the flowchart analysis in Figure 19-8, which describes the problems of a nursing unit that chronically received and had to send back to the dietary department trays for patients who had already been discharged.

Clearly, the problem here is one of timing. The flowchart presents the system dispassionately and demonstrates at least two

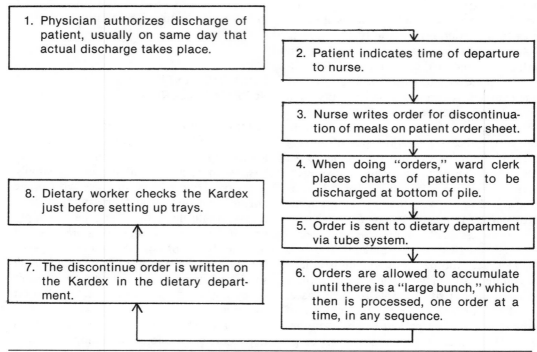

Figure 19-8. Flowchart Analysis of the Problem of Unneeded Dietary Trays

slowdown points. First, there is a slowdown at step 4. The ward clerk who delays handling of charts of patients to be discharged might be reeducated concerning her sequencing of tasks; alternatively, the nurse might use a different system for issuing stop orders on meals. On the dietary side of the system, it is obvious that another slowdown occurs at step 6. If orders are ignored until "a large bunch" have accumulated, orders that arrive during a relatively quiet period are necessarily delayed. Perhaps a reorganization by which orders are attended to every 15 or 30 minutes no matter how many or how few have accumulated would decrease the slowdown. This example illustrates how a rational approach to supply problems can work to the advantage of both parties, acquainting each manager with the problems and goals of the other department or division.

A second type of supply system in a health care institution is one that works on usage norms rather than on individual requests.

The laundry service is an example of this sort of system. When problems arise in a system based on usage norms, the manager needs to inquire how the norms are set. For example, the laundry might calculate linen supply according to number of beds per unit, daily census, average yearly or monthly census, or past linen usage practices of a unit. A unit of 30 patients who are up and about will require fewer linens than a unit of 30 bedbound patients, hence even an accurate census is not a direct predictor of linen usage; perhaps this system problem could be solved by deriving linen requirements on the basis of the patient classification system rather than the census. In other words, some systems problems can be solved by establishing a norm that is more reflective of the supply in question.

Any system based on norms should have a means of flexibility built into it for instances when the units being supplied are above or below the norm. Often a flowchart will show that the norms are acceptable but that the system lacks flexibility.

When dealing with her delivery system, the nurse executive must ensure, through the necessary negotiations with others, that the right equipment and supplies are where they are needed when they are needed. The systems that control movements of materiel must be efficient, economical, and designed to control accountability.

BIBLIOGRAPHY

Allen, R.W. Renovation saves hospital landmark. *Hospitals* 53(4):175, 1979.

Ashley, I.E., and Mann, G.J. Abandoned air force base redesigned as rehabilitation center. *Hospitals* 53(4):181, 1979.

Berg, N.H. Medical center applies financial strategies to renovation project. *Hospitals* 53(4):147, 1979.

Blair, B.J. Air force hospital expands physical facility and mechanical systems. *Hospitals* 53(4):187, 1979.

Blumenkranz, J., and Weber, R. From custodial to rehabilitation facility. *Hospitals* 49(10):66, 1975.

Brors, D.P., and Mullin, K.R. Cluster clinics create flexibility. *Hospitals* 50(3):117, 1976.

Buckley, D.M. Two HMOs retrofit buildings in historic and commercial downtown. *Hospitals* 53(4):155, 1979.

Burgun, J.A. Construction considerations for ambulatory care facilities. *Hospitals* 50(3):79, 1976.

Cook, H.S. Interior design sets cheerful, calming mood. *Hospitals* 50(3):87, 1976.

DeNyse, R.A. Hospitals meet space and HSA criteria through merger. *Hospitals* 53(4):137, 1979.

Edge, D.R. A hospital must study cost, codes, alternatives to decide on reuse or new building. *Hospitals* 53(4):109, 1979.

Fox, D.H. A contemporary organizational design for maternal and infant care projects. *J.O.N.A.* 5(4):26, 1975.

Green, A.C. Changes in care call for design flexibility. *Hospitals* 50(3):67, 1976.

Grubbs, J., and Bobrow, M.R. Centralized ambulatory care unit convenient and efficient. *Hospitals* 50(3):127, 1976.

Haselhuhn, G.R., and Grapski, L. Rebuilding for the future: a forward-looking master plan. *Hospitals* 53(4):167, 1979.

Hyman, R. Choosing art for your hospital: some basic do's and don't's. *Hospitals* 53(6):95, 1979.

Levitan, M.S. To reuse or reconstruct: that is the question. *Hospitals* 53(4):93, 1979.

Mountz, W., and Falick, J. New facility emphasizes efficient care, positive image. *Hospitals* 50(4):57, 1976.

Oberlander, R. Beauty in a hospital aids the cure. *Hospitals* 53(6):89, 1979.

Parker, W., Jr. Flexible designs are key to reuse projects. *Hospitals* 53(4):125, 1979.

Reingold, J. A master plan approaches its goal. *Hospitals* 50(11):55, 1976.

Ryan, J.L. The nursing administrator's growing role in facilities planning. *J.O.N.A.* 5(9):22, 1975.

Sprague, J.G. How to get health facilities built. *Hospitals* 50(3):73, 1976.

Sprague, J.G. Is recycling of buildings a health alternative for the hospital industry? *Hospitals* 53(4):82, 1979.

Thier, L. Facilities planning: a discussion. *J.O.N.A.* 6(5):29, 1976.

Turner, W.W. Tri-unit complex effects economy. *Hospitals* 49(17):49, 1975.

Tusler, W., Jr. Could two-level process eliminate costly planning problems? *Hospitals* 53(4):85, 1979.

Velsey, D.W., and Tobey, P.E. Space allocation based on levels of care. *Hospitals* 50(3):109, 1976.

Zilm F. Computer simulation model provides design framework. *Hospitals* 50(16):79, 1976.

Zimmerman, J.P. Service areas and their needs must be reassessed. *Hospitals* 49(17):46, 1975.

Chapter 20   Labor Law and Legal Considerations in Nursing Management

Many domains of law enter into the work of the nurse executive. The following represent only a few of these domains:

1. *Laws impacting on the hiring, promotions, and firing of personnel, their use while employed, and their recompense as wage earners.* Employment of personnel is affected by several bodies of law. Labor law is one such body of law, and it will be discussed in detail in the second half of this chapter. Other laws apply to this domain also, e.g., constitutional law and federal laws impacting on employment—for example, the Fair Labor Standards Act. The nurse executive also must be aware of her state's work laws. These may identify how many hours an employee may work, how many days in a row may be worked, and how many hours off must occur between shifts. Copies of relevant laws are available from appropriate state agencies.

2. *Laws impacting on the work environment.* The Occupational Safety and Health Act (OSHA) illustrates this legal constraint. This law is designed to protect workers from injury by environmental hazards. In addition, a health institution will have regional or local controls on its environment, such as inspections by the local board of health. The nurse executive must be aware of environmental protection mechanisms operating on federal, state, and local levels.

3. *Laws impacting on the practice of professionals.* Legal constraints also dictate who may do what in relation to skilled health care practices. The nurse executive not only must make judgments concerning what constitutes lawful practice for

all employees in her division, but she must be responsible for seeing that all employees have satisfactorily proven their licensure, certification, or registration for assigned work.

4. *Laws protecting patients.* Patients' rights may be protected by state laws or, more commonly, by case law, which has grown as the result of suits against health care workers and health care institutions. The nurse executive needs to know her organizational responsibilities as to patient protection, patient experimentation, and informed consent of patients to their treatment. Patients' rights will affect decisions in complex situations such as treatment of unconscious, unidentified persons; treatment of persons accused of (or subjected to) crimes; and treatment of persons who reject life-preserving therapies.

5. *Laws impacting upon the organization itself.* In addition to laws concerning persons in and the environment of the organization, there are laws that affect the organization, itself, as a legal entity. There are laws regulating nonprofit corporations, laws specific to health care institutions, special building codes for health agencies. The nurse executive must be aware of these legal constraints.

Because of the diversity of legal domains the nurse executive may encounter, expert legal advice should be available to her whenever she needs it. It is not enough to have access to the institution's counsel. The individual so named often is an attorney skilled in corporate law and specializing in the laws that affect the organization as a legal entity. At present the legal profession has few official specialties, and it is rare for a corporate lawyer also to be skilled in malpractice law and labor law, so the nurse executive should seek counsel appropriately skilled in dealing with malpractice suits, labor relations, and every other type of legal-administrative problem that may arise in the day-to-day nursing environment.

Legal assistance does not relieve the nurse executive of her responsibility for knowledge of statutory and administrative law. Every nurse executive should refresh and update her legal background at frequent intervals. This chapter will not attempt to deal with the varied and diverse bodies of law that the nurse executive must know, for even a whole book could not do justice to the subject. Instead, the purpose here is to make the nurse executive aware of her legal responsibility for this aspect of her practice. Ultimately, the decisions made in her division will be her responsibility. Since not all decisions will be made by the nurse executive herself, she must be responsible for seeing that staff have clear directives concerning legal matters that affect decision making. Some areas of nursing practice may involve more decisions with legal implications than others—emergency room practice can be expected to bring up more legal issues than practice on an orthopedic unit, for example—nevertheless, no nursing staff member is totally free of situations with potential legal implications.

LAW AS A RESOURCE AND A CONSTRAINT

It usually is easy to recognize law as a constraint; the law tells what one may or may not do. But the law is also a resource, because it protects one's right in domains that are legitimately one's concerns. Labor law, for example, grants certain areas of practices as being the proper and exclusive concern of management unless management voluntarily agrees to bargain within those domains. And labor law identifies those rights of workers which cannot be abridged.

The nurse executive will be involved with legal resources and constraints on at least three levels: federal, state, and local. Further, she will be concerned with rules and regulations from three sources: 1) enacted laws themselves, 2) rules and regulations that have been established to administer complex laws, and 3) case decisions which set precedent for future actions. She also will need to be aware of constitutional rights of individuals.

One reason that laws presently are seen by nurse executives as constraints, rather than resources, is the many and conflicting rules and regulations on the federal level. Since these dictates require significant use of other resources in compliance, and since they often conflict so that conformity to one regulation means nonconformity to another, it is not surprising that the nurse executive perceives much of law to be an administrative burden. Nevertheless, there are signs that this problem is being attacked nationally (administratively) and in courts—witness, for example the cases being brought by the American Hospital Association for the specific purpose of laying bare the overt contradictions in many federal guidelines and regulations.

There are now many instances of management taking active positions and going to court on issues where managerial rights have been abridged. This is particularly noticeable in the area of labor law. Further, there is aggressive legal opposition to laws whose rules and regulations require massive outlay of resources for minimal gain in human protection; many regulations of the Occupational Safety and Health Act presently are being challenged on this ground.

At any one time, however, the extant law provides a framework for the operations of the health care institution and for the nursing division. It draws boundaries and protects the rights of the organization, its officers, employees, and associates.

LABOR RELATIONS IN NURSING

Labor law has been selected as one illustration of a legal process which has an impact on nursing management. Labor relations is a growing area of concern to more and more nurse executives as nursing workers in ever greater numbers unionize nationwide. Let us focus upon the organizing of workers into unions, the negotiation of a labor contract between employees and management, and the administration of a contract by the nurse executive.

Stevens makes a point of differentiating personnel relations and labor relations, with the former based on constitutional law and the latter originating in contract law[1]. While good personnel relations do not necessarily protect an institution from unionization, it is certain that poor personnel relations leave an institution ripe for unionization. It is important, therefore, to identify the major errors in personnel relations that make an organization vulnerable to unionization.

Errors in Personnel Relations

Three critical systems in personnel management affect staff attitudes toward unionization: the wage and salary administration system, the performance appraisal and disciplinary system, and the supervisory system. There are major errors possible in each of these systems, errors that will encourage unionizing activities.

The Wage and Salary Administration System

Inequitable salary distribution is one of the major factors inciting unionization. The issue is equity, not absolute amounts of money. A worker may be drawing a high salary, but if a coworker with less seniority and less responsibility draws a higher one, the first worker will be discontent. In a nursing division, inequity often attaches to seniority. If the nurse is not rewarded for years of service, she will perceive this as inequity. Not only is it the case that length of service is minimally rewarded in some nursing divisions, but there are numerous cases where beginning salaries actually are higher than the salaries of employees of the same class already working in the institution. The reason for this policy is obvious: it is an attempt to attract newly graduating nurses to an institution which has great staffing needs. Nevertheless, the natural response of the employee with longer tenure who becomes aware of this practice is either to resign from the institution or to seek employee protection through unionization. Either of these acts is detrimental from the perspective of the nurse manager. Some institutions caution employees not to share information concerning their pay rates, but this tactic is singularly unsuccessful, and workers soon make it their business to learn the salaries of peers. Given human ingenuity in finding out such information, it is better for an institution to act in a straightforward manner, publishing and following equitable pay scales.

Inequitable pay patterns occur not only among workers of the same job classification but between job classifications. For example, if the RN and the LPN jobs differ significantly in responsibility, then their pay scales should reflect that difference. The pay vis-à-vis responsibility for nursing positions should be comparable, moreover, with the pay vis-à-vis responsibility for other positions in the rest of the institution. There are instances in which professional staff in nursing divisions are paid less (have lower pay scales) than nonprofessional staff with restricted responsibilities in other divisions, an unconscionable practice.

Having clear and equitable pay scales does not imply the absence of merit pay. Certainly, within the constraints of a pay scale, distinctions may be made among workers based on quality of work. Such differences, however, should be clearly defined as attributable to merit. Indeed, it means little to have a merit system if it is not used, openly, to encourage better performance.

The wage and salary administration system, then, should have clear and equitable salary ranges and pay scales, and personnel should be placed fairly on those scales and recompensed accordingly. Within the given salary ranges, it is possible to have a merit system functioning. The pay system should not be covert because employees soon defeat such attempts at secrecy anyway and may find them offensive.

Performance Appraisal and Disciplinary System

Performance appraisal is discussed in detail in Chapter 23. What is important here is that the performance appraisal system actually function to rate and rank employee performance fairly. Regular evaluations should take place according to policy, and the employee should be made aware of how his performance measures up to the standards set for his position. Ironically, performance appraisal becomes an issue, not when employees are rated strictly under the system, but when good employees see mediocre or poor employees receiving the same ratings and benefits as themselves. A fair performance appraisal rating system will produce a satisfied staff.

In looking at employee ratings, it is important that all nurse managers in an institution apply a comparable degree of stringency in their ratings. For example, if the head nurse of 5 West always rates more strictly than the head nurse of 5 East, her employees may receive a less-than-equitable portion of merit increments or may not be considered for advancements even though their actual performances equal those of employees on the other patient unit.

The same point applies in relation to the disciplinary system. If some employees constantly ignore policies (such as those relating to tardiness and absenteeism) without any penalty, while others are penalized according to the rules, then morale sinks and the situation is ripe for unionization. Since inequity of treatment is a major factor inciting unionization, nurse managers simply cannot afford to implement policies discriminately. For example, the head nurse cannot dis-

cipline the alcoholic aide for tardiness, while failing to discipline a nurse aide who is similarly tardy due to babysitter problems.

It is important that an institution have a good grievance procedure available to the employee who feels he has been unfairly judged or disciplined. The grievance procedure itself should be clearly described and simple to follow; it should not have too many steps until final resolution is achieved. If an LPN has a dispute at the unit level which is not settled to her (or her union's) satisfaction, it should not be necessary that it be heard at every intervening level—head nurse, supervisor, department director, vice president for nursing, and president. When an employee must go through so many different hearings, too much time passes with the issue still unsettled. Most grievance procedures sidestep the usual chain of command to shorten this procedure. Often the final hearing officer is appointed from the personnel department, though this is not invariable. The nurse managers of an institution must be careful to try not to deviate from the established pattern for grievance hearings. In one case the director of nursing stepped in and held a hearing for an employee on an issue that first should have been heard by that employee's own head nurse; because of having bypassed the regular policies for grievance, the director lost this case at a higher level due to procedural deviation.

The nurse manager must be careful to apply the grievance procedure precisely. One important factor is timing. Most grievance procedures have time limits for how soon after an incident a grievance must be filed and for how soon after a hearing the hearing officer must respond. Other time factors may be included. Often a well-meaning nurse manager will want to extend the time limits in a grievance procedure. However, to do this is to set a dangerous precedent. For example, if the nurse manager allows a given employee a week's grace in filing a grievance that she thinks the employee should win, then she has no justification for not extending the same favor to all subsequent grievants. A nurse manager who hears a grievance must recognize that the employee automatically "wins" a case if she fails to respond with her decision within the set time frame as well.

Because the hearing officers in grievance cases always are managers of the institution, it is important that the hearings be fair, not "loaded" in favor of management. If the grievance is merely a *pro forma* event, with the outcome easily forecast, then the procedure will cause more discontent than would exist without it. Where there is a contract, such *pro forma* hearings will result in a large number of expensive arbitration cases. Where there is not a union contract, unfair grievance hearings may result in moves to unionize. Unfortunately, some hearing officers are so threatened by the thought of employee action that they are prejudiced in favor of the grieving employee. In this case, the institution makes a travesty of management by undercutting the power of its own managers. The aim of any grievance hearing should be that of fair resolution; neither party should be automatically favored.

The Supervisory System

Since one of the chief sources of employee dissatisfaction is inequitable and prejudicial supervision, today's supervisor, on whatever level, simply cannot afford to play favorites. Employees must be judged on their performance, not on their personal appeal. Further, all supervisors of a division must apply that division's policies with equal stringency to avoid a secondary source of inequity. It is important that the nurse executive back up her subordinate managers. This means she is responsible for teaching them how to make sound managerial decisions in the first place and how to collect evidence to support those decisions. Nothing is more demoralizing to a supervisory staff than a nurse executive who, in an attempt to relate personally to staff members, counteracts their valid managerial decisions. The nurse executive should never overturn a decision by a subordinate manager without seriously considering the implica-

tions of that act. If the supervisor really is making decisions that cannot be supported, then she should either be adequately educated or be replaced. All too often the fault lies in the nurse executive who believes the first interpretation she hears of an event—that offered by the employee who has run to her for counsel. Employees soon learn if a nurse executive is a "soft touch," and the director should be suspicious if many employees seek her out "over the heads" of their immediate supervisors, for it indicates a severe problem—either with the supervisors or with the director herself. A director who fails to set such a situation right is herself creating serious problems for her division.

Managerial Principles for Labor Relations

When the nurse executive is dealing with a situation where contracts already exist or where the potential for contractual relations exists, there are several important principles that may assist her. First, she must know what laws are applicable and she must know them not just in name but in content. At present all private hospitals, both profit and nonprofit, fall under the provisions of the Labor Management Relations Act (LMRA). The act incorporates the National Labor Relations Act (NLRA), the Wagner Act of 1936, the Taft-Hartley Amendment of 1947, and the Health Care Amendment Act of 1974. Often one hears the LMRA indiscriminately referred to by the title of one of its components, but it is essential that the nurse executive recognize the full extent of the law under which she functions. If the nurse executive is in a federal institution, then labor relations are covered by executive order 11491 as amended and the Federal Personnel Manual. This order functions in the federal public sector much as the LMRA does in the private. However, the provisions of the two documents are not identical, so the nurse executive will need copies of the legislation which affects her institution. If the nurse executive is in an agency in the public sector but under a state or political subdivision rather than in a federal institution, then she must check on the laws of her state to find out the status of collective bargaining. About half of the states have legislation mandating collective bargaining in the public, nonfederal sector; about half lack such mandatory legislation. Both the LMRA and the aforementioned executive order make collective bargaining mandatory. Where collective bargaining is *not* mandatory, the agency still may elect to enter into bargaining on a voluntary basis, though this is seldom a wise managerial decision.

It is essential for the nurse executive to know whether or not she must bargain with an elected union and what enabling rules she must follow. She should have access to an expert labor relations consultant if she is new to the collective bargaining process. She needs consultation long before negotiation begins, and should seek consultation at the start of any unionizing activity. Even though some institutions claim to handle unionizing and unionizing activities within the personnel department, the nurse executive will be better off if she has a voice in the matter. If part of the nursing staff are involved in unionizing, there will be impacts on her division that will go beyond the interests and attention of the typical personnel department. Seldom is the personnel manager or the institution's lawyer able to provide the advice that the nurse executive needs in relation to this special domain.

All too often the nurse executive seeks expert help after a contract has been negotiated that is virtually impossible to execute. One director who had relied on the personnel department to negotiate a contract without her called in a labor relations expert to help determine what to do about the contract, which allowed all vacation time to be chosen at the employees' discretion. But she called for help too late: the contract had already been signed and she was forced to let employees determine their own vacation times, even though it ended up costing her thousands in replacement salary, since too

many employees selected the same vacation times.

In another case, a nurse executive was involved in negotiations without counsel, and she agreed to guarantee her LPNs so many days of "charge duty" weekly. She made this agreement in a time of RN scarcity without foresight that the situation might change. Now she has RNs working under LPNs because that contract is still in effect though she no longer has an RN deficit in staffing. An expert consultant could perhaps have prevented this short-sighted agreement.

Finally, the nurse executive must realize that labor relations are bilateral: they divide people into two camps—managers and employees. Labor relations work on the principle of balance created by the push and pull of the vested interests of the two sides. Many nurses and even nursing organizations are hesitant to admit to this division between worker and manager. Many a nurse executive offers the rationalization that even bedside nurses are managers; they "manage" the care of patients. Attempts to ignore the bilateral nature of labor relations only create confusion. The labor laws of the land are based on a bilateral system, and nursing must accept the laws as constructed. Indeed, the sophisticated nurse executive recognizes that her role of manager necessarily gives her a unilateral position at the negotiating table in favor of management. If she tries to "play both sides" in an attempt to show her indivisibility from the nursing staff, all sides will suffer from an imbalance in the bilateral relationship. The nurse executive must realize that labor relations are based on the principles of conflict and negotiation, not on principles of synergism and cooperation. If she enters negotiation in the wrong spirit, she is likely to give away vital managerial prerogatives without realizing that she is actually losing in a competitive situation.

Phases in Labor Relations

For simplicity, the process of establishing a labor contract will be reviewed in a sequence of four steps: the organizing phase, the recognition phase, the contract negotiation phase, and the contract administration phase. Each of these steps will be examined.

The Organizing Phase

The organizing phase takes place when a union builds a base of support among workers. Managerial responses to this activity depend on whether or not the institution legally must bargain with a duly elected union, whether or not the management favors unionization (or *this* union), and whether or not unionization is perceived as inevitable or preventable.

The typical management response to incipient union organizing is to try to defeat the movement. Counteractions may take two forms: correction of wrongs—if any—that led to the activity and attempts to counter the notion of unionizing. Often, if an organization waits until the threat of unionization to correct blatantly unfair policies, the action may come too late. There are instances, however, when such belated action does ward off unionization. When a nurse executive is involved in an antiunion propaganda campaign, she must be careful not to overstep legal boundaries. Under the LMRA, she cannot institute employee surveillance (such as photographing employees entering a meeting on unionizing), interrupt employees promoting unionization on their free time and on property where the work of the organization is not being disrupted, nor allow biased disciplinary action against leaders of the unionizing movement.

Even here the nurse executive needs to see the law not only as a constraint on her actions but also as a resource: under the law, she can stop unionizing activities when they impinge on the work of the institution and when they use the work hours of employees. She must draw a fine line, however, defending her rights to support and maintain the work process, without jeopardizing the legal rights of employees to unionize.

The organizing phase of unionizing includes solicitation (oral encouragement to form a union) and distribution (written encouragement to form a union). Groups organizing under the LMRA are able to demand an election if they can produce signed cards showing that 30 percent of the employees of the given class are interested in holding an election. While such an election cannot be held more than once a year, any group with a constituency can constitute a "union." Where more than one union is interested in representing a group, the winner of the election will get sole representation rights (providing that unionizing is not voted down).

The Recognition Phase

A union is recognized as the sole representative of an employee group if it wins the majority of votes in an election. This is true no matter how many or how few qualified voters actually vote; representation is determined on the total number of votes cast. The nurse executive may want to educate employees to this fact if there is a significant group who do not want to unionize. Often such employees feel that not voting is a move against unionizing; given the way that votes are counted, failure to vote does not represent a move against the union. (As phases of unionizing are discussed throughout this section, the reader may assume that the discussion refers to procedures under the LMRA.)

Some issues of significance must be decided in relation to the recognition phase. First, who is to be recognized? Typically a "group" is considered to be formed by a "community of interest." In the health field, it is typical that groups divide between professional and nonprofessional roles. Professionals cannot be forced to join in a union with nonprofessionals, though they may elect to do so if they choose. Ideally each small group would like to have its own union; this is because each group feels that its issues and needs are, to some degree, unique. However, if each and every group were granted the right to bargain separately, management would be forced to spend unreasonable time and resources in the bargaining act. One can imagine the problems in the nursing division alone if groups such as the following each had their own unions: operating room technicians, intravenous technicians, critical care nurses. For this reason the National Labor Relations Boards will make decisions concerning who must be in the same union so as to limit the numbers of unions that are legitimate bargaining agents with a single institution.

The National Labor Relations Boards also interpret the LMRA, and make determinations such as which positions are management jobs and which are labor in borderline cases. At the moment there is much unrest because of the varied and dissimilar decisions made by local labor relations boards. More and more often their decisions are being challenged (particularly by management) and taken to court.

In nursing, there is much confusion over manager/staff placements. This is because of several factors. First, it may be difficult to identify where "management" responsibility starts and employee functions leave off. Is the team leader a manager? This is a difficult determination because she does have responsibility for subordinate staff members, yet that responsibility in many cases is transient. The nature of the nursing work world makes it difficult to pass judgment on the locus of given jobs. Further, employees may fill a managerial function (team leading) one day and a clearly staff position (bedside care) the next. The situation is further complicated by the fact that among RNs who seek to unionize, the most popular representative union is that of the state nurses' association. The problem is that most nurses, managerial and staff, belong to this organization and pay dues into common coffers, and hence it is difficult to claim that such a union is not "tainted" by the presence of managers. Some court cases have dealt with this issue, and at least one major case excused an institution from bargaining with a state nurses' association because of this "contamination"[2]. Further, some chief officers have refused to hire a nurse executive who "belongs to the union"—that is, belongs to her professional organization. It is really critical that nursing settle these issues so that both nurse managers and nurse employees are not caught in the middle in unclear situations.

Unlike most other organizations, some health care institutions now are bargaining with managers who have collected and formed their own unions (or have joined in unions with staff nurses). There is no legal necessity for an institution to bargain with such a group, and it is surprising that so many voluntarily agree to bargain with their own managers. This breaks with a long tradition, that managers are the representatives of the organization and that the organization has the right to have full confidence in its managers. It is for this reason that managerial jobs seldom involve any guaranteed tenure such as one finds under labor contracts.

Under the LMRA a supervisor (a manager) is anyone with the authority to make personnel decisions such as assignment, hiring, suspending, promoting, and firing, or even anyone who has the right *to recommend such actions*. Certainly most job descriptions would place head nurses in the category of managers. Some might extend the title of manager to a permanent charge nurse, as have several actual cases.

In any case, in the recognition phase, the institution must recognize as the bargaining agent any legitimate union that wins election under the appropriate procedures and laws. When an agent is recognized, under the LMRA, the institution cannot legally refuse to enter into the next stage: collective bargaining.

The Contract Negotiation Phase

For negotiation in the health care field, the major issue, from the manager's perspective, is not wages but managerial rights. In truth, there is only so much money to be distributed in wages; unlike General Motors, the hospital cannot easily raise its prices to cover agreements for increases in wages. Third-party payers will pay only a given amount for a given service; many states have rate review boards which must pass on any proposed increase in rates; all kinds of constraints prevent excessive gains in salaries of health care workers.

Given this situation, workers in a health field will try to win concessions in nonsalary issues. Such items as every other weekend off or greater medical benefits or more paid education days may be proposed by the union. These are not really divorced from cost; obviously all these items ultimately cost the health care institution money. Many proposals limit managerial flexibility. If the nurse executive must allow one-half of her staff off every weekend, for example, she is unable to distribute staff according to patient need. It is logical to assume that patients are just as sick on weekends, and therefore a reduction in staff probably will involve either a decline in quality of care or an increased cost for bringing in part-time workers for weekends only.

Unions will try to limit management as to reassignment of staff. If the nurse executive agrees to a contract which does not allow her to move staff from 5 West to 5 East in emergencies, she will have to hire larger staffs for each floor to make up for the inflexibility she has incurred. In an era when cost containment is so important, the nurse executive must look at the real cost when she gives up such managerial prerogatives as scheduling and assigning of staff. Obviously, as nursing moves into an age of specialization, flexibility naturally does decline. For example, one cannot assign a regular medical-surgical nurse to a specialized intensive care unit and expect her to be able to assume responsibility for the specialized care that goes on there. One can, however, assign such a nurse to such a unit if she is to work there under the supervision of a nurse who knows that specialty and if the transferred nurse is accountable only for performance of those routine nursing acts with which she is familiar.

The nurse executive herself or her agent should sit at the bargaining table so to ensure that others do not give away nursing managerial prerogatives without recognizing that they are doing so. The personnel manager may not recognize the potential impact on care of an every-other-weekend-off policy. Certainly, the contract should not be agreed to and signed without the approval of the nurse executive if it deals with nursing personnel. The nurse executive will want to watch developments as contracts are negotiated outside of the nursing division as well. If another group of workers "bargains" out of a given duty or task, the assumption may be that the nursing division will pick up the task. The wise director keeps up with any and all negotiations underway in her organization. Nursing is the hub of the organization's services; it is usually affected by changes made in any other section of the institution.

Dynamics of Collective Bargaining. The nurse executive who sits on a negotiating team for the first time needs to be prepared for the negotiating process itself. She must recognize the process as an adversarial one, and one in which the other side may use unpleasant tactics so as to put the managerial team at a psychological disadvantage. Of course, both sides have been known to use such tactics in the negotiating process. Unfortunately, personal attacks are used at times because of their effectiveness at putting the party in a less than coolheaded state. The nurse executive should be prepared to cope with such tactics, and she should try to develop an ability to deal with such attacks from a psychological distance. Of course, this is easier to say than to do, and many nurse executives refuse to sit at the negotiating table because these tactics tend to alienate them from their nursing staff. It is a difficult problem, and the director who cannot deal with such tactics with a cool head probably does not belong at the table. Nevertheless, it is important that nursing top management be represented and that the nurse executive follow the happenings in the negotiations in detail.

In principle, negotiations take place with each side giving up some lesser goals so as to achieve its major goals. The give and take of the negotiation must take place if both sides actually negotiate in "good faith." Give and take does not mean, however, that management must give in to unreasonable demands of labor. Management must consider labor's demands; it need not cave in to them. And certainly, management should get something for every item it gives to the other side.

In nursing there is much rhetoric about the "professional union," and the ability to negotiate in cooperation. Although it certainly is possible and desirable to negotiate in a calm and logical manner instead of in an emotionally charged one, it is not really logical to assume that two sides will agree to a contract by the cooperative mode. Union leaders are elected on the basis of what benefits they are able to obtain for their membership. Has a union official ever been reelected because she gave up the union members' weekends (or other benefits) for the sake of better patient care? Although the "professional union" claims it is bargaining for patients' rights as well as staff members' benefits, it is typical that when those rights and benefits clash, the union opts to support staff benefits, claiming that it is management's job to find a way to achieve high-quality care. This is an instance where the ideal—professional negotiation—and the real—member benefits—cannot always be simultaneously achieved.

The Contract Itself. In constructing the contract, the nurse executive should be sure to have expert help. If she fails to have advice, she may underrepresent management by what is included in the contract or by what is excluded. For example, if the contract inadvertently mentions certain personnel documents, a director may subsequently find herself unable to change even a job position description without agreement by the union because those outside documents are legally included in the contract by reference. Conversely, an inexperienced management nego-

tiating team might fail to include some critical clause, such as a managerial rights statement, a scope clause, or an exclusionary clause. Particular components of a good contract will not be discussed here because they are too specialized but the director who endeavors to negotiate a contract on the basis of "good sense" without the added special knowledge of labor negotiation will have problems—unless her opponents on the other side of the bargaining table are as ignorant as she is, and that situation is rapidly vanishing. Much nursing negotiation is being taken over by groups that have been in the union business a long time—from teamsters to teacher's organizations. Even the state nurses' associations have by now acquired expertise in negotiating. The nurse executive who allows a lesser degree of skill on her side of the table ultimately will pay the price.

The contract itself primarily covers such items as salaries, fringe benefits, and working conditions. Some nursing contracts also refer to controls on patient care quality which may be exerted by the employee. Here is a problem area for nursing, because this is an infringement on the basic rights of management to control the processes of production. Of course, there are different levels of employee participation when employees are allowed in on the setting of standards for care: consultation only, required mutual agreement between management and labor, or approval by labor. The nurse executive will need to be very careful if she negotiates in the domain of responsibilities that usually are managerial.

Clear language is essential in a contract. The function of a contract is to prevent disagreements between management and labor concerning the issues included, but if the contract's language is ambiguous, the contract may present as many problems as it solves. The contract must be carefully checked for contradictory clauses, another potential source of future problems.

One important clause in almost every contract is the arbitration clause. In exchange for a guarantee of no strike during the life of the contract, management agrees to arbitration of disputes that are not satisfactorily resolved in the grievance procedure. In an arbitration, an outside party makes the judgment in a dispute, and both parties—labor and management—agree to abide by the arbitrator's decision. Two methods are used in seeking an arbitrator: either an arbitrator is sought for each separate case, or the two sides agree on a permanent arbitrator to hear all cases within the institution. The second method allows the arbitrator to become more familiar with the institution and thus more likely to be able to resolve disputes to everyone's satisfaction.

The Contract Administration Phase

Once a contract has been negotiated, the administrator is responsible for seeing that its provisions are upheld. The nurse executive will need to know intimately any contract that she administers as well as to educate new managers to the necessity of preserving the contractual agreements. The nurse executive cannot afford to keep a manager who fails to implement the contract carefully for consequent grievances and arbitrations would be too costly.

In the day-to-day relations with the union during the life of the contract, the nurse executive must remember that certain actions which she might think of as merely cooperative are actually illegal. For example, to "support" the union by providing phones, offices, or meeting rooms for union activities is illegal under NLMRA. There is a question of legality concerning collecting dues for the union by payroll deduction plans; some questions also are raised concerning the sending of employees to continuing education programs which will put money into union coffers.

In contract administration, the nurse executive must remember that she does not derive her right to make managerial decisions from the contract; it is her obligation to make such decisions. And her relations with union representatives should only concern those matters legitimately within the contract. Two major responsibilities, then, fall to the nurse executive: to see that the contract provisions are upheld, and to provide the appropriate grievance channels where there are disagreements as to whether or not the contract was enacted. Where grievances are not satisfactorily resolved through the usual channels, most contracts provide for arbitration. The nurse executive must remember that only matters contained within the contract are subject to this route. She should never agree to arbitration on an issue not contained in the provisions of the contract. Any items not contained within the contract should remain a managerial prerogative. There are at least two major sources of arbitrators: the American Arbitration Association and the Federal Mediation and Conciliation Service. Both will provide lists of possible arbitrators and their qualifications. Ideally, an arbitrator with previous experience in the health field would be selected.

The objective in contractual relations should be to define relationships clearly so that disagreements are minimized during the life of the contract. The latter is certainly the objective of the nurse executive in the administration phase.

SUMMARY

A brief review of labor relations has been given in this chapter as illustration of one of the aspects of executive role performance where legal structures, resources, and constraints are involved. At present most nurse executives will find that they work in an environment where there are many legal dictates and requirements. Often a bureaucratic style of management will be required to deal with such issues accurately. Given the demands of the impinging legal structure, it behooves the nurse executive to acquire personal knowledge and the help of experts in the important domains of legal practice that affect the work of the nursing division.

REFERENCES

1. Stevens, W.L. Labor Relations and Personnel Administration. Speech on September 27, 1978, at First National Conference, Journal of Nursing Administration, Dallas, Texas. (Available on tape)
2. See *National Labor Relations Board v. Annapolis Emergency Hospital Association, Inc., d/b/a Anne Arundel General Hospital,* No. 76-1166, United States Court of Appeals for the Fourth Circuit.

BIBLIOGRAPHY

Amundson, N.E. The rules of the game are changing. *J.O.N.A.* 1(3):45, 1971.

Amundson, N.E. Labor relations and the nursing leader. *J.O.N.A.* 4(5):10, 1974.

Amundson, N.E. Alternatives to the strike in collective bargaining. *J.O.N.A.* 5(1):11, 1975.

Beletz, E.E., and Meng, M.T. The grievance process, *Am. J. Nursing* 77(2):256, 1977.

Bickford, J. The crisis. *J.O.N.A.* 9(1):28, 1979.

Bloom, I. Strike with honor *J.O.N.A.* 5(4):19, 1975.

Bryant, Y.N. Labor relations in health care institutions: an analysis of Public Law 93-360. *J.O.N.A.* 8(3):28, 1978.

Cleland, V.S. The supervisor in collective bargaining. *J.O.N.A.* 4(4):33, 1974.

Cleland, V.S. Shared governance in a professional model of collective bargaining. *J.O.N.A.* 8(5):39, 1978.

Connelly, C.E., et al. To strike or not to strike. *J.O.N.A.* 9(1):52, 1979.

Dankmeyer, T. Collecting the parties on collective action. *Hospitals* 51(15):52, 1977.

Dempsey, P. Strategy and tactics in collective bargaining. *Professional Management* 6(4):22, 1974.

Emerson, W.L. Appropriate bargaining units for health care professional employees. *J.O.N.A.* 8(9):10, 1978.

Epstein, R.L. Guide to NLRB rules on solicitation and distribution. *Hospitals* 49(16):47, 1975.

Epstein, R.L., and Stickler, K.B. The nurse as a professional and as a unionist. *Hospitals* 50(2):44, 1976.

Erickson, E.H. Collective bargaining: an inappropriate technique for professionals. *J.O.N.A.* 3(2):54, 1973.

Fleishman, R. Living with a contract. *Hospitals* 47(22):51, 1973.

Fralic, M.F. The nursing director prepares for labor relations. *J.O.N.A.* 7(6):4, 1977.

Hershey, N. Nursing practice acts and professional delusion. *J.O.N.A.* 4(4):36, 1974.

Herzog, T.P. The National Labor Relations Act and the ANA: a dilemma of professionalism. *J.O.N.A.* 6(8):34, 1976.

Hush, H. Collective bargaining in voluntary agencies. *J.O.N.A.* 1(6):55, 1971.

Jacox, A. Conflicting loyalties in collective bargaining: an empirical illustration. *J.O.N.A.* 1(5):19, 1971.

McIsaac, G.S. What's coming in labor relations? *Harvard Business Rev.* 55(5):22, 1977.

Metzger, N. The arbitration procedure—part one. *Hospitals* 48(8):47, 1974.

Metzger, N. The arbitration procedure—part two. *Hospitals* 48(9):45, 1974.

Miller, H.J., and Dodson, L. Work stoppage among nurses. *J.O.N.A.* 6(10):41, 1976.

Miller, M.H. Nurses' right to strike. *J.O.N.A.* 5(2):35, 1975.

Miller, R.L. Anticipate questions, seek answers for adept labor relations efforts. *Hospitals* 50(13):50, 1976.

Perry, S.E. Managing to avoid malpractice: part I. *J.O.N.A.* 8(8):43, 1978.

Perry, S.E. Managing to avoid malpractice: part II. *J.O.N.A.* 8(9):16, 1978.

Reece, D.A. Union decertification and the salaried approach: a workable alternative. *J.O.N.A.* 7(6):20, 1977.

Rosmann, J. One year under Taft-Hartley. *Hospitals* 49(24):64, 1975.

Rothman, D.A., and Rothman, N.L. The nurse and informed consent. *J.O.N.A.* 7(10):7, 1977.

Sargis, N.M. Will directors' attitude affect future collective bargaining? *J.O.N.A.* 8(12):21, 1978.

Stevens, W.L. Arbitrability and the Illinois courts. *Arbitration J.* 31(1):1, 1976.

Wagner, E. Avoiding illegal employment practices. *Hospitals* 49(12):45, 1975.

Werther, W.B., Jr., and Lockhart, C.A. *Labor Relations in the Health Professions.* Boston: Little, Brown, 1976.

Werther, W.B., Jr., and Lockhart, C.A. Collective action and cooperation in the health professions. *J.O.N.A.* 7(6):13, 1977.

Part V

Controls of Nursing Management

Part V examines the major control systems of the nursing division. Control systems are perceived as having two major components: the feedback-assessment component and the adjustment component. The systems discussed in this part of the book are those that have regulative impact on the total nursing management.

Chapter 21 develops a basic systems model which may be used to interpret various nursing control systems. Chapter 22 examines quality control mechanisms devised to evaluate patient care, with emphasis upon differentiating systems according to whether they evaluate patient outcomes, nursing processes, or organizational structure. The necessity for corrective action subsequent to evaluation is stressed.

Chapter 23 examines the performance appraisal system—the system that regulates employee behaviors. Management focus is

again shifted from evaluation for its own sake; a principle of coaching for improved performance on the basis of the results of evaluation is described.

Chapters 24, 25, and 26 focus upon three elements of inservice education; inservice as a department, inservice as a constellation of actitivities and services, and inservice as the preparation and performance of an individual project. Inservice is perceived as a major control element because it is frequently the mode of adjustment used in other systems, to correct poor staff performance, for example.

Chapter 27 summarizes the administrative communication and control systems that regulate management acts. These include controls exerted by external accrediting and licensing agencies as well as control devised within the nursing division itself.

Chapter 21

Development and Use of Control Systems

Delivery of nursing care calls for the conscious, planned application of resources, processes, and structures, by the nurse executive, to the achievement of desired goals. These goals include desired patient health outcomes, effective and efficient nursing processes, as well as effective and efficient patterns of organization. In order to evaluate success in achieving nursing goals, it is necessary to devise mechanisms for feedback of results and adjustment of resources, processes, and structures where necessary to better achieve goals. These two mechanisms, feedback and adjustment, comprise the control element of nursing management.

Because it is useful in explaining control phenomena, a systems model will be used as the basic theme of this chapter. A system is a set of interrelated and interdependent parts (such as nursing's resources, processes, and structures) designed to achieve a goal or set of goals. The goal dictates the system's central processes, that is, the activities that turn the raw material (input) into the finished

product (output). In Figure 21-1, the system gets its raw materials from the surrounding environment and returns its finished product to that environment.

A system is differentiated from its environment and that which is external to its environment. A system's environment surrounds the system, and the system interacts with it. An element is part of the environment, not of the system, when the system can do relatively little about the element's characteristics or behavior, and when the element determines, in part, how the system performs. That which is external to the system has no interaction with it.

Some systems are "closed," that is, they do not interact with an environment. Such systems supply their own energy for continuation. Since closed systems are rarely seen in the nursing division, the reader may assume that subsequent discussion refers to open systems, which interact with their environments.

Virtually any phenomenon can be viewed

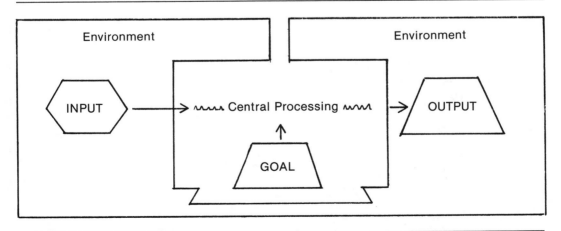

Figure 21-1.   Basic Systems Model

from the systems approach. Indeed, a component of one system may itself be viewed as a system, or as a subsystem of the larger system. Within the total system of the nursing division, one can identify subsystems for patient care, employee performance, administration, and education. It is possible to relate these subsystems to each other by viewing the nursing system as a whole, thus producing a better mechanism for control in the nursing division.

It is logical to assume that patient care is the major subsystem of the nursing division. Improved patient health may be assumed to be the major nursing goal, with ill persons as the system input, well or improved patients as the output, and the nursing actions that effect the change as central processing, sometimes called "thruput." See Figure 21-2 for an illustration of the patient care system.

Other nursing goals for other nursing subject matter may be viewed similarly in a systems model. Figure 21-3 illustrates an instance when staff behavior is the subject matter.

An effective systems model requires still another component—a cybernetic loop to establish communication and control. (See Figure 21-4.) The properties of a cybernetic system can be summarized as follows:

1. *The system has the capacity to sense departures from the desired output.* For this to happen, the system first must know what output is desired. A clear description or measure of the goal is necessary in order to have a basis for comparison. Second, the product of the system must be assessed, measured, or described in a similar manner. If the product cannot be characterized in the same way as the goal, there is no way to compare them. Finally, one must be able to tell how the two items (goal and product) differ.

2. *The system is able to prescribe action to correct deficiencies in the product.* Where differences between the product and the goal can be identified, the system must be able to determine or hypothesize the source of that difference, and it must formulate a decision strategy to correct the disparity. In other words, the system must relate the outcome to the processes (central processing or thruput) that caused it. The cybernetic system, therefore, prescribes corrective actions. In some cases those actions may be obvious; in others, the system may have to explore proposed alternative actions until successful ones are discovered.

3. *The system allocates resources and efforts to implement the proposed corrective actions.* The proposed corrective actions must be feasible, and they must be implemented. Otherwise, the prescription is meaningless.

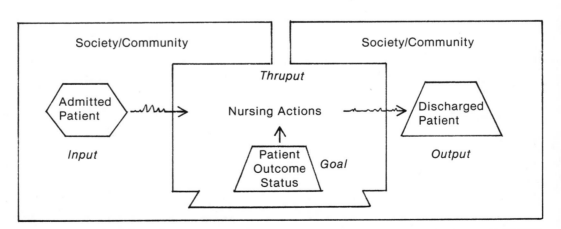

Figure 21-2. Patient as Input to the Nursing System

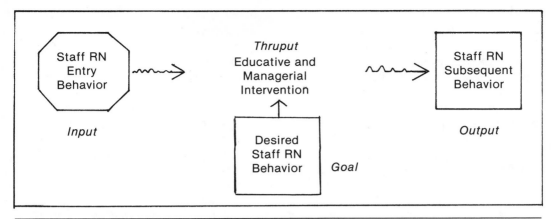

Figure 21-3. Staff as Input to the Systems Model

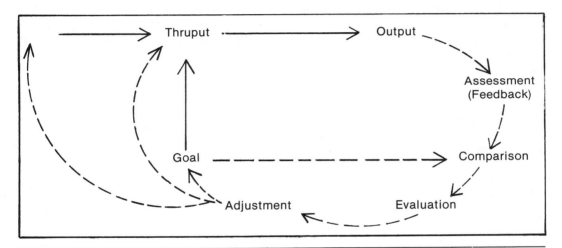

Figure 21-4. Systems Model with a Cybernetic Loop

4. *The system has the capacity to sense results of the change in processing.* Here one is back to the first step; for the system again measures output (the new output) against the original goal.

Notice in Figure 21-4 that control can be exercised so as to make the product and goal correspond in three different ways: The thruput may be altered so as to produce a product as desired. The goal itself may be altered to more closely resemble the product; this might be done if it were determined that a goal originally had been set too high or too low. The input may be altered so it responds more adequately to the available processes. As illustration, only nurses' aides of a certain IQ would be admitted to a training program if those with lower IQs habitually failed the program. Hereafter, illustrations will deal with the most common condition: alteration of thruput.

One may illustrate the cybernetic function in relation to an inservice education program. Suppose that a given patient outcome, such as safe use of crutches, is measured by numbers of falls and accidents suffered by patients while using crutches. Suppose, also, that the set standard has been exceeded: more falls and injuries are occurring than should be tolerated. The cause has been diagnosed as staff ignorance of procedures for safe use of crutches. The relevant systems model, including a cybernetic loop, might look like Figure 21-5.

In this example, the change in central processing (offering an educational program) improved the output, but did not succeed in causing the goal to be met. Hence the cybernetic system calls for still further changes in the central processing. For example, the instructor might change the content of her course, the method of instruction, or she might monitor attendance. If these steps of control prove ineffective in decreasing the number of injuries on crutches, then one would consider further factors of education or, perhaps, other factors not related to education (perhaps some factors in the environment contribute to falls, for example, poorly kept crutches).

Another example will illustrate *alternate paths*, different modifications of the central processing component of the system. Suppose that two head nurses are finding an undesirably high number of geriatric patients falling out of bed and suffering injury at night. One head nurse might choose to reduce injuries by requiring that siderails be in place and elevated for every geriatric patient every night. She might combine this requirement with a request for increased frequency of nightly rounds by the nurse in charge. The second head nurse might try a different process alteration; she might have carpet installed in patients' rooms, lower each bed nightly, and use few if any siderails. Obviously, this head nurse is hypothesizing that many falls are due to confused patients trying to climb over siderails. She further hypothesizes that lower beds and carpeting will reduce incidence of injury in

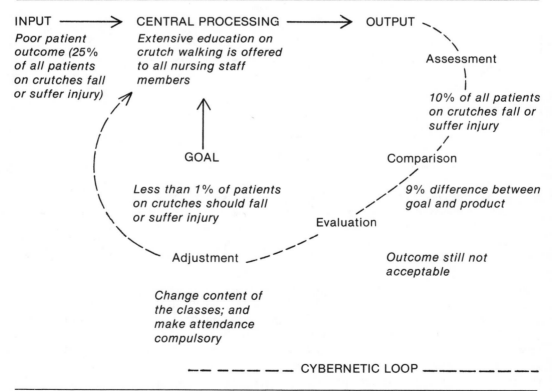

Figure 21-5.   System with Cybernetic Loop to Manage Falls and Injuries of Patients on Crutches

such cases. The first head nurse is working toward the goal from different premises, trying to prevent falls rather than to lessen their impact.

Suppose that both head nurses bring their injury rate down to the acceptable level. How does one judge which approach was best? Other values, both human values and managerial, will serve as criteria for the judgment. If one places a high value on human autonomy, the solution that restrains fewer patients will be selected. If, however, the expense of carpeting is an imposing cost, then economy may be the deciding factor. Further considerations might include the kinds of patients admitted to the two units. Perhaps the solution for one unit would be unsuccessful when applied to the patient population of the other unit.

This incident describes an important fluctuation in a systems model. It may be the case that where the *input differs* the processes also must differ in order to reach the *same output* goals. Figure 21-6 illustrates this point. Suppose that the goal is the same: no development of hypostatic pneumonia following surgery, for example. Suppose, however, that Patient A is a 95-year-old man admitted from a nursing home with a pathological fracture of the hip. Suppose

Patient B is a 17-year-old young man who sustained his hip fracture during participation in a football game. Medical therapy for both patients involved surgical hip pinning. Obviously, neither patient should fail to meet the standard (no hypostatic pneumonia) but the nursing care (thruput) probably will not be the same, one patient needing more special care than the other for achievement of the standard.

These examples illustrate the use of a systems model with cybernetic controls in nursing management. Such a model enables the manager to relate outcomes to central processing in a significant way. If the central processes are unsuccessful in producing the desired goals, they are systematically modified until a sequence of processes is found that achieves the desired outcome.

When a desired goal has been achieved, the management job still is not complete. Even where nursing values have been satisfied and the goal has been effectively reached, management values of efficiency and economy still must be addressed. The manager now applies the same model, asking in each case whether the product (the desired goal) can be achieved with less expense, fewer resources, or in a shorter time. Where two processes are equally successful in

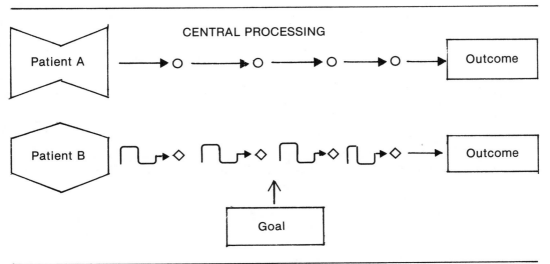

Figure 21-6. Different Central Processing to Assure Same Product when Input Varies Significantly

achieving the desired goal, the less costly process usually is to be preferred. Figure 21-7 illustrates an instance where the *same input* is handled in *diverse ways* so as to produce the *same goal*. Such an illustration might represent staff education in a given procedure, some learning by attending a class while others learn by viewing an audiovisual tape. Or the alternate path model might represent two different nursing plans to achieve the same patient health outcome for similar patients. In this case, the deviation might be due to different resources available at two different points in time.

SYSTEM ERRORS

A systems model is useless if any part of the system is missing or inaccurate. The success of the system can be assured only by careful design of the elements. What can go wrong with the components? It is useful to consider each element separately.

First, what can go wrong in setting *goals*? A goal is useless if it is set too high. A goal which cannot be met makes staff members feel like failures. Similarly, if a goal is set too low, it is meaningless. If everyone reaches the goal as a matter of course, it hardly can

be directive for practice. In addition, goals may be inappropriate or just plain wrong for this system at this time or in this setting. Goals set for matters not within the control of the nursing division also are useless.

A good goal, therefore, is one that represents the best realistic outcome that can be achieved through the influence of nursing care or nursing administrative processes in a given institution. It is a sign of institutional health when the nursing division is able to identify realistic goals for all its activities.

What about *input*? The level of control over input may vary radically among nursing systems. For example, where the patient is the system input, the nursing division may perceive that it has no control since it does not regulate patient admissions to the institution. In other cases, however, nursing may have total control. For example, the nurse executive may set her own standards for each class of employee hired, and she may refuse ''input'' of a candidate who does not meet the qualifications. Sometimes the nursing division may wish to control the input to one system by acts in another system. For example, a home care program may decrease numbers of admissions of geriatric patients who have limitations in self-care abilities.

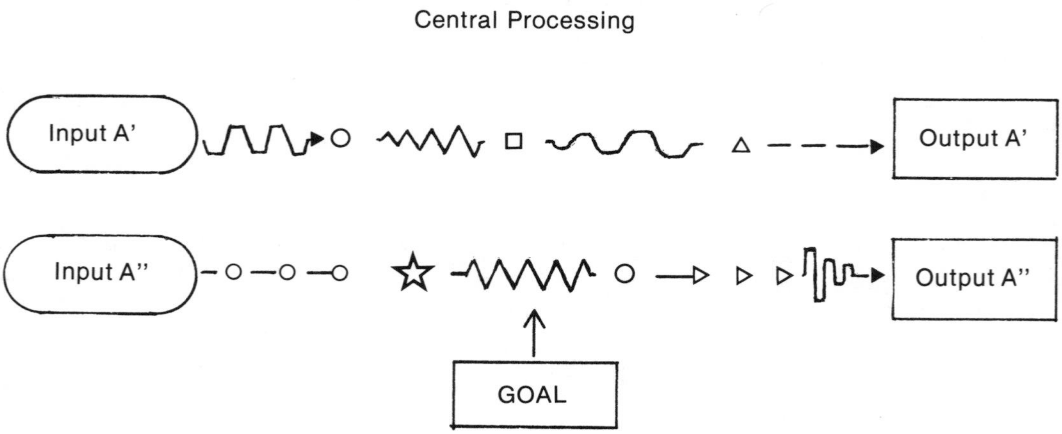

Central Processing

Figure 21-7.   Alternate Routes of Central Processing, with Similar Input and Same Goal

Figure 21-8 illustrates another important relation: the one between *input* and *environment*. In this instance the input is the battered child. Since the system in this model only considers itself to cover the hospitalized care, it is obvious that the environmental effects are self-defeating. In this illustration the system reaches the desired output (a child with physical injuries healed), only to have the environment return that output to its original detrimental state. Obviously, one could construct an image of a larger system, one that includes the aspects labeled "environment," the parents and home situation; the output desired might then stipulate psychological elements as well as physical ones.

What about *central processing*? Errors here tend to be those of traditionalism, clinging to a process that either does not achieve the goals or is unrelated to goals, or else achieves goals at too great a cost. Another error in nursing related to central processing is that of covert processing. As illustration, when nurses fail to identify and keep records of the plan of nursing care, it is not even possible to *know* the processes and hence never possible to make reasonable judgments concerning what processes are effective in producing what outcomes.

What about the *feedback* and *comparison* phases of control? What can go wrong in the control process? Clearly, control cannot succeed unless the goals can be operationalized so as to lend themselves to careful and consistent measurement. Similarly, control will fail if for some reason there is no way to apply these operationalized goals to the output. Feedback and comparison are not enough if one cannot make a *judgment* as to whether or not the reality has missed or conformed with the goal. Usually this means that the system has mini-max levels of acceptable conformity, but one must be sure when that leeway has been overextended.

Feedback and comparison are only as good as the tools which allow one to collect and analyze the data. Hence, if a format is devised to measure a given output, it is important that the form be both valid and reliable. A tool is *valid* if it measures what it purports to measure. A tool to measure mental status of patients in a psychiatric unit, for example, should not primarily ask questions dealing with physical status, as a recent one did.

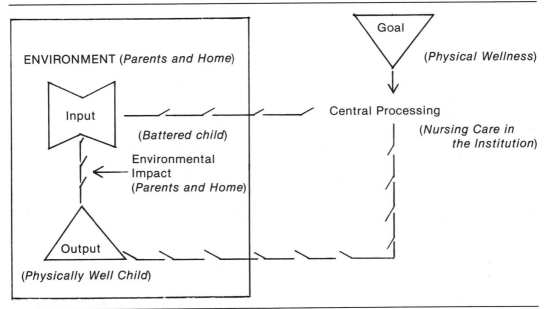

Figure 21-8.   Impact of Environment on System Output

A tool lacks *reliability* if different persons using the same tool come up with different ratings or scores on the same subject matter. Suppose a quality control tool asks nurses to judge the muscle strength of patients yet fails to give adequate criteria to make such a judgment. If the tool just says to rate muscle strength as excellent, good, fair, or poor, these terms are not definitive enough and are too subjective to assure that any group of nurses would rate a group of patients similarly.

Another deficit in reliability occurs when a tool can call forth different responses from the same rater at different times. A supervisor using the same evaluation tool she used a month or more ago to rate an employee whose performance has not changed in any significant way should not come up with a radically different score. If the tool did not help the supervisor to interpret a similar performance in a similar manner, then that tool lacks reliability.

What about the *adjustment* element of the control system? What can go wrong in making adjustments? There can be no intelligible adjustment if the processes (thruput) and the output have not been properly associated. Hence if the thruput varies from day to day, there is no way to establish correlations between thruput and output nor to control thruput for a systematic change. Thruput, then, must be known and repetitive before one is ready to make any adjustment in it.

The adjustment component must allow for a reasoned change. In some systems, the needed change will be evident. In other systems the nurse executive may postulate and test alternatives. And in some cases change may be trial and error—or nearly that—until a successful methodology is discovered. Obviously, this aspect is where nursing research and nursing administrative research fit in. Research becomes the adjustment phase when one is unsure of the proper changes to make in a system to produce the desired goals.

The adjustment component also requires an environment in which controlled change is possible. Where rigidities in the nursing division prevent the adjustment phase, it is a waste of time to evaluate carefully; evaluation for its own sake produces no improvement in patient care. Adjustment must be possible for a systems model to work. Stability after an adjustment is essential if the worth of the adjustment is to be assessed. Many people make the mistake of measuring an adjustment before it is fully integrated into the norms of the system. Judgment of a given adjustment should not be made until it has become part of the standard operating procedure.

What errors can be made in the *output* of the system? Many of the problems already have been discussed as the output relates to the goal of the control system. One other element may be mentioned here, however. Many people determine to measure all aspects of the "output" for a system. Every nurse executive has seen at least one measurement tool which has hundreds of standards for numerous parts of a given output. Often such a detailed tool defeats its own purpose. If the testing mechanism involved in measuring the output is too complex, it is not likely to be used for long. Instead of aiming for comprehensiveness in measurement, the nurse executive will be wise to encourage the development of measurements which address the critical elements of a given output, ignoring the less critical elements. In this way, indices are developed which give quick and relatively accurate information on a given output. Nursing education uses the critical index approach when it teaches diabetic foot care. Though foot care is only part of the care required by a diabetic, it is assumed that if the feet are properly cared for, it is likely that the rest of the body will be in a similar state. The foot has been picked as the index because of its vulnerability; if there is a deficit in the body or its care, it is likely to be reflected first in the foot.

DIVERSE NURSING SYSTEMS

The systems model may be applied to diverse phenomona in the nursing division; for several major applications see Table 21-1.

Table 21-1.   Major Systems of the Nursing Division

System	Input	Thruput	Goal	Output	Feedback	Adjustment
Patient Care	Individual patients	Nursing interventions	Set in care plans	Meets goals, Patient satisfied	Case assessments	Care plan modification
	Patient groups (by need, problem, or disease category)	Nursing interventions	Patient care standards, Quality control criteria, ANA standards	Meets goals, Patient satisfied	Patient opinionnaires, Quality control audits	Change in nursing interventions
Employee Performance	Employee skills, knowledge, attitudes, actions	Supervision, Inservice education, Peer pressure, Self-assessment, Rewards/punishments	Job descriptions, Quality control criteria, Policies and procedures, ANA standards	Nursing acts, behaviors, attitudes	Supervisor's observations, Performance appraisal	Coaching and counseling, Education
Nursing Division	Organization structures and processes of the division	Nursing management	Own objectives, External standards of JCAH, ANA	Direction and control of division	Summaries of performance of major nursing systems	Reorganization, Changes in systems
Inservice Education	Staff ignorance, lack of skills	Education, Orientation, Information, Departmental programs and projects	Divisional objectives, Department objectives, Quality control standards, Job functions	Knowledge, Skills, Attitudes	Quality control audits, Performance appraisal results, Tests subsequent to educational projects	Education, Orientation, Information

The nurse executive will note that certain elements in each of these total systems are more "popular" in the literature, receiving more attention than other elements. Ironically, these elements seldom are the goals of the system. Performance appraisal (the form-to-be-filled-out) often is seen falsely as an end in itself; in some places quality control formats are treated in this manner. The nurse executive will want to maintain her overview of the nursing division so that she keeps in balance all the components of the major nursing systems, so that *instrumental* components achieve the *ends* of the systems. Further, the nurse executive will see that the systems receive appropriate balance in relation to each other, since together they comprise the major control systems for the division.

Notice that each of these major systems deals with one mode of quality control, controlling quality of patient outcomes, of staff behavior, of organizational effectiveness, or of educational output. In each case, the system must be developed as a totality if it is to be effective. Standards must be determined, methods selected for implementation, feedback information collected and analyzed, and adjustment in the thruput must be made where results differ from goals set.

In order to effect a control system, the nurse executive must see that three steps are followed for each system:

1. Setting standards
2. Developing or selecting measuring tools and/or indices
3. Developing a surveillance process to carry out measurements, analyze data, recommend or implement corrective actions

SURVEILLANCE PROCESS

There are numerous decisions to be made in developing a surveillance process for any major nursing system. The following questions must be answered in each case:

1. Who should participate in the surveillance process? What should their role be? Evaluator? Data collector? Interpreter? Data distributor?
2. What sort of monitoring does the surveillance process implement? *What* is to be measured? *How often*? Using *what tools* or *indices*?
3. How are judgments to be made when multiple tools and indices are used in the surveillance process?
4. What is the appropriate distribution for surveillance data once interpreted? Who needs the information and why?
5. How is accountability placed for change when deficiencies occur?

Sometimes a surveillance process will be devised to cover all or many subsystems of a major nursing system. A quality control committee may be in charge of evaluating the care given to 20 different groupings of patients, including cardiovascular patients, obstetric patients, postoperative patients, patients with sensory deprivation. Such a committee will have to make many decisions for each subsystem group, and if resources are limited, will have to assign priorities to various surveillances activities. It might be decided, for example, to collect data frequently in an area known to suffer deficiencies but only infrequently in an area which usually maintains excellent control.

The advantage of having a single surveillance committee for each major nursing system is that the system then is viewed as a whole. The surveillance committee in the preceding example will have a good idea of the total quality of patient care in the institution and will be able to compare the care in the different nursing arenas, identifying weakness and strengths in the system.

Some institutions prefer to set up a separate surveillance process for each subsystem, perhaps a surveillance process for care of cardiovascular patients and another for care of obstetric patients. When many different surveillance processes exist simultaneously, the comprehensive view of the total system may reside solely with the nurse executive or her top management team. If separate surveillance processes are used, it may be only at the top level that such separate data are brought together for comprehensive and interrelated interpretation.

Other nursing divisions have evolved a combination of surveillance processes—some for total nursing systems, others for smaller subsystems. What matters is that surveillance processes be carefully thought out by the nurse executive to achieve her managerial goals. The control systems of the nursing division should not simply develop happenchance. Furthermore, all control systems need to be considered as a totality at some point in the evaluative cycle.

In order to process the extensive data derived from the surveillance systems of the nursing division, it is necessary that data be cumulated and summarized in meaningful ways. This will enable all nurse managers to process and interpret more information in a more significant manner. The nurse executive of a large, major university hospital might waste many valuable hours if she insists on reading every incident report in her division. Here reports of accidents and injuries constitute part of the patient care nursing system control. Instead of reading every incident, the nurse executive would get a better picture of the errors occurring if she requires a monthly report which classifies and categorizes errors according to type, unit where incident occurred, type of worker involved in bad judgment—or other summary categories according to the specific needs of the executive.

SUMMARY

The nurse executive and her top management staff assume responsibility for maintaining the view of the whole. One way that this responsibility is fulfilled is through careful monitoring of the division's major control systems, which should be organized so as to provide meaningful feedback on the state of the systems. The systems should be organized for action, so that corrective measures are determined and implemented when a deficit is identified by the control system. The nurse executive will want to balance her activities and those of her staff over the major control systems of the division in such a way that attention is given to each system in proportion to its significance to the whole. Top management also must consider the performances of the major nursing systems as they relate to each other. This synthesis of data and response is one of the major responsibilities of executive management.

BIBLIOGRAPHY

Ackoff, R.L. Toward a system of systems concepts. *Management Science* 17(11):661, 1971.

Aiken, L., and Aiken, J.L. A systematic approach to the evaluation of interpersonal relationships. *Am. J. Nursing* 73(5):863, 1973.

Archer, S.E. PERT: a tool for nurse administrators. *J.O.N.A.* 4(5):26, 1974.

Camman, C., and Nadler, D.A. Fit control systems to your managerial style. *Harvard Business Rev.* 54(1):65, 1976.

Henn, C.L. A last plea for logistics. *Distribution Worldwide* 13(11):60, 1974.

Miller, F.G. Applying systems analysis. *J. Systems Management* 24(10):24, 1973.

Nadler, G. *Work Systems Design.* Homewood, Ill.: R.D. Irwin, 1967.

O'Malley, C.D. Application of systems engineering in nursing. *Am. J. Nursing* 69(10):2155, 1969.

Chapter 22   Quality Control of Patient Care

The patient care quality control system resembles a quality control system for any other field, occupation, or subject matter. It is a system set up to measure the quality of the product of the organization; in this case the product is patient care. Slee identifies three essential components of any quality control program: standards, surveillance, and corrective action[1].

SELECTING THE SUBJECT MATTER FOR QUALITY CONTROL

Quality control of patient care is best accomplished when data are gathered from diverse sources of evidence. This chapter will consider the three most common sources: the organization, the nursing care, and the patient outcomes. As indicated in Chapter 4 the nursing organization usually is assessed on structure standards, nursing care activities usually are assessed on process standards, and patient status usually is assessed on outcome standards. For simplicity, these common linkages will be used, recognizing that they are not invariable; one *can* assess factors of structure, process, and outcome for each of the three subject matters, organization, nursing process, and patient.

It is important to gather data from all three arenas when evaluating patient care because of the interlinkages among them. For example, the structures of the organization affect the type of nursing care that is offered, and the type of care affects the patient outcomes achieved.

SELECTING THE FORM OF STANDARD TO BE USED

The setting of standards is, of course, the first step of structuring quality control systems. In setting standards, one can choose to appraise patient care from the perspectives of structure, process, or outcome[2], and from the subject matters of organization, nursing, or patient.

Structure Standards

If one looks at the standards used by most accrediting or standards-setting agencies in nursing, such as the American Nurses' Association, the National League for Nursing, and the Joint Commission on Accreditation for Hospitals, it is apparent that these groups have selected structure as the area of concern. The following questions and statements compiled from accreditation questionnaires and lists of standards from these three sources will illustrate the point:

1. Is a registered nurse responsible for planning, evaluating, and supervising the nursing care of each patient?
2. Are written care plans used?
3. The nursing department provides training programs and opportunities for staff development.
4. There is a system for recording accurate and objective observations of patients in the clinical record.

One can see that these questions and statements are directed toward assessing the structures by which nursing care is organized and managed, the arrangements by which nursing care is delivered. These arrangements represent the uniform organizational structure in which each nursing employee functions. They are the established frameworks for the patient care delivery system. It is logical that accrediting bodies would focus on structure because it is a single entity and stable, whereas nursing processes and patient outcomes are numerous and require an extensive sampling if one wishes to make a judgment concerning them. An accrediting body seldom has the time for such an extensive survey. For this reason, it will concentrate on structure, the only aspect of patient care which is singular and relatively stable.

Structure-based criteria are designed to identify necessary, but not sufficient, conditions for good-quality care. It might be *necessary* for a registered nurse to plan patient care, but the fact that such care is planned by a registered nurse is no assurance that the planning is well done. Written care plans may be *necessary* for good care, but that such plans are written does not, in and of itself, assure that they are good plans. Criteria based on structure give conditions under which it is likely that good nursing will take place, but such criteria do not assure that the good care does in fact take place. Structure criteria address themselves to the way in which the subject matter is systematized; they evaluate the organizing frameworks.

The following statements illustrate *structure* standards for the organization, for nursing, and for the patient, respectively:

1. Organization. There is a fail-safe system for removing outdated supplies from nursing units.
2. Nursing care. The nursing process is applied in the derivation of patient care plans.
3. Patient. The amputee has the capacity, motivation, and opportunity to learn ambulation.

Process Standards

Process standards provide a second perspective; they measure the actions of the subject matter. Typically, in nursing, process associates with direct nursing care actions. Nursing process here will refer to the activities of the individual nurse—actual interactions between the nurse and the patient. The nursing process takes place within the providing structure; it is the *action* rather than the structure in which that action takes place that constitutes process.

The primary difference between process and structure standards can be demonstrated by the conversion of two of the previously quoted structure standards into representative process standards.

Structure Standard. Are written care plans used?

Related Process Standards. Is the written care plan appropriate for the patient? Does it demonstrate consideration of his personal needs, disease-related needs, and therapy-related needs?

Structure Sample. There is a system for recording accurate and objective observations of patients in the clinical record.

Related Process Standards. The charting shows evidence of relevant observations of patient progress, of patient response to therapy, and of completion of physician's orders. Evidence of the patient's psychic state is present where relevant.

A process standard tells how accurately a performance is enacted. A critical difference between structure standards and process standards is that the process standards require a professional judgment to determine whether each criterion has been met. Whereas anyone can determine whether care plans are used, a structure standard, only a nurse can judge whether a plan represented a proper care plan for that patient, a process standard. Judgment does afford possibility for some differences in rating, but such differences can be decreased by writing each criterion in clearly defined behavioral terms, to make the judgment less subjective.

The following illustrate *process* standards for the organization, for nursing, and for the patient, respectively:

1. Organization. The nursing division reassigns staff on each shift according to the classification system data.
2. Nursing care. The nurse turns the unconscious patient every two hours.
3. Patient. The diabetic patient accurately tests his urine for sugar and acetone.

Outcome Standards

The outcome standard takes yet another perspective; it measures the result rather than the process used. The difference between a process standard and an outcome standard can best be illustrated by conversion of a process standard to an outcome criterion:

Process Standard. Nurse applies dressings with appropriate sterile technique.
Related Outcome Standard. Patient does not develop a wound infection.

Patient outcome standards represent the ultimate goals of nursing measurement, for, if the patient outcome is unsatisfactory, it matters little what nursing processes were used or what organizational arrangement (structure) supported that therapy. Nevertheless, outcome alone is not sufficient as a sole criterion. Outcome represents effectiveness. Ultimately in nursing management, one must look for efficiency as well as effectiveness. This means that one also must look for the least costly ways of achieving the desired outcome.

The following illustrate outcome standards for the organization, for nursing, and for the patient, respectively:

1. Organization. Absenteeism is reduced 50 percent.
2. Nursing care. A program for diabetic teaching is designed and implemented.
3. Patient. Normal peristalsis is returned by the second postoperative day.

Patient outcome standards can be difficult to isolate. Ideally one would like to be able to determine how much of the patient's health outcome is due to nursing, how much is due to medicine, and how much to other factors. Typically the patient's health outcome is the result of multiple interacting factors of which nursing only is one. Even where the effects of the nursing component cannot be isolated, its significance still can be assessed by changes in statistical outcomes which correspond with specific, identified nursing processes.

For the majority of patients, treatments are mixed and outcomes are complex or highly individualized. To use outcome standards given these conditions means that one accepts the following assumptions: 1) there are some health outcomes primarily attributable to nursing, 2) there are some health outcomes partially attributable to nursing, and 3) regulation of nursing actions can produce statistically improved health outcomes for patients in these categories.

The statistical concept is important here, for no single outcome can be assured. For example, suppose it is determined that nursing makes a critical difference in the number of surgical wound infections. This does not mean, of course, that nurses are responsible for all wound infections. Nor does it mean that the infection of any given patient can be attributed to nursing. The patient might acquire such an infection from a variety of sources: the physician's poor technique during surgery, the intern's technique in changing the dressing, ineffective sterilization of dressings, his own interference with the dressing, or nursing technique. Changing that nursing technique to a better one should produce a statistical change in number of wound infections but not an elimination of all infections.

In addition to the problem of multiple causation of health effects, there is a difficulty in establishing desired patient outcome standards that have significance for multiple patients. At one extreme, if patient outcome standards must be developed singly for each patient, then there is no generalized standard against which the nurse may measure her patient's outcome. With individualized standards, there is no constant measure against which to compare end results for various patients receiving different nursing managements. Some individualization of patient outcomes is done in the nursing care plan document. Even here, however, judgments are based on norms modified to take into account individual patient motivation, capacity, and opportunity.

At the other extreme, some institutions have tried to solve the standards problem by identifying universal standards applicable to all patients. Such a universal standard might read, "that each patient return to the optimal physiologic health possible within the constraints of his disease process." Though worthy as goals, such statements are meaningless as operational criteria against which to measure and compare outcomes.

The most useful solution to the outcome standards problem is the middle road, the classification of patients into groups that logically may be expected to have similar desired outcomes. For example, one can easily set a standard that all obstetric patients learn appropriate techniques for feeding and handling the newborn infant. Similarly one might set a standard that all

amputees learn the procedures of safe crutch walking. For all patients with surgical incisions, one might set a standard of first-intention-wound-healing.

Common standards can be developed for patients grouped by similar diseases and conditions or by similar incapacities. They can be identified for all juvenile diabetics (similar disease) or for all paraplegics (similar incapacities) regardless of the source of their disease process. A taxonomy for the selection of patient groups for quality control measures is shown in Table 22-1.

RELATION AMONG THE THREE TYPES OF STANDARDS

As indicated earlier, the relation among the three perspectives of evaluation—structure, process, and outcome—is important. Failure in meeting an outcome standard may indicate a need for a change in the nursing process; failure in meeting a nursing process standard may indicate a need for changing organizational structure. For example, if several patients develop postoperative infections, a negative *outcome,* it may be that the staff needs to examine the *process* of caring

Table 22-1.   Taxonomy for Selection of Patient Groups for Quality Control

Grouping Criterion	Examples
Disease	All new diabetic patients Cardiac patients
Like treatment	Preoperative patients All patients on renal dialysis
Like needs	Patients with immobility Patients with decreased vision
Geographic criterion	All patients in the outpatient clinic All patients on this unit
Life stage	All geriatric patients All teenagers
Illness stage	All patients needing intensive care All self-care patients

for wounds. If nurses are lax in techniques of dressing wounds, it may be that the nursing *structure* creates pressures causing shortcuts in the proper process. Thus results of assessments from one of the three perspectives may have implications for another perspective.

The following evaluations of a cardiac resuscitation illustrate that all three perspectives can be used to describe the same event.

Evaluation 1. Patient survived, suffered no irreversible brain damage, received no physical trauma such as cracked ribs. Patient understands what happened to him and has worked through his reaction to the event.

Evaluation 2. Appropriate verification of the state of cardiac arrest was made. Patient was placed on a hard surface. Air passages were checked for obstruction. Cardiac massage and resuscitation were begun immediately.

Evaluation 3. Cardiac board and mechanical respirator were ready at hand in the treatment room. Respirator was equipped and ready for immediate use. Cardiac resuscitation team arrived within three minutes. Prearranged standing orders enabled them to provide defibrillation and medication at once.

CONSTRUCTING STANDARDS

After the subject matter to be measured and the type of standard (structure, process, or outcome) have been selected, the next step in quality control is to construct the relevant standards. Since outcome standards are the most difficult to compose, these will be reviewed in detail.

The first problem in setting outcome standards is that of reaching consensus on the meaning of a standard. Two contrasting definitions are frequently used in nursing literature: 1) A standard is a criterion of excellence or attainment. 2) A standard is a baseline against which to measure the event or behavior. In the first concept, a standard

is written in terms of the optimally desired outcome; in the second concept, the lowest acceptable level of outcome is described. While there is no "right" or "wrong" definition of a standard, it is essential that a group reach a consensus on the definition of a standard it chooses to use.

When composing outcome standards it is important to set realistic goals for realistic time frames. Standards set for specified time periods must represent accurate nursing prognoses for the given patient base. One problem in constructing outcome standards is that health outcomes change over time. For certain impairments there are stages of illness; for others there is a gradual progression from the initial illness to the final outcome. The setting of standards requires that one determine when outcomes will be measured.

To deal *only* with final outcome criteria begs the question. Even if a patient ultimately reaches the desired final outcomes, one cannot claim good nursing process if he suffered unnecessarily, had unnecessary side effects, and took longer to achieve the final outcomes than would have been the case with more expert nursing.

Some conditions virtually set their own critical measurement points. For example, most nurses would agree that postpartum patients should be assessed at the completion of the delivery phase, on the first postpartum day, and at day of discharge. Other conditions may require more arbitrary setting of times for outcome assessments.

It has been suggested that measurement take place at the end of a certain phase of illness rather than at a given time. The problem here is that the criteria for assessment may be identical to the criteria that mark the end of the given phase of illness. When this is the case, evaluation becomes a tautology: the patient is not out of the phase until he meets the criteria, therefore he will always meet the criteria if he is measured at "end of phase." This is one of the big problems in the evaluation of quality control for psychiatric patients—a problem yet to be satisfactorily resolved.

In formulating outcome standards, it is helpful to classify them on three different axes: 1) attainment or avoidance option, 2) performance or state of being option, and 3) absolute or relative option. Consideration of these axes can help in planning adequate and uniform measurement tools.

On the first axis an outcome standard is either a state to be attained or a state to be avoided. The standard "maintains normal urinary output" gives a desired attainment, whereas the standard "does not develop a bladder infection" represents an avoidance standard. Some nurse authors prefer to deal strictly with attainment standards; others use both types. Avoidance standards can be converted into attainment standards. The avoidance standard given above can be converted into a statement such as "maintains bladder's normal microbial status," an attainment standard.

The second axis for outcome standards indicates whether the outcome is something the patient does or a state he exhibits. For example, the standard "walks on crutches with a four-point gait" is a performance standard. "Maintains intact skin surfaces," on the other hand, is a state-of-being standard. Note that when a desired outcome is a performance (process) then there is a conformity of a patient process objective with a patient outcome objective.

When using performance, it is necessary to differentiate between standards that indicate an ability to perform and those that require the performance itself rather than the ability. Ability to demonstrate full range of motion of the shoulder joint is adequate measurement of shoulder mobility. The patient's *ability* to administer insulin to himself accurately, however, may not be an adequate measure if he tends to ignore some doses. Here the action itself rather than the ability must be measured.

The last axis determines whether the standard is absolute or relative. The standard "all skin surfaces remain intact" is absolute. In contrast, a relative standard may show progression rather than absolute attainment; for example, "The patient, following a cardiovascular accident, increases his ability to depress a hard rubber ball with the weakened hand." This standard is relative because it is measured in relation to the patient's past performance rather than in relation to a particular and absolute measurement of strength. Such a standard could be quantified—the percent of strength increase per week could be given—but this would not change the fact that the percent increase would be relative to the patient's past status.

Every outcome standard can be classified along three axes: attainment or avoidance, performance or state of being, and absolute or relative status. It often is useful to classify the standards of a given measurement tool in order to find the biases and predilections of the tool's author. Many such tools have a disproportionate number of *performance standards* with an inadequate number of *state-of-being standards*. Perhaps this can be traced to the fact that most nurses are comfortable with behavioral (performance) objectives, but state-of-being standards cannot conform to the same grammatical pattern. Some nurse authors insist on calling states of being performances even though they are not events or voluntary acts.

One basic problem in composing outcome standards is to know when one really has a *patient* standard rather than one directed to another agent. Probably the easiest way to judge whether or not a standard is a patient standard is to apply two rules that tell when one *does not* have such a standard. When the understood or stated subject of the standard is the nurse, the organization, the patient's family, an event, or anything other than the patient himself or some aspect of his being, it is not a patient standard. When the statement says what someone other than the patient does (e.g., "Patient is turned frequently"), the standard is not a patient standard.

Another problem in composing standards is deciding how specific they should be. There is no absolute answer to this question. The specificity of standard statements is closely related to the scope of content covered in the evaluation tool as well as the nature of that content. For example, if the evaluation tool is measuring all alcoholic patients in the stage of delirium tremens, it is possible to state the desired outcomes with great detail. Similarly, if the subject matter lends itself to easily quantifiable measures (e.g., blood pressure), then standards can be concrete and specific.

For performance standards, the format for behavioral objectives can be used (see Chapter 4). State-of-being standards cannot be stated with action verbs, as are performance standards, but they can be given equal specificity and concrete description.

As the scope of content of the evaluation tool broadens, the nature of the standard must change. Suppose one were to try to write outcome standards using the Mager form (see Chapter 4) for obstetric patients on the third postpartum day. One could easily produce a list of 200 to 300 such standards; clearly, this form of evaluation is unwieldy and impractical, and so, for situations such as this, it behooves the evaluator to reduce standards to a manageable number, even if they are less complex.

There are several different ways to form standards for a given objective. One may divide the subject matter into its component parts, forming one or more standards for each component. Not every subject matter lends itself to this treatment. Another alternative is to select indices of the whole. In this case, standards are addressed to critical points, rather than to the totality of components. For example, one might consider feeding, diapering, and handling to be critical points in the mothering of a newborn infant. Although these are not the only elements in care of the newborn, they would be sufficiently significant indices where it is not practical to measure all potential aspects of mothering. A third alternative for the formation of standards involves the use of illustrations rather than indices or components. This method is used when the objective is a principle which has many different instantiations. By using examples rather than components or indices, the reader is taught to recognize an instantiation

of the principle, even if it differs somewhat from those of the multiple illustrations. Consider a standard such as, "Patient shows positive response to staff interaction." Since there are many diverse ways in which a patient could show a "positive response" and it is not possible to identify each potential behavior, a list of illustrative responses can alert the evaluator to look for certain kinds of response.

Standards should be few enough in number not to overwhelm the evaluator and should be worded so as to encourage similar interpretations by different evaluators. Behavioral objectives are appropriate for some cases but will not suffice where differences in performance are allowable or where states rather than performances are the subject matter of inquiry.

Frequently a standard is accompanied by the statement of a rationale. Unfortunately, so-called rationales often turn out to be merely explanations of the standard. Appropriately used, a rationale is a justification, not an explanation; it should tell why the preceding statement is important enough to be chosen as a standard and should not merely restate the standard.

FORMATS FOR QUALITY CONTROL TOOLS

Once the standards have been determined, a general format for the tool itself must be prepared. The principal rule to follow is to keep the format simple, easy to use, and easily interpreted by all users. Some common formats are shown in Figure 22-1.

Format 1 is less likely than others to produce diverse opinions among raters, but it requires each standard be defined precisely. Format 2 has the disadvantage of eliciting greater variation in raters' responses. Format 3 has the same disadvantage but may be useful if the institution wants to quantify the answers. Quantification has the advantage of promoting competition among nursing units or of permitting the nursing unit to surpass its previous grade. When offering a

1. Standards	Met	Unmet	Not observed	Comments
Long-range goals written on Kardex				

2. Standards	Excellent	Good	Fair	Poor	Not applicable

3. Standards	1	2	3	4	5

4. Standards	Above Average	Average	Below Average

5. Standards category	First descriptive statement	Second descriptive statement	Third descriptive statement
Patient teaching	Patient has received no teaching	Patient has received some teaching, but does not adequately understand material	Patient has received thorough teaching and understands what was taught

6. Standards	Frequently	Infrequently	Never

Figure 22-1.   Formats for Quality Control Tools

scale for numerical rating, one should not exceed the number of differentiations that can be made accurately; if a scale has 10 categories, it is unlikely that an evaluator can actually differentiate level 7 from level 8 performance.

Format 4 has the advantage of stability, for as the "average" improves in an institution, the form is still applicable. Format 5 is the most difficult to construct, but permits identification of specific levels of nursing care. Notice that in this particular example, two elements rather than one are combined in the standard: teaching and learning. Often attempts to combine two or more elements fail. One can identify options that are not given in the illustrated format, for example, such as, "Patient receives poor teaching but learns anyway," or "Patient has received thorough teaching but adamantly refuses to learn." For the evaluator who is constructing her first set of descriptive standards, it is suggested that each standard deal with a *single* element as it varies over the continuum of gradations.

Format 6 is used when the quality of the standard is not as important as the frequency with which it is carried out. Sometimes when an element can be measured with great specificity, percentages of time may be substituted for descriptive terms such as "frequently," "occasionally," "seldom."

SOURCES OF EVIDENCE

Once the standards and format for the quality control tool have been determined, the next step is to identify the sources of evidence. Primary and secondary sources are usually combined, but, where possible, primary sources are preferable. (Often secondary sources are substituted because of the cost of obtaining primary data.) A primary source gives the rater direct knowledge concerning the standard. For example, if a standard states, "Patient receives adequate oral hygiene," the rater goes to the source, the patient, to observe whether this standard is fulfilled. For the standard, "Emergency equipment is complete and ready for use," the observer again goes directly to the source, evaluating the equipment firsthand.

Not all standards lend themselves to immediate observation. "Promotion of independence" might require a careful evaluation of nursing notes over a period of time. Some standards combine primary and secondary sources: "Adequate hydration is maintained," might combine direct observation of the skin turgor with secondary observation of the intake and output records.

The patient's chart is such a frequent secondary source that evaluation of nursing via the chart often is either included in the quality check or developed separately as a nursing chart audit. But a chart is not an entirely reliable secondary source, for it is possible that nurses write things they do not do—or do things they do not write. Nevertheless, the chart is a popular secondary source because of easy access to it, and because it is relatively easy to evaluate.

Another source of evidence is the patient's response to (satisfaction or dissatisfaction with) his nursing care. It is important that a group forming a quality control system determine ahead how relevant patient satisfaction is as evidence of professional care. Wording of questions to patients is quite important. Some questions can be worded so as to give primary responses: "Did the nurse discuss your surgery with you the day before the operation?" Others cannot be given similar weight: "Are you generally pleased with your nursing care?" The following sources are the most frequently used in quality control checks: charts, rounds, records, nursing care plans, interviews of patients, interviews of nurses, interviews of other health personnel or of patient's family.

It is important that methods of evaluation be specified for each standard. If five evaluators were told to rate blind patients in a rehabilitation unit according to the following standard: "Ambulates safely in known territory," it is conceivable that without further direction the evaluators might use five different methods to rate a patient. These methods might include:

1. Noting the patient's performance on the standard as recorded in his chart.
2. Asking several nurses about the patient's ambulation.
3. Asking the patient about his ambulation
4. Observing the patient for several days as he ambulates on the unit and grounds.
5. Giving the patient a specific test, such as telling him "Go to the solarium and get X".

Clearly some of these evaluation methods are better than others, but the point is that uses of evidence must be identified if standards are to be judged equitably. The selection of methods often is a compromise between the ideal and the economic in time or effort.

FACTORS THAT INFLUENCE THE QUALITY CONTROL SYSTEM

The nurse executive needs to define precisely her purposes in using a quality control system. Typical purposes include:

1. Obtaining accurate patient care feedback.
2. Correcting care deficits.
3. Motivating nursing staff to improve patient care.
4. Verifying effectiveness of established nursing processes.
5. Conducting nursing research relating structure, process, and outcome elements and seeking to identify effective nursing methods.

Another factor that may influence the formats of the quality control system is the division's concept of nursing and of the patient. The following samples represent divisions of nursing care that could be used as a basis for structuring a quality control form:

1. Nursing care
   a. Sustenal
   b. Remedial
   c. Restorative
   d. Preventive[3]
2. Nursing problems
   a. Preserve body defenses
   b. Prevent complications
   c. Reestablish patient in outside world
   d. Detect changes in the body's regulatory system
   e. Implement prescribed therapeutic and diagnostic activity
   f. Provide comfort[4]
3. Nursing care as process
   a. Observation
   b. Inference
   c. Validation
   d. Assessment
   e. Action
   f. Evaluation[5]

Concepts of the patient, rather than of nursing care, also may be used as a basis for a quality control format and standards. The following structures could serve such a purpose:

1. Man as subsystems
   a. Physiologic needs
   b. Self-concept
   c. Role function
   d. Interdependence[6]
2. Man as behavioral subsystems
   a. Affiliation
   b. Aggression
   c. Dependence
   d. Achievement
   e. Ingestion
   f. Elimination
   g. Sex[7]

Which particular structure is selected as a background for the development of a quality control system or project is not so important as that a structure *be* selected. Too many control checklists lack organization and simply present a random list of standards. A nursing division may determine to use a single conceptual framework for many quality control tools in order to evaluate diverse subject matters from the same perspective. (ANA in effect recommends a singular approach by advocating "the nursing process" as a uniform approach to nursing.) Alternately, a nursing division may determine to plan each quality control project around the construct that seems most relevant to the given topic. Often the approach selected will be affected by whether the institution has accepted a single nursing theory or whether it has an eclectic approach to nursing practice.

SURVEILLANCE AND FEEDBACK SYSTEMS

Once the standards have been completed for a project, consideration is given to setting up the surveillance system. It is important that the quality control form be used in a systematic way. One needs to determine who will evaluate what at what times. Answers to these questions must be based on the institution's needs, but the following guidelines have proven useful in some organizations:

1. Schedule evaluation visits at periodic, unannounced intervals. The unexpected visit is more likely to reflect the normal quality of nursing care.
2. Not all patients of a given class need be evaluated; a sampling technique is quite adequate in most cases.
3. Patient sampling may be done at random, or patients may be selected on the basis of which require challenging nursing care.
4. Persons should serve on the evaluation team long enough to become thoroughly familiar with the evaluation process.
5. If evaluation team members split the work, each member should grade the same portion of the checklist on all units evaluated.

6. Where a surveillance system monitors several quality control projects, the evaluations of a given subject matter should be recycled according to need.

The final component of quality control is that of corrective action. A quality control system is useless if proper and immediate feedback is not offered to the nursing units involved. It is more productive, however, to have the staff view quality control as a challenge than as a threat. Supervisors and head nurses can be counseled to see the program as a diagnostic tool more easily if they have an integral part in its use.

For the nurse executive, measurement of the quality of nursing care gives a scientific basis on which to calculate needed nursing personnel. She can measure the point at which increased staffing alone fails to improve care quality as well as the point at which care begins to decline due to personnel shortages.

The feedback from process and outcome standards differs. Process standards immediately identify the deviant nursing process, the practice that fails to conform to the practice described in advance. That is not the case with outcome standards. Outcome standards tell what is going wrong in the patient's progress, but they do not tell what is wrong in the nursing process or how to correct it. The outcome standards, therefore, serve as starting points for research into nursing process because they do not assume that traditional nursing measures are the proper solutions to patient outcome problems. The research design for determining the cause of an undesirable patient outcome requires use of the scientific method, formulation of hypotheses, identification of possible variables, and systematic manipulation of variables until the cause of the undesirable outcome is identified and a corrective solution is found.

When the same subject matter is subjected to both outcome and process standards, it may be possible to establish correlations between them. Figure 22-2 illustrates a tool in which outcome and process have been systematically correlated.

In this tool the nursing processes which have been deduced to have impact on each desired patient outcome have been systematically correlated. Here, as is probably the case with much tradition-based nursing care, it has been determined that the supposed relations are not always the accurate ones. In Figure 22-2, there is a start of data collection that may lead to some nursing research. Note that some interesting conclusions can be drawn from data such as that collected in Figure 22-2. Note that in this illustration the processes that were assumed to be critical to Patient Outcome A were not all essential since the patient goal was achieved even though nursing process standard 3 was not met. Processes 1 and 2 alone seem to be adequate for achievement of the goal. (Of course these data do not guarantee that processes 1 and 2 are actually required for goal achievement, which could have been due to variables not identified at all in this tool.)

Note that Patient Outcome B is achieved when all the identified nursing processes are supplied. Here, again, we can assume that these processes are *sufficient* to achieve the outcome, though we cannot assert that all are *necessary,* or that any particular one is necessary. In Patient Outcome C, we appear to have identified a nursing process which is associated with the outcome: even when all the other nursing processes required were provided, the desired patient outcome was not reached in the absence of Nursing Process 2. Process 2, therefore, appears to be necessary for goal achievement. While such conclusions only can be tentative since unidentified variables may enter the situation in each case, it is still likely that such correlated quality control forms will lead to identification of valuable hypotheses for nursing research.

Where nursing is approached as an attempt to correlate patient outcomes with nursing processes, a new ideology of nursing care evolves. It is important to compare this ideology to the ideology of the recent past, as is done in Table 22-2.

QUALITY CONTROL TOOL SUMMARY SHEET

STANDARDS	MET	NOT MET
Patients Outcome Standard A	X	
Related Nursing Process Standard 1	X	
Related Nursing Process Standard 2	X	
Related Nursing Process Standard 3		X
Patient Outcome Standard B	X	
Related Nursing Process Standard 1	X	
Related Nursing Process Standard 2	X	
Related Nursing Process Standard 3	X	
Related Nursing Process Standard 4	X	
Patient Outcome Standard C		X
Related Nursing Process Standard 1	X	
Related Nursing Process Standard 2		X
Related Nursing Process Standard 3	X	
Related Nursing Process Standard 4	X	

Figure 22-2.   Quality Control Relating Outcome and Process

The types of quality control now common in nursing have significant effects on the nursing ideology. One major effect is that professional autonomy is no longer falsely correlated with mere whimsy or ability to do what one elects apart from the decisions of others. If data are to be kept on the success of nursing regimens, it is required that all nurses caring for a given patient follow a prescribed protocol since inconsistent care will not permit correlating care and outcome. Such necessary cooperation and agreement should go far to remove some of the present distrust among nurses. Further, a coordinated approach to nursing regimen derivation and delivery will force nursing to move from a primarily oral tradition to a written tradition—a necessary step in the scientific advancement of the profession.

COMPARISON OF QUALITY CONTROL AND TASK ANALYSIS SYSTEMS

Task analysis is the second assessment technique presently being used in nursing. The task analysis method of measuring reveals the influence of systems analysis on nursing. This system is used only for measurement of nursing process. With this technique systems analysts, using time studies, establish time norms for most common nursing tasks. These norms are specific for the institution under investigation. Thus, logically, the average bathing time in a research hospital with critically ill patients might be longer than that in an average community hospital.

Such studies are of practical value in establishing criteria for distribution of staff

Table 22-2.   Nursing Ideologies

Old Ideology	New Ideology
Nursing acts are judged by their conformance to standard practice.	Nursing acts are judged by their ability to produce desired patient outcomes.
Each nurse has complete autonomy to devise her own care plans, to "do her own thing" with her assigned patients.	Care protocols are frequently used in order that large numbers of nurses will give standardized care in order that statistical data may be collected to correlate nursing regimen and patient outcome.
Data are not important: nursing care plans and nursing orders—if any—are discarded when patient is discharged.	Data are important; longitudinal data is kept on nursing care plans and nursing orders so that they may be correlated with patient recovery trajectories.
Nursing rewards are primarily affective; the nurse is rewarded by the affection and gratitude from the patient.	Nursing rewards are primarily intellectual; the nurse is rewarded by her ability to devise and implement effective care plans for a statistically significant number of patients.
Nursing answers to problems are assumed to be known; tradition is accepted as "correct." The nurse who does not know the answers is seen as deficient.	Most of nursing action is seen as problematic, unresearched, unknown. A questioning attitude prevails and is the accepted form.

or of patients. Nurses have always known that the same unit of 30 patients may be extremely busy one month and not so busy the next month, but never before have they had a scientific base to use as a distribution criterion. Time studies usually reveal that certain tasks are significant in determining patient nursing care hours and that other tasks are inconsequential. Drug distribution, for example, seldom affects patient care hours, while presence of a Levine tube usually is related directly to increased nursing hours.

Quality control and task analysis are useful tools for the nurse administrator, provided their purposes are not confused with each other. Quality control identifies instances when particular nursing teams are more productive of good care than are similar teams in similar circumstances. It may recognize appropriate nursing models for study and imitation. The task analysis method defines all nurses as interchangeable. While it will indicate failures of a nursing team to carry the expected number of tasks, it has no means of identifying group excellence in care. Table 22-3 compares some of the critical differences in purpose between the two systems.

Nursing measurement systems are the necessary basis for evaluation, research, and change in nursing practice. They are the basis of systems that will enable the profession to compare nursing from one institution to another. Quality control systems and task analysis systems are the beginning of a real data base for nursing. Every nurse manager should know how such systems work and what they can accomplish.

SUMMARY

Creation of a quality control system, while oversimplified, can be summarized in the following steps:

1. Have a purpose — WHY
2. Decide what areas to evaluate — WHAT
3. Identify standards — HOW MUCH
4. Select a format and construct the tool — HOW
5. Set up a surveillance system — WHO, WHEN, WHERE
6. Set up a feedback system — HOW
7. Develop a system for change — WHY

Table 22-3.   Comparison of Task Analysis and Quality Control Systems

Points of Comparison	Task Analysis System	Quality Control System
Aim of the system	Fairly distribute nursing tasks	Evaluate the quality of care
Basic criterion	What *is* being done	What *ought* to be done
Concept of nursing	Nursing is a series of specific tasks	Different theories can be used
Deviations from the norm	Instances when a team completes more or less tasks than the norm	Instances of exceptional nursing, both good and bad
Perspective	What happens in the delivery system	What happens to the patient

REFERENCES

1. Slee, V.N. How to know if you have quality control. *Hospital Progress* 53(1):38, 1972.
2. Donabedian, A. Some issues in evaluating the quality of nursing care. *Am. J. Public Health* 59(10):1833, 1969.
3. Pardee, G., et. al. Patient care evaluation is every nurse's job. *Am. J. Nursing* 71(10):1958, 1971.
4. Brodt, D.E. A synergistic theory of nursing. *Am. J. Nursing* 69(8):1674, 1969.
5. Carrieri, V.K., and Sitzman, J. Components of nursing process. *Nursing Clinics of North America* 6(1):115, 1971.
6. Roy, C. The Roy Adaptation Model. In Riehl, M.P., and Roy, C. (Eds.) *Conceptual Models for Nursing Practice*. New York: Appleton-Century-Crofts, 1974, p. 135.
7. Johnson, D.E. One Conceptual Model of Nursing. Paper presented at Vanderbilt University, Nashville, Tenn., April 25, 1968, p. 3.

BIBLIOGRAPHY

American Nurses' Association. *Standards of Nursing Practice*. Kansas City, Mo.: ANA, 1973.

American Nurses' Association. *Standards for Nursing Services*. Kansas City, Mo.: ANA, 1973.

American Nurses' Association. *A Plan for Implementation of the Standards of Nursing Practice*. Kansas City, Mo.: ANA, 1975.

American Nurses' Association. *Standards of Cardiovascular Nursing Practice*. Kansas City, Mo.: ANA, 1975.

American Nurses' Association. *Standards of Emergency Nursing Practice*. Kansas City, Mo.: ANA, 1975.

American Nurses' Association. *Standard for Orthopedic Nursing Practice*. Kansas City, Mo.: ANA, 1975.

Bailit, H., et al. Assessing the quality of care. *Nursing Outlook* 23(3):153, 1975.

Commission for Administrative Services in Hospitals, *Quality Control Plan for Nursing Service*. Los Angeles: CASH, 1965.

Clark, E.L., and Diggs, W.W. Quantifying patient care needs. *Hospitals* 45(18):96, 1971.

Davidson, G.E. Collaborating with the medical staff in developing standards of care. *Nursing Clinics of North America*, 8(2):219, 1973.

Davis, A.I. Measuring quality: development of a blueprint for a quality control assurance program. *Supervisor Nurse* 8(2):17, 1977.

Diddie, P. Quality assurance—a hospital meets the challenge. *J.O.N.A.* 6(6):6, 1976.

Donabedian, A. Patient care evaluation. *Hospitals* 44(7):131, 1970.

Donovan, H. The personalized nursing audit. *Supervisor Nurse* 2(12):37, 1971.

Ethridge, P.E., and Packard, R.W. An innovative approach to measurement of quality through utilization of nursing care plans. *J.O.N.A.* 6(1):25, 1976.

Etzioni, A. Alternative concepts of accountability—Part I. *Hospital Progress* 55(6):35, 1974.

Etzioni, A. Alternative concepts of accountability—Part II. *Hospital Progress* 55(7):56, 1974.

Felton, G., et al. Pathway to accountability: implementation of a quality assurance program. *J.O.N.A.* 6(1):20, 1976.

Finkelman, A.W. The standards of nursing practice and the supervisor. *Supervisor Nurse* 7(5):31, 1976.

Hagen, B. Conceptual Issues in the Appraisal of the Quality of Care. In *Assessment of Nursing Services*. Bethesda, Md., Department of Health, Education and Welfare, 1975, pp. 49–75.

Hanson, S. Ambulatory nursing standards. *Supervisor Nurse* 6(12):10, 1975.

Hegedus, K.S. A patient outcome criterion measure. *Supervisor Nurse* 10(1):40, 1979.

Hegyvary, S.T., and Chamings, P.A. The hospital setting and patient care outcomes. Part I. *J.O.N.A.* 5(3):29, 1975.

Hegyvary, S.T., and Chamings, P.A. The hospital setting and patient care outcomes. Part II. *J.O.N.A.* 5(4):36, 1975.

Hegyvary, S.T., and Haussmann, R.K.D. Monitoring nursing care quality. *J.O.N.A.* 6(9):3, 1976.

Hegyvary, S.T., and Haussmann, R.K.D. The relationship of nursing process and patient outcomes. *J.O.N.A.* 6(9):18, 1976.

Hegyvary, S.T., and Haussmann, R.K.D. Correlates of the quality of nursing care. *J.O.N.A.* 6(9):22, 1976.

Hurwitz, L.S., and Tasch, V. Developing a quality assurance program. *Supervisor Nurse* 8(2):17, 1977.

Joint Commission for Accreditation of Hospitals. *Standards for Accreditation of Hospitals*. Chicago: JCAH, 1969.

Joint Commission for Accreditation of Hospitals. *Accreditation Manual for Hospitals*. Chicago: JCAH, 1973.

Lang, N. Quality assurance in nursing. *AORN J.* 22(2):180, 1975.

Langford, T. The evaluation of nursing: necessary and possible. *Supervisor Nurse* 2(11):64, 1971.

Lindeman, C. Measuring quality of nursing care. Part I. *J.O.N.A.* 6(5):7, 1976.

Lindeman, C. Measuring quality of nursing care. Part II. *J.O.N.A.* 6(7):16, 1976.

McCain, R.F. Nursing by assessment—not intuition. *Am. J. Nursing* 65(4):82, 1965.

Moore, M.A. The Joint Commission on Accreditation of Hospitals: standards for nursing services. *J.O.N.A.* 2(2):12, 1972.

Nicholls, M.E. Quality control in patient care. *Am. J. Nursing* 74(3):456, 1974.

Phaneuf, M. *The Nursing Audit: Profile for Excellence.* New York: Appleton-Century-Crofts, 1972.

Ramey, I.G. Setting nursing standards and evaluating care. *J.O.N.A.* 3(3):27, 1973.

Routhier, R.W. Tool for the evaluation of patient care. *Supervisor Nurse* 3(1):15, 1972.

Rubin, C.F., Rinaldi, L.A., and Dietz, R.R. Nursing audit—nurses evaluating nursing. *Am. J. Nursing* 72(5):916, 1972.

Sanazaro, P.J., and Slosberg, B. Patient care evaluation. *Hospitals* 40(7):131, 1971.

Schmadl, J.C. Quality assurance: examination of the concept. *Nursing Outlook* 27(7):450, 1979.

Selvaggi, L., and Eriksen, L. Implementing a quality assurance program in nursing. *J.O.N.A.* 6(7):37, 1976.

Vincent, P.A., Broad, J.E., and Dilworth, L. Developing a mental health assessment form. *J.O.N.A.* 6(4):25, 1976.

Wandelt, M.A., and Ager, J. *Quality Patient Scale.* Detroit: Wayne State University, 1970.

Wandelt, M.A., and Stewart, D.S. *Slater Nursing Competencies Rating Scale.* New York: Appleton-Century-Crofts, 1975.

Watson, A., and Mayers, M. Evaluating the quality of patient care through retrospective chart review. *J.O.N.A.* 6(3):17, 1976.

Zorn, J.M. Relationship of nursing process and patient outcomes. *J.O.N.A.* 6(9):18, 1976.

Chapter 23   The Performance Appraisal System

The performance appraisal system is one of the major control systems of the nursing division. It controls individual employee behaviors by measuring them against specified job standards. In order for the performance appraisal system to be effective, the nurse executive must think of it in its entirety: 1) input—the employee's behavior upon hire or before evaluation; 2) thruput—those structures designed to modify and/or direct his behavior; 3) output—the employee's behavior after exposure to the thruput; and 4) feedback and control—the performance appraisal and the subsequent employee coaching and counseling.

This chapter will review the performance appraisal system, the formats used for recording performance, the techniques of interview, and discipline elements in appraisal.

THE STAFF BEHAVIOR SYSTEM

Following the literature of the nursing community, the term performance appraisal system is used here although performance appraisal is only part of the cybernetic function of the staff behavior system. It is an interesting comment on the discipline that one component of the total system has been selected for focus of this sort. In order to look at the total system in which performance appraisal plays a part, it is necessary to use a systems approach. The reader is referred to an excellent article by Haar for a well-detailed systems model for staff behavior[1]. In the staff behavior system, it is important to identify the system goals. What does the nurse executive expect from the system, and in what way does performance appraisal contribute to those goals?

Almost any nurse executive would be delighted if her staff behavior system accomplished the objectives of making satisfactory workers better, ridding the system of unsatisfactory workers, and improving the distribution of merit pay.

Most present performance appraisal systems accomplish few if any of these objectives. Where are the problems? How can the leaks in the system be plugged? Often the first problem is that performance appraisal is seen as an isolated entity. Most nurse managers think of a performance appraisal as a form which is filled out once a year for employees with seniority, more frequently for those who are new to the institution. A better view of performance appraisal is to see it as one component of a larger system designed to accomplish ends outside of itself. When delivering the form to the personnel department becomes an end in itself, it is no wonder that performance appraisal and the system of which it is a part are ineffective.

Suppose the nurse executive views performance appraisal as a system designed to accomplish the three stated objectives. How would a system be designed to reach these goals? An appraisal system rightfully is more than a form: it tells who will do what, with whom, in what manner, when, and to what purpose.

Making Satisfactory Workers Better

The first stated purpose, to make satisfactory workers better, is a good place to start. What system is likely to make this happen? "Satisfactory workers" include everyone from employees who are just meeting baseline performance standards to those employees who give an exceptional level of performance. The objective of making all these workers better is an optimistic one, for it assumes that everyone can improve. Not only that, this objective assumes that these persons never will reach a limit, but that they can continue to improve year by year. There is both truth and fiction in this assumption. Theoretically it is always possible to conceive of one more ability a good employee might acquire even though he may already be excellent. On the other hand, managers talk about persons who ''are working at their maximum capacity.'' The real question is not whether the assumption of continuous improvement is true or false, but whether it is an assumption effective for improving the work of most or even many workers.

This assumption has one important virtue: it treats everyone alike. If everyone is expected to set goals and work toward improvement, no one can say that it is unreasonable that improvement is expected of him. In one stroke, this assumption of ongoing improvement becomes the underpinning for a complete system in which workers expect their faults and deficiencies as workers to be a focus of attention. And it is expected that improvement of faults or acquisition of new capabilities will be goals for all employees.

If the goal of making satisfactory workers better is to serve as a goal for a total system, what components must that system contain? The following are logical components in such a system:

1. The employee and his immediate supervisor must know what behaviors are expected of the employee. (Goals)
2. The employee and his supervisor must know what behaviors the employee exhibits. (Feedback)
3. The employee and his supervisor must be able to see where the employee's behavior fails to meet the requisite behavior pattern. (Assessment and evaluation)
4. The employee and his supervisor must explore ways to change the employee's behavior. (Adjustment)
5. The employee and his supervisor must agree upon a plan for altered behavior. (Adjustment)
6. The employee must put the plan into action. (Adjustment)
7. The employee's changed behavior must be compared to the original expected behaviors. (Feedback)

In a system designed to make satisfactory workers perform better, performance appraisal is a means rather than an end. Appraising the performance is only part of the cybernetic loop for the total system, the assessment/evaluation part. The loop also includes an adjustment component, otherwise control is never instituted. For this purpose the system might use a coaching process of employee counseling much like that used in training athletes: careful study of the employee's present behaviors and purposeful, practiced change in behavior to improve performance.

If such a system is to be effective, what are the responsibilities of the nurse executive, the evaluating supervisor, and the employee? First, it is the responsibility of the nurse executive to see to it that adequate *job descriptions* exist which identify desired behaviors. It also is up to her to see that adequate orientation to the requirements of each job is provided to all nurse managers, and their employees so that employees are made aware of the goals of the staff behavior system from the start.

The nurse executive has the responsibility for seeing that her nurse managers learn and consistently use the coaching process. Coaching requires greater skills than does the typical appraisal process. One way for the nurse executive to teach the coaching process is through her own use of it with the employees she evaluates. But since example is seldom an adequate teaching mechanism, supervisors probably will need educational programs that include role play practice in recognizing and assessing work behaviors in subordinates and in using the coaching process itself.

In additional to showing how to coach, the nurse executive must show that she is serious about the use of coaching as a control measure. This may mean that nurse managers who fail to develop coaching skills will have to be removed from managerial positions. If this measure seems harsh to a nurse executive, then she is not genuinely committed to the objective of improving worker performance.

What are the responsibilities of an evaluating supervisor in this system of performance appraisal? They are knowledge of the job requirements for each employee under her direction and initiation of upward mobility for workers if warranted by improved performance. If promotion is not possible, given licensure and certification laws, and the employee has met all required job behaviors, then the supervisor is responsible for helping the employee determine appropriate new behavioral goals to enhance performance of the given job.

The need for developing skill in assessment and interview techniques also is a supervisor's responsibility. Within the performance appraisal system, each supervisor must take time to create the opportunity for close observation of each employee immediately under her direction; she must know the performance patterns of each employee she is to evaluate. Consequently, no supervisor should have to manage more persons than she can observe and assess. Where coaching is not based on accurate assessment, it should not be used. If a nurse executive expects coaching to be done, then she must plan for a reasonable span of control for each manager.

Many nurse executives have middle managers evaluate their head nurse's employees. Such distortion of management lines does not fit the coaching concept. The head nurse is the immediate supervisor of her staff, and she should do the coaching of her own personnel. Coaching must be done by the manager who is most familiar with the worker's behavior; this manager is the employee's immediate supervisor, whatever title that supervisor holds.

Most employees enjoy coaching-based evaluation. Usually it is rewarding to the employee to see himself continuously acquiring new skills and abilities. Some employees, however, will resent this approach. When a competent employee is unwilling to put more effort into self-improvement on the job, he may see the coaching process as an unwarranted intrusion. In this case the supervisor may need to use a different approach in managing this employee.

As a general rule, however, the coaching process is a singularly effective means of making satisfactory workers better. In the coaching process, performance appraisal is an essential step, but it is only one step. Performance appraisal is subordinated to the setting of behavioral standards and the planned alteration of work behaviors in order to meet those standards.

Dismissal of Unsatisfactory Workers

What about the second objective? How would a performance appraisal system be designed to get rid of unsatisfactory workers? The coaching process is a good start in this process, for it documents and compares required and exhibited behaviors. Also, it offers the worker an opportunity to change his behavior by setting specific behavioral goals with target dates and review periods. The coaching process alone, however, is only part of a dismissal system.

It is important not to overlook the legal, contractual, or quasilegal considerations involved in firing an employee. Today the employer virtually has lost his historical right to be capricious and arbitrary in dismissing an employee. Many health institutions now are functioning under negotiated employment contracts; many more institutions will be unionized in the near future. Even where there are no negotiated contracts to protect the worker who faces dismissal, he is not likely to submit meekly. Indeed, even where there is no contract to be administered, the nurse executive may have to substantiate her dismissals thoroughly—either to her own boss or to the personnel department.

When a dismissal case goes to grievance or arbitration, what errors will cause the nurse executive to lose the case? The following conditions are the most common sources of failure:

1. When the charges upon which the dismissal rests are not proved
2. When the charge is not sufficient to warrant the severity of the punishment, i.e., dismissal
3. When the cause of the firing is unrelated to job performance
4. When the proper disciplinary procedures were not followed

How can these four errors be avoided? The simplest answer, of course, is not even to try to get rid of the poor employee. One hears supervisors all over the country claim, "It is not possible to get rid of a poor employee here." In most cases this is another way of saying that the supervisor is not willing to go to all the trouble of getting rid of a poor employee. Unfortunately, in some cases, this claim is the truth. Where every fired employee can convince the nurse executive that he is simply misunderstood and deserves another chance, the supervisor is substantially correct: firing is impossible.

Often the supervisor perceives lack of support by the nurse executive when, in fact, she has placed the nurse executive in a position where the only reasonable action is to rescind the dismissal. No intelligent nurse executive is going to let a losing case go to grievance or arbitration. What is really needed between supervisor and nurse executive is a tacit agreement. The supervisor must do her homework on a firing: none of the four common errors must occur. In return, where the supervisor has followed appropriate channels and procedures, the nurse executive must support her decision and her managerial right to make that decision.

Failing to Prove Charges

What is necessary to prevent the four errors which will cause the nurse executive—or her boss or the arbitrator—to reverse a firing?

The first error occurs when a supervisor fails to prove the charges upon which a dismissal rests. Proof for a firing need not be as explicit as proof in a court of law, but there certainly must be a preponderance of evidence supporting the supervisor's position.

There are two kinds of issues to be settled in most cases. The first is the question of facts. What really did happen? Most firings are the result of cumulative poor performances rather than the result of a single dramatic error. This means that the supervisor must be able to prove past as well as present poor behavior; there must be documented proof of past behaviors.

In addition to proof of facts there may be questions of interpretation of the facts. The wise supervisor will have elicited the interpretations of all parties involved so that she may be able, if required, to substantiate her own interpretation and to refute those interpretations which label the offending behavior as acceptable.

The wise supervisor bases her case upon the employee's actions and their consequences, not on the employee's intentions. One can be certain that a malicious intention will have become a benign one by the time it is explained to a third party. Therefore, the supervisor should not focus on an employee's intentions. She should stick to the behavior and its consequences.

In order for discipline to be implemented, the supervisor must learn to document her judgments and actions and those of her employees. It is up to the nurse executive to demand this level of performance from supervisory staff. Each supervisor must be held accountable for accurately, objectively, and consistently documenting poor performance.

Mismatch between Charge and Punishment

The second error occurs when the charge is not judged sufficient to warrant dismissal. It is hardly a new principle that the punishment should fit the crime. There are two ways in which this error is likely to occur. The first is when the supervisor does the firing in a temporary rage without weighing the punishment and the crime. Obviously, if the nurse executive is wise, she will eliminate a supervisor whose actions chronically are based on spontaneous emotions.

The more common cause of an apparent injustice occurs when the employee's provoking behavior was simply "the last straw." If previous poor behaviors have not been documented adequately in the disciplinary record, however, the single "last straw" is not likely to stand on its own. It is particularly frustrating when one looks back at the problem employee's record and finds that he always was rated as average or above average on performance appraisals. Such appraisals inevitably will cause a hearing officer or arbitrator to reverse a dismissal decision which appears to rest on a single incident. Typically, the supervisor has only herself to blame for not recording past deficiencies accurately.

The nurse executive should make herself familiar with the performance rating habits of each supervisor. When a supervisor turns in an evaluation which the nurse executive thinks is inaccurate, she should ask the supervisor to explain it. Often the supervisor needs education in how to evaluate employees, or she simply may need to understand that the nurse executive will not tolerate inflated performance appraisal reports.

One may respond that the supervisor pays for her inflated evaluations by having to live with her mistakes, but this is not the end of it. Patients and good staff members also pay a price for carrying along poor performers. When a supervisor has a pattern of overrating employees, it is up to the nurse executive to hold her accountable for changing this behavior. Her practice of inflating employee ratings is unfair to other employees whose supervisors are grading them fairly within the system.

Firings Unrelated to Job Performance

The third major error is firing unrelated to job performance. One sometimes sees supervisors who are new to unionization dismiss employees who are troublesome in their roles as union stewards or leaders. Occasionally a supervisor will fire an employee whose private life-style is considered to be deviant. Obviously, there is no way a nurse executive can support such dismissals; the public relations aftermath can be disastrous for the reputation of the nursing department. Of course, the opposite condition does not hold: these employees should not be protected if they actually are failing at the work; the supervisor must have good evidence of the employee's failings to be able to refute a claim that the firing was performance-related.

Often a firing for cause unrelated to job performance is disguised: the supervisor looks for job-related failures upon which to justify the dismissal. The nurse executive must suspect an apparently weak case for dismissal of a person whose nonjob-related activities are known to create prejudicial attitudes.

Failure to Use Disciplinary Procedures

The last common error occurs when proper disciplinary procedures are not followed. The nurse executive must demand that supervisors know and use the steps for discipline. Also, she must see that the discipline and dismissal policies are written, formal policies. Where a disciplinary system is not formal, an arbitrator usually will accept the following series of actions as reasonable. The series also can be used as a protocol for a formal policy.

1. Verbal warning. Anecdotal notes to be kept by the supervisor.
2. Written notice. On a standard form, with a copy to the employee.
3. Suspension. Usually two days to two weeks. This should not be given at the time of the offense, but later, so that the employee has time to submit a grievance over the suspension if he desires to do so.
4. Dismissal.

Failure to follow the appropriate disciplinary procedure as published and practiced in the institution, or failure to follow a reasonable course of action as outlined above, will leave the executive or arbitrator no choice but to rescind a dismissal.

This disciplinary sequence may be bypassed in exceptional cases; some behaviors warrant immediate dismissal. These include instances in which the employee's behavior presents a clear danger to patients and other employees, involves illegal acts, or presents a case of insubordination.

Many employees and supervisors fail to understand the concept of insubordination. Employment is a quasicontract in which the employee agrees to perform assigned tasks that fall within the scope of his job description. In return the employing agency agrees to give him remuneration. The employing agency retains the right to select those assigned tasks; after all, that is what the agency is paying for. Provided these acts fall reasonably within the scope of the job description, the employee has no right to refuse to do the tasks. Refusal constitutes a breaking of the contract between the two parties. Thus insubordination, the refusal to carry out a legitimate assignment, is a case of self-firing. The employee breaks the contract and has no right to expect further benefit from the employing agency.

Probably the most common case of insubordination in nursing occurs when an employee refuses assignment to a floor other than his regular one. If the assignment is substantially the same, as when an employee is moved from one medical-surgical floor to another medical-surgical floor, the employee has no right to refuse the assignment. Nor can the supervisor afford to yield management prerogative because an employee refuses to accept a legitimate assignment. Many employees are unaware that a refusal of this sort constitutes grounds for immediate dismissal. It is up to the supervisor to inform the employee of the nature and seriousness of his proposed refusal.

Cases tried under the Labor-Management Relations Act have established that "An employer has a fundamental right to assign employees to positions which he deems, in the exercise of his managerial discretion, to be most expedient"[2]. The supervisor cannot let patient needs take a back seat to employee preferences or perceived rights. The employer has the right to move any personnel. From the employee's narrow perception, colored by self-interest, movement to another floor may appear unfair, but the supervisor cannot let such special interests work to the detriment of the organization.

Nor do employees have the right to change their work performance in rebellion to placement changes: "Employees have the right to strike, but they have no right to continue working on their own terms while rejecting the standards desired by their employer"[3]. Thus there is legal support for the supervisor's position in maintaining control of assignments and in demanding that standards be met.

Where disciplinary policies are not followed closely, one is certain to lose disputed cases of dismissal. In addition, if common practice in an institution is to be more lenient than the written policy, then a nurse executive may lose a dismissal case that follows the official policy. *Common practice* is the standard to which the supervisor and nurse executive will be held. Suppose, for example, the nurse executive wishes to "get tough" and begin implementing a discipline policy strictly, when past supervisory policy has been lax. She first must notify every employee of the intention to enforce the policy. This must be done in a way that ensures calling the change to everyone's attention. A notice on an overloaded and ignored communal bulletin board will not be accepted as proper notification in any subsequent grievance or arbitration case.

Uniformity of practice presents another problem. Suppose a nurse executive has four supervisors, one who runs a "tight ship" and three who are lax. If the disciplinarian fires an employee who fails to measure up to her standards, the employee will be back the following week if an arbitrator finds that other supervisors would *not* have fired him.

What rules in any hearing is *general practice*, and if general practice is a low standard of work, the well-intentioned supervisor who is trying to improve standards will lose every time.

Thus it is the obligation of the nurse executive to see that a uniform high standard of practice is enforced. The nurse executive cannot afford to keep inefficient supervisors; their inaction may tie the hands of the effective supervisors.

Nurse executives often bemoan the poor performance of supervisors in disciplinary action as if it were an event beyond their control. Certainly effective discipline is one of the principal job behaviors required of supervisors. The nurse executive who uses coaching with her supervisors must set disciplinary control as a behavior target for all supervisors.

It should console the nurse executive to know that she has an easier job in removing poor managers than does the first-line manager. For a head nurse to get rid of an unsatisfactory worker, she must fire him. For a nurse executive to get rid of an ineffective supervisor, she need only reduce the supervisor to staff status. There are many employment contracts that protect a worker's job, but few that guarantee him a managerial position.

Another problem with uniformity of practice is the fact that no arbitrator will uphold a disciplinary action against an employee for a fault he shares with the supervisor. For example, if a supervisor is chronically late for work, she cannot discipline an employee for tardiness. The supervisor is supposed to be a role model, and her own record must be good before she can criticize a subordinate.

What, then, are the requirements of a performance appraisal system which works to get rid of unsatisfactory workers? The nurse executive needs a disciplinary policy which is: clear and unambiguous, effectively communicated, and uniformly and consistently applied. Where such a policy and its implementation are combined with accurate assessment of employee behaviors and coaching toward required behavioral change, then the performance appraisal system will accomplish the objective of eliminating unsatisfactory workers.

Improving the Distribution of Merit Pay

In order to talk about merit pay, it first must be differentiated from a yearly increment, a cost of living raise, or any other salary adjustment based upon a principle other than merit. Incidentally, to call a yearly increment a merit raise does not make it so. Arbitration cases have ruled in favor of employees where supervisors have tried to withhold yearly raises on the grounds that the employee does not "merit" it. If it is practice for every employee to receive a yearly raise, then it is *not* a merit raise.

What is a merit raise? It is a financial reward for performance above and beyond expectations. It may take the form of a one-time-only bonus or it may be in the form of an addition to the hourly, weekly, or monthly earning rate of the employee. When a merit raise takes the latter form, the nurse executive must realize that even a minimal merit award can be a substantial financial increment, for that award will be paid every subsequent year in which the worker is employed by the institution by virtue of its incorporation into the base pay rate.

In addition to being an addition to the yearly base pay, a merit raise also tends to increase other increments. When the yearly increment or the Christmas bonus or any other award is calculated as a percentage of the base salary, the merit raise will help to increase these awards. In other words, merit raises are serious business and they should not be handed out without careful consideration.

What performance appraisal system would help in the fair distribution of merit pay? Since a merit increase is a reward for service above and beyond that expected or required on the job, the first requirement is a system that identifies employees who do exceed the expected job behaviors. Once again the careful appraisal, which is part of the coaching process, can provide the answer. It is important that merit raises be tied to specific and identified job behaviors and accomplishments. Otherwise they tend to become popularity awards. Most unions are suspicious of variable merit raises for just this reason.

Hence, merit awards should require documented proof of superior performance just as discipline requires documented proof of performance below the standards. Identification of employee behaviors which exceed behavioral standards will not solve all the problems of merit pay. The nurse executive still must weigh the nature of each outstanding performance and the concrete accomplishments that can be attributed to that performance. She also must determine how to distribute merit pay among outstanding employees in all job classifications. Performance appraisal of job-related behaviors will provide a logical and defensible basis for making fund distribution decisions.

APPRAISING PERFORMANCE

In appraising performance of a subordinate, it is important to use as many sources of evidence as possible. Selected sources should be easy to use, valid, reliable, and objective. For this discussion, the evaluation of a staff nurse will serve as illustration. This level of evaluation is selected because it presents more problems in gathering of evidence than does evaluation of a higher-level employee. Managerial employees are easier to evaluate because they provide multiple sources for evaluation in their recording and reporting and in their overt managerial decisions. Further, the problems that nurse executives typically encounter in the performance appraisal system, have to do, not with their own evaluations of subordinate managers, but with the ineptitudes of inexperienced subordinate managers in evaluating staff members. The principles of data collection are the same on any level, however.

Before identifying sources the head nurse might use to collect evidence of performance by a staff nurse, one must ask *what performance* is to be identified. Is it the performance the staff nurse evidences at *this time*? Or the performance norm that she has demonstrated *over the last six months or year*? Obviously, the data will differ depending on the answer to this major question. Both time frames have advantages and disadvantages. While an evaluation of present performance is a more contemporary measure, there are some employees who are lax 9 months out of 12, only giving performance of quality around the time of evaluation. On the other hand, a normative judgment over a sustained period of time does not give recognition for real learning and improvement that is ongoing. An employee who has worked sincerely to improve performance may be discouraged when his rating is a gradation between past poor performance and present good performance that he has worked hard to achieve.

Most performance appraisal systems are designed to report normative behavior over a span of time. This perspective will be used here; it requires systematic appraisal throughout the performance period. Indeed, this is the major managerial responsibility: to collect sample behavior over time, not to try to remember performance patterns once an external constraint (such as a personnel form deadline) sets evaluation into effect. If evaluative data is seen as control data, the manager will not wait for some formal evaluation occasion to use performance data. The effective manager will provide informal feedback on performance during the year, six months, or two years when performance data are being collected. This continuous, ongoing feedback with recommendations for improvement is a major managerial responsibility. Feedback and correction should be ongoing, spontaneous, and to the point. There should be no delay, no waiting for an "official" evaluation date.

In order to provide feedback one must gather evaluative data on performance. If the manager allows such evaluative work to wait for an unbusy time, she probably will never gather data. She probably will do better to plan ahead for evaluation time. There are two basic approaches to evaluation. In one, the manager selects a particular class of employees—all staff nurses, say—and evaluates them on one evaluation day on a selected key job function from their mutual job description. Observing a number of employees on the same dimension makes for better comparison. It enables one to eliminate false shading that often occurs because of personality and character differences. In the second approach, the manager tries to evaluate a single employee on all key functions of her job on a given evaluation day. There also is some merit to this, in that the employee may manifest behavior relevant to several key functions simultaneously.

There are numerous sources of evidence, but direct observation is always the best. The head nurse or a manager of any other level must reserve some time for seeing the employee in action. Direct observation may be complemented by peer evaluation and employee self-evaluation if the manager so chooses, but the manager should keep in mind the weaknesses and limitations of these two methods.

Peer evaluation places fellow employees in great stress. If a worker knows that his raises depend upon the judgments offered by his peers, then he is certainly aware that those peers are looking carefully at his own evaluations of them. It is not unusual for an employee who has received a low rating to take revenge upon those peers whom he surmises have marked him negatively—even if the reports are kept confidential. Like it or not, the worker must depend upon his fellow workers for assistance on the job, and employees know that it is not to their advantage to mark their fellow workers poorly, whatever their actual performance.

Indeed, employees often rebel at the notion of peer evaluation, recognizing that it is shifting the managerial obligation from their boss to themselves. If one assumes that the manager is at a higher level of awareness than the subordinate staff, it is actually possible that the manager will recognize some productive work patterns in some employees that are not fully appreciated by their less astute peers.

Where the phrase peer evaluation is used to mean the evaluation of how a given case was handled, rather than how a peer performed, then the task so described *does* fall within the obligation of the professional staff. This is not a managerial task but a professional one, and it is an appropriate task for peers.

Self-appraisal also is a limited tool for performance rating. The good performer typically is astute and recognizes his limitations, but the not-so-good performer may not have the insight to see his faults. Ironically, then, the better worker may be harder on himself in evaluation than is the less competent worker. If the manager allows these judgments to become part of the final evaluation judgment, then the system often will penalize the most capable.

Many managers rely on nurses' basic honesty and willingness to reveal faults as a substitute for managerial observation. After the employee recognizes one of his own revealed "faults" carrying heavy weight in the final appraisal, he will soon cease helping his supervisor to downgrade his performance. Where self-rating is used, it should be considered only as a measure of the degree of self-insight manifest by the employee, not as a measure of the facts of performance.

When making observations of staff members for evaluation purposes, the manager should resort to anecdotal notes, simply because what seems clear today inevitably will have faded if the supervisor tries to recall six months to a year later. Two types of observations usually are combined when arriving at a performance appraisal: routine behavior samples and critical incidents. The routine samples are those behaviors noted when the manager goes out to check on behaviors related to key job functions as part of the routine collection of performance data. Here the attempt is not to get anything unusual. Indeed, the attempt is just the opposite: to record the average behavior, be it good, bad, exciting, or mundane. It is important to collect enough such samples so as to be able to assert that they do in fact represent the average, typical behavior.

A critical incident, on the other hand, is a single observed event that is so good or bad that it reflects upon the total performance of the employee. For example, if the manager observes a staff nurse break all the rules of aseptic technique in applying a dressing to an open wound, this single incident tells the manager much about the nurse. Similarly, if a nurse is observed to react to a subtle patient problem in a resourceful manner, the effect is the same in that a single event reveals sensitivities and abilities, or insensitivities and inabilities, as the case may be.

In collecting observations it is important that a manager preserve actual descriptions of the behavior exhibited rather than just judgments about that behavior. Later that manager may have to substantiate her judgments if an employee contests the evaluation or action subsequent to the evaluation.

Secondary sources of evidence of performance may be used to supplement judgments drawn from direct observation. For evaluating the staff nurse, her nursing care plans may be excellent secondary sources. Although it is possible that a nurse may derive excellent care plans without following through on them, it is more likely that the care she gives is good if she is able to specify it in care plans than if she is not able to do so. Other documents such as incident reports and illness and tardiness records may be taken into account in deriving a performance appraisal. Professional activities (speaking, writing) also may be considered in the case of professional nurses. Participation in institutional, divisional, or departmental committees may be considered—especially if the nurse has made significant contributions to such committees. In evaluating a manager, the superordinate manager will also consider the manager's reports and her attainment of objectives set for her department or unit.

Where an institution has an effective clinical ladder, the ladder must be tied to the appraisal system in a meaningful way. Both a good clinical ladder program and a performance appraisal system attempt to rate the nurse behaviors. Ideally the nurse will be rated as to how she performs on the step of the ladder where she is placed. A performance appraisal might indicate the misplacement of a nurse, and a supervisor might well use the performance rating to initiate reclassification of a nurse.

Placing Judgments on Data

When placing judgments on performance data, the nurse manager should be careful to avoid such common errors of judgment as the following:

Halo effect. The individual whose performance in several known areas is good is assumed to be able to perform well in other, unknown areas. Sometimes this error is termed, "trait carryover."

Recency effect. Recent issues weigh heavier with the rater than do events that occurred earlier in the evaluation period.

Problem distortion. One poor performance weighs heavier with the rater than do 20 good performances that went unnoticed since they created no problems.

Sunflower effect. Rater may grade all her employees too high because of a feeling that she has a "great team."

Central tendency. Evaluator may tend to mark everyone as average, especially if she is unsure of the real performance on a particular criterion.

Rater temperament effect. Different raters may have differences in the strictness or leniency with which they rate employees.

Guessing error. Some raters guess rather than record that particular observations were not made.

Feasible versus Ideal Observation

While the manager must set aside time for evaluation, there is never enough time to do all the evaluation that one might choose.

Since the manager cannot evaluate everything, it is important that she evaluate the key functions of an employee's job. Also, it is important that the employee be evaluated in any domain where he previously was found to be deficient. Specific assignments to individual nurses help in evaluation; where accountability is assigned, then evaluation can be similarly individualized. In contrast, if any nurse may revise a care plan any time, then the head nurse is unable to assess the care planning ability of any one nurse.

The head nurse role is identified because of the evaluation problems at that level. Often the head nurse has an extensive number of employees to evaluate—usually more than any other manager. This problem is further accentuated where the head nurse has 24-hour responsibility for staff on three different shifts. Simply because anything else is impractical, the head nurse may have to settle for coordinative evaluations of staff—a less than ideal situation.

PERFORMANCE APPRAISAL FORMATS

There are many common formats used for performance appraisal. They include essay, ranking systems, rating scales, and checklists. Each format has advantages and disadvantages and may be adapted for different purposes.

Essay

Essay has the advantage of being free-form; it allows the rater to respond in ways that capture the unique performance of the employee. The disadvantage of essay is that it makes it difficult to compare performances across groups of workers.

Free-form essay can be improved if the rater uses a common list of critical topics to be addressed for every worker in a given classification. In this way, the subject matter corresponds from evaluation to evaluation, but the rater still is free to individualize comments on different subjects. The key job functions as reflected in the job description should be identified. Consistent use of the same categories also will enable the employee to compare his performance at any one time against his past performance.

Where essay is used, the manager must be clear and definite in her description of the employee's behavior. She cannot let the meaning be lost in polite phrasing. Look, for example, at the following essay, taken from an actual performance report:

> Miss M. conducts herself in a professional manner. She is an active member of the ANA. Her attendance is very good, and she remains flexible about time changes in her schedule. She is knowledgeable about hospital policies.
>
> Her rapport with nonprofessionals continues to improve. We established, together, the following goals: 1) become proficient in the role of primary nurse, 2) become accountable for documentation on progress notes and care plans, 3) follow through on goals set for assigned patients.

Ironically, the supervisor and the employee came away from the conference at which this essay was discussed with radically different notions of the nurse's performance. The staff nurse reported to colleagues that the supervisor had no complaints about her performance. The supervisor was astonished to hear this because, as she reported, one could infer many faults in the practice from the nature of the goals set. Since the goals set would not be needed in the face of good nursing practice, she had anticipated that the nurse and others would "see" that the report was negative. Indeed, when the supervisor later produced this document at a grievance hearing, she lost the case because her "warning" to the employee was too disguised to be taken as a warning.

An essay is poor if it: 1) is noncommittal, 2) addresses insignificant topics, 3) alludes to faults in a way that is indirect, or 4) speaks through "omission" rather than by explicit statement.

Ranking Systems

Ranking systems compare employees to each other by placing them in order according to their performances on the given dimensions. Often the ranking of employees on specific job dimensions will help the manager to overcome prejudices and biases that may be related to personal factors.

A ranking system alone does not make a statement concerning the overall quality of the group or of any individual in the group being ranked. It merely reveals how the employees compare with one another. Although ranking has little use for day-to-day evaluation of individual performance, it is a useful technique for considering candidates for promotion or for distributing merit pay fairly.

Summary judgments may be made about ranked candidates by scoring each dimension upon which candidates are ranked according to its overall importance. This factor may be multiplied by the candidate's rank, as in Table 23-1.

Notice that in Table 23-1 three nurses are being compared and ranked on dimensions

of the nursing process and the recording accompanying that process. Weights have been assigned to each component and have been multiplied by the rank of the nurse in each instance. Notice that the nurse that ranked highest was given a 3, not a 1, in order that the mathematics could be calculated per highest score. In this instance, Nurse A's is considerably higher than her two colleagues' scores.

Rating Scales

A rating scale allows the evaluator to make a choice from among a quantitative or qualitative range of options for every criterion being assessed. Such options may include, for example:

1. Excellent – Good – Fair – Poor
2. Above Average – Average – Below Average
3. Yes – No
4. Always – Frequently – Occasionally – Seldom – Never
5. 1 – 2 – 3 – 4 – 5
6. 0-25% – 26-50% – 51-75% – 76-100%

Table 23-1.   Ranking System, Quantified

Key Functions	Weight	Rank			Item Score for Nurse		
		A	B	C	A	B	C
1. Assesses patient needs	3x	3	2	1	9	6	3
2. Sets appropriate goals	2x	3	1	2	6	2	4
3. Formulates good nursing care plans	3x	2	3	1	6	9	3
4. Implements care plan successfully	3x	2	1	3	6	3	9
5. Evaluates and modifies plan	2x	3	2	1	6	4	2
6. Documents care	1x	1	3	2	1	3	2
Total Score:					34	27	23

Sometimes the same range of options is given for each criterion, with an attempt to further describe the meaning of each option. In other cases, the options vary for different criteria; one criterion might be answered in terms of frequency, while another might be answered in terms of quality or degree of excellence.

In more sophisticated rating scales, the options may be descriptive statements, as in Figure 23-1.

Most rating scales force the rater to select one or another of the given options. Some few scales are constructed on a continuum so that the rater may use more discretion. A continuum may allow the rater to make more subtle differentiations among candidates who rank close to each other. The continuum, however is subject to the same problem as is a scale with too many options. It becomes difficult to justify the degrees of differentiation that such scales offer.

The checklist is an alternative format for an evaluation system wherein each standard is checked either as met or not met. Checklists also may be given numerical values, either by a simple counts of yes and no items or by weighting items as in a rating scale.

Whatever format is used, anecdotal notes and critical incident reports are used in determining the placement of the employee on each item. Some managers elect to have the employee fill out a similar tool and then negotiate a final judgment between the two reports, comparing that of the employee with that of the manager. The employee is likely to have an advantage, for by marking himself highly, he is in a position to nego-tiate his evaluation upward. This practice is not to be recommended.

Whatever reporting method is used—essay, ranking, rating, or checklist—the format should provide room for supporting evidence for the judgments made. Clear, concrete illustrations should be given of the behaviors that led to the judgments. These become particularly important when coaching employees to improve or when an employee submits a grievance over the grade assigned him or over subsequent action based on the grade. The more concrete the illustrations of behavior, the better.

The format also should provide a place to record when and where the evaluation conference took place at which the report was shared with the employee. Most forms have a place for the employee to sign indicating that he has seen the report. Sometimes, if he disagrees with the judgment, an employee may refuse to sign the report. When this occurs, the manager may stress that the signature only indicates that the report was seen by the employee, not that it was accepted. If the employee still refuses to sign, the manager will do well to have a witness sign that the conference did in fact take place.

Tool Deficiencies

Performance appraisal tools may suffer from many deficiencies. When the nurse manager is forced to use a poor tool, say one prescribed for institutionwide use by a personnel department, her job is made more difficult. Many a nurse executive has created

STANDARD	CRITERIA				
Supervisor's use of research	No apparent use or knowledge of recent research	Applies research findings on her units	Makes her units available to researchers	Devises and implements nursing research on her units.

Figure 23-1. Descriptive Rating Scale Sample

her own tools just to overcome the defects in such a universal form. Even where use of such a form is required, there is no reason the nursing division cannot supplement evaluation with tools that provide meaningful records of employee behavior.

The problem with a universal tool used for all employees is one of *validity*. A single tool cannot possible evaluate every employee based upon his job description. And if one is not evaluated on performance of the job he was hired to do, then the evaluation is invalid. The universal tool, since it cannot address performance, usually addresses personality traits and/or broad generalities of more or less importance in various jobs. Items typically include appearance, loyalty to the institution, quantity of work, quality of work, cooperativeness with others, professional manner, and tardiness or absenteeism. Indeed these few aspects are the only ones shared by all personnel. Such a form is incapable of capturing the essence of each job and cannot accurately evaluate job performance. Each job classification should have a separate performance appraisal tool, one adapted to the key functions of the particular job.

The performance appraisal tool also can be made invalid—fail to measure what it purports to measure—if the items it comprises are poorly chosen. For example, if more items reflect incidentals and few items reflect the major substance of the job, the tool will give a false measurement. Similarly, if weighting of items does not reflect their actual significance in the job performance, then the tool will be invalid. The rating scale or checklist is made representative by either balancing the original selection of items or by weighting items so as to create a balance that reflects the job requirements. The essay is balanced by identification of specific categories to be addressed. (Ranking systems will not be considered here because, as already indicated, they cannot give an absolute but only a relative measure.)

Some tools err by failing to identify the acceptable level of performance. If a rating scale uses a range of 1 to 5 the evaluator and the employee need to know what number represents baseline acceptable performance. Is it 2, 3, 4? If one uses such terms as excellent, good, fair, and poor, the same question arises. Is "fair" baseline performance? Or is "good" the acceptable level? For a checklist, it is assumed that each item itself is a baseline element and that a positive score is required as evidence of acceptable performance. In an essay the evaluator must identify whether or not the performance in each instance is at an acceptable level.

Not only must one be able to interpret each item as it relates to baseline acceptable performance, but one must be able to place a summary judgment on the total performance as indicated in the tool. First, one must be able to arrive at a final judgment that considers the criteria and their marks. Where each item in a rating scale has a score, then these scores may be added together and divided by the number of items to derive a total score. Where weighting is used, additional mathematics is required, but the score still is a mathematical derivation, not a judgment. Where descriptive scales are used, one must equate terms with values. Supposing, however, that "fair" is taken to be baseline acceptable performance. There are still questions to be answered. How many items may fall below the acceptable level before discipline or dismissal occur? On how many performance appraisals will substandard performance be tolerated? Are there certain critical items which *must* be at acceptable level, while there may be some room for deviation on other, less critical items? These same quesions apply also to checklist items.

Simply put, the decision rules for how to interpret a summary score must be determined before the evaluation process begins. For essay, it is more difficult to draw a summary conclusion from the previous materials, but it must be done. Otherwise the essay is not really an evaluative tool; it must place a summary judgment on the employee's performance as it relates to the job standards.

Appraisal tools also may suffer from deficits in *reliability*. When standards are poorly operationalized or when grading criteria are poorly described, different raters may use the tools in different ways. Precision is needed in both elements: constructing standards open to a single interpretation and describing judgments, be they numerical or verbal, so that they cannot be misinterpreted.

Criteria for an Evaluation Tool

A good evaluation tool meets the following requirements:

1. Utility. The tool actually is useful in promoting change in employee behavior.
2. Simplicity. It is easy to use, not requiring complicated procedures.
3. Validity. It reflects the key job requirements.
4. It defines minimal acceptable levels of performance.
5. Real behaviors, not employee traits comprise the items.
6. Differentiation. The tool allows one to differentiate among performances of various employees, without requiring an unrealistic, unfeasible degree of differentiation.
7. Appropriate weighting. The tool balances categories on the basis of their importance.

While all of these criteria are important, it is necessary to review the criteria concerning behaviors in detail. This is required because so many performance appraisal forms still deal with personal traits rather than work behavior. Since this procedure passes judgment on the character of the individual being evaluated, it is not surprising that the employee finds it threatening to his self-esteem. Categories such as initiative, appearance, problem-solving ability, competence, interpersonal relationships, and the quality of judgments are statements about the individual, not about the *events* in which he participates. Poor markings in such traits inevitably result in the employee's adopting a pattern of self-defensiveness and self-

justification or in his withdrawal from real communication.

Use of trait categories also places the evaluator at a disadvantage, for trait language represents a summary opinion derived from the observation of multiple behaviors. If the employee disagrees with the judgment of the evaluator, his typical response is to ask for examples that form the basis of the judgment. If the evaluator is unable to recall specific incidents, he looks inept. If the evaluator is able to identify events, there is still no guarantee that he and the employee will place the same interpretation on those events. For example, what the evaluator sees as behavior that shows failure to apply basic nursing principles may be interpreted by the employee as creative behavior. In trait language there is no way to resolve different interpretations of the same behavior. This produces the undesirable interview which ends in a mutual stand-off.

The solution to this problem is to revise evaluation systems so as to use event language rather than trait language. Employee behaviors can be compared with stated criterion behaviors. Criterion behavior statements take forms such as "evolves appropriate care plans for assigned patients," "prepares patients for discharge by adequate teaching programs," and "assigns team members according to their credentials and abilities." This form of statement obviates the necessity of interpreting behaviors into traits. The evaluator need only compare the actions of the employee to the actions described in the desired criteria. Fewer disagreements occur between employee and evaluator when the only question is about what did in fact happen rather than about what that event "meant."

Identification of criterion behaviors is the first of several steps required for structuring the evaluation system that is to use event language. Criterion behaviors will not be the same for individuals filling two different positions. The staff nurse and the nursing assistant are expected to demonstrate different behaviors; therefore, they would have to be measured against different criteria. Their criterion behaviors should be included in the job description as well as in the evaluation form as behaviors most important to the role performance. The behaviors also should be realistic in terms of measurability.

In wording, the behavior statements should be explicit so that they will have the same meaning for all readers. Each statement should identify the expected level of performance in precise behavioral terms. Both the job description and the evaluation tool, if well constructed, will reveal what is considered most important by nursing management.

The following statements give an example of some criteria selected by one institution for evaluation of the staff nurse:

1. Accurately assesses patient care needs
2. Sets realistic short- and long-term patient goals
3. Plans appropriate nursing care measures to reach identified goals
4. Documents nursing care plans
5. Demonstrates competency in implementing nursing care
6. Documents nursing care given
7. Evaluates effectiveness of nursing care in relation to goals
8. Modifies care plans as needed to reach goals

Some institutions prefer greater detail in their criteria than that given here. In any case, the criteria are stated as desired behaviors, not as traits of the individual.

THE APPRAISAL INTERVIEW

There are many different aspects of the appraisal interview. This chapter will look at the context in which the interview takes place, the content of the interview, and the interview process.

Who, When, and Where

The ideal evaluator is the manager to whom the employee reports. For a staff nurse or a nursing assistant, this manager usually is a head nurse. For a head nurse, the rater usually is a supervisor. Evaluation is best handled at the management level closest to the employee, because this manager has firsthand knowledge of the employee's performance. This rating system also helps reinforce the appropriate lines of authority. If a supervisor evaluates the employees who work under a head nurse, for example, this undermines the head nurse's authority.

Another issue is the question of how often to evaluate personnel. The more often evaluation can be performed, the less stressful the situation becomes, and the more evaluation takes on the nature of guidance rather than of judgment. Yearly evaluations, for example, are too far apart to have vital impact on behavior patterns, yet the very rarity of the event causes high anxiety levels in both employees and supervisors.

One need not and should not wait for an official evaluation time, such as the employee's anniversary date if the employee's performance is problematic. Evaluation should take place whenever an employee's performance warrants it. If an employee's performance is stable and good, the official evaluation times may be adequate. When an employee has been evaluated as unsatisfactory, it is legitimate to increase the frequency of evaluation, otherwise it would take years to get rid of an unsatisfactory worker. The repeat evaluations should be scheduled at intervals long enough to allow the employee time to develop new desired behaviors.

The setting for the performance appraisal interview also is important. The place of interview should be quiet and private. If a supervisor uses her own office, her secretary or the switchboard operator should be notified to hold phone calls. Nothing is more fragmented than an interview which takes place piecemeal between phone calls; both parties are so distracted that the interview is less than useless.

Not only should care be given to selecting the physical setting, but the psychological setting should also be prepared by planning ahead for the interview time. The employee should be notified in advance so that he may plan for the conference; he may be asked to come prepared to discuss his performance, its strengths and weaknesses, his performance problems, and any needs for supervisory help in relation to performance. The psychological tone is carried over into the conference itself, with the supervisor making it evident that the conference is serious and formal business by telling the employee, "We are meeting here today to review your performance for the last six months and to see how it might be improved." The conference neither begins nor ends as if it were a social occasion.

Content of the Interview

Evaluation interviews will differ in content depending upon the specific purpose behind the interview. The interview discussed here will be the one primarily aiming at improving employee performance. Such an interview is future-oriented, change-oriented, and does not focus on placing blame but on correction. A prerequisite for such an interview is that the employee be acquainted with the desired work behaviors. A good way to accomplish this is to begin an evaluation interview by reviewing the employee's job description in order to locate and explore differences in interpretation and attitude concerning the job. Even when an employee has been in a position over a long period of time, mutual exploration of his role and its expected behavioral components can be useful.

Another useful technique for discovering different job interpretations is for the manager and the employee each to prepare for the interview by listing and ranking the key functions of the employee's job as they see them. Comparing and discussing differences between key function lists, as well as comparing them to the job description, will help the manager and the employee to understand each other better. Differences in both content and priorities will help the employee see

what functions the manager views as most important. Seeing the employee's list will help the manager to understand the employee's work behavior.

Another prerequisite for a productive evaluation interview is to help the employee learn in what way his own behaviors fail to match those desired by the manager. In the average employee appraisal, judgment of the employee's behavior is the real focus of the interview process. The employee sits passively while the manager tells him what things he did right and what things he did wrong. In this context, hearing what he did right merely sugarcoats hearing what he did wrong. The "right versus wrong" mechanism forces the evaluation process into a trial-like judgment in which the employee simply hopes that the good will outweigh the bad. This type of evaluation will not change employee behavior, because the total interest of the employee is focused on the judgment, on how well his performance balances out. The most he can do is accept or reject the judgment.

The employee needs to be oriented to the nature and purpose of the interview. He needs to know beforehand that the purpose of this interview is to improve his job performance, not to congratulate him on his successes though that may occur incidentally for the good performer. Thus the best employee and the least effective one will experience similar interviews: both will be structured around a probe for ways to improve performance.

How that purpose is managed in the interview will depend on the insight, objectivity, and motivation of the employee. If the employee is capable of objective self-evaluation, his performance deficiencies may be identified in a mutual interaction between manager and employee. In instances when an employee is not capable of objective self-evaluation, it is up to the manager to specify the behavioral deficiencies.

One of the ironies of the system is that the better the employee, the more likely he will be able to identify his deficiencies; the less capable the employee, the less likely he will be to see his defects. The capable employee usually knows what performance areas can be improved. This type of person measures himself against internalized standards he has set for himself. The less capable employee is likely to need assistance in identifying his deficiencies; in some instances, the manager will have to assert that specific behaviors must be changed.

It is not prudent to go into detail about all the deficiencies of an employee if he has many. It is better to focus only on those that most urgently need changing, since it is unlikely that an employee will be able to work effectively on more than one or two behavioral changes at a time.

With the employee whose performance is satisfactory, the manager may find it most productive to let him select the behaviors he will try to improve. With another employee, the manager may have to specify which particular behaviors are major impairments in the employee's work. An exceptionally poor employee may have more than one or two behaviors that must be changed immediately if he is to be retained in his position. Although it is unlikely that the individual will be able to make so many behavioral changes at once, at least the interview serves to document that need for the changes has been communicated to the employee. In most cases, this will be documentation toward an eventual firing. In some rare cases, where the employee actually has the capability, he may show extensive improvement in numerous areas of practice after such an interview.

Like any other system, change-oriented employee evaluation must be used with judgment. The system works best with two types of employees: self-motivated achievers, who enjoy working toward a goal, and workers who clearly need guidance and direction from an authority figure. It is always possible, on the other hand, that a very good employee is not interested in making any further adaptations in his performance. In this case, the manager will be wise to alter the evaluation system if she wants to retain the employee. When an employee has in effect announced that he will go this far for the job and no farther, then the manager should accept that stand and decide whether or not to keep the employee on that basis.

In identifying behaviors to be changed, it is also important that the manager not be overzealous in trying to inflict some "ideal employee image" on each worker. It is unrealistic to expect exactly the same behaviors from all employees. The manager who aims for this will rob herself of many of the best talents of her staff. For example, one nurse may approach her work with zest and enthusiasm and another may approach her work with cautious, steady planning. Both of these contrasting behaviors may be valuable contributions to the total work group. The manager should focus on developing the talents and abilities inherent in the employee's make-up. If the manager and the employee together identify the behaviors to be improved, these individual considerations will be taken into account.

A third prerequisite for the productive employee interview is for the manager to see that the employee learns how to change his behavior toward the desired pattern. Too often the manager thinks that the job is done by pinpointing an undesirable behavior and directing the employee to change it. This approach is seldom effective. It is important that the employee and the manager identify together the new behaviors the employee will be expected to exhibit. These behaviors must be stated, action by action. For example, for the manager and the nurse employee to agree that the nurse will now distribute her medications on time does not give the nurse any help. It does not tell her how to modify the behaviors that now cause her always to distribute drugs late.

A time limit should be set by which the employee can be expected to have practiced and habitutated the new behavior. Of course, some behaviors cannot be allowed to develop gradually, but these are in the minority. Usually the employee can be given a grace period during which he can concentrate on effecting the change in behavior.

The last prerequisite of the successful

employee interview is that the employee leave the conference determined to change his behavior. For many individuals, participation in setting the behavioral goals alone will provide this motivation. If the process of employee evaluation is seen as a means whereby the manager assists her employee to find easier ways to function, then the process is seen as assistive, not judgmental. If the employee feels that the manager sincerely is trying to help him, this will serve as motivation to adopt the agreed upon behavioral changes.

There are many false conceptions about motivation. The worst is that it can be supplied from the outside. Motivation is an internal principle; an individual either is or is not motivated in relation to something. It is not possible for a manager to motivate a person who does not want to be motivated. Threats of punishment or promises of rewards do not motivate, they manipulate. Some individuals can inspire others in such a way that they become motivated, but the manager should not have to rely on charisma.

Although it is not possible to motivate, it is possible for the manager to require certain behaviors as conditions of holding a job, getting a raise, or getting a promotion. Thus, control mechanisms can be used so that the employee will leave the interview with the knowledge that to be able to hold his job or obtain a raise or promotion he must change his behavior. The employee now has an exact idea of what to do. Setting time limits for the behavioral change also lets him know that the conversation has not been mere rhetoric. To assure that these time limits have meaning, it is important that the manager have one or more follow-up conferences during and at the end of the time frame. It is a good idea to close the evaluation interview by setting the date for the follow-up conference and by affirming that the purpose of that conference will be to evaluate progress toward the changes in behavior.

The evaluation interview designed to improve deficient employee performance is only one kind of appraisal interview. For some employees, the manager will prefer to build on strengths rather than to correct weaknesses. This is one way a successful employee sincerely can be commended. When a manager is interested in the special knowledge or abilities of an employee to the extent that she helps the employee build on these talents, there is no question of employee recognition. The manager's interest provides much more employee satisfaction than does the abstract "reading off" of a list of virtues in the typical employee evaluation interview.

Processes of the Interview

The manager is likely to have four objectives for the interview: 1) to convey information, 2) to foster actual behavioral change, 3) to keep the interview situation itself comfortable and as free of tension as possible, and 4) to maintain control of the situation. Several suggestions can be offered to the manager with these objectives in mind. First, it is important that the manager go into the interview with clear purposes in mind. She should know specifically what kinds of change she wishes to bring about in the employee; she should know how she will suggest those changes be implemented. It helps if the supervisor has some strategies for the interview prepared in advance. By thinking ahead into the interview situation and anticipating the employee's responses, the manager can prepare her own tactics for dealing with the anticipated responses.

The manager knows that in a situation where criticism of performance is necessary, the following defense mechanisms may be invoked in the employee: withdrawal, denial, excuses, or challenge and confrontation. She should be prepared for any or all of these responses. Indeed, she must be prepared to get beyond these immediate responses if the employee's behavior is to be improved.

Keeping control involves several aspects of managerial behavior. First, the manager must use introspection during the process of the interview. She must try to be both an involved participant and a disinterested, removed judge of what is going on. She must watch for power shifts between herself and the employee. Sometimes she can allow the employee to take control of the interview, but not if such control threatens the purpose of the conference. The manager can reassert control when required if she has clearly asserted her prerogatives at the start of the conference. She can indicate verbally or by her attitude that as manager, she has the prerogative to listen, but that she has no need to negotiate. Ultimately, as manager, she will determine the significance of the situation, including the final judgment of the subordinate's behavior.

The manager will more easily keep control if she is sensitive to both the facts and the feelings that make up the interview. Again, she can interpret these if she mentally steps "outside" the interview situation as an impartial judge. (Perhaps this is to say that the successful manager must be somewhat schizophrenic in the interview situation.) At one instance, she may find it appropriate to focus on the facts being discussed; at another time it may be advantageous to be aware of (and possibly discuss) the feeling tone of the interview.

The greatest asset of the manager is the knowledge that she does not have to stick to any particular response pattern when dealing with an employee in interview. She can keep her response options open. If she is to respond thoughtfully to the employee, however, she must actually listen to what the employee says and she must dare to take the time to think rather than rushing into an unconsidered response. Both take more skill than one might assume. Listening to the employee means letting him do most of the talking, letting him finish sentences, not thinking ahead into one's response while he is still talking and checking to see if the message he was trying to convey was actually received. Taking time to think before responding may be even harder, for it means that the supervisor will allow herself to break

the time norms for response that dominate in this society. Nevertheless, it is the supervisor's inalienable right to think before she speaks—even if it does break a social norm.

Another bit of advice for the supervisor is that she hold a two-way communication. This means that the interview must be planned to involve active participation from the employee, not just "tell and sell" from the evaluator. The manager can assure two-way communication by preparing a number of pivotal questions to ask the employee—questions that require thought and discussion, questions that cannot be answered by a "yes" or a "no."

The key function comparison scheme mentioned earlier is an example of an activity that creates two-way communication. In order to make the interview two-way, the employee should be advised to prepare for the evaluation just as adequately as does the manager. Both parties should not only identify key functions and work problems but also make suggestions and pose relevant questions. Another way to establish two-way communication is for the two individuals to discuss their mutual expectations of each other.

Where possible, the manager seeks agreement concerning deficiencies and goals. However, the interview should not be reduced to a bargaining session. The manager may need to assert her authority when the employee is not in agreement; employee acceptance is desirable but not always possible.

Another principle for the interview is that the manager make absolutely clear what she means. For example, if this interview is a last warning before a potential dismissal, she must make certain that the employee understands the situation. Some employees use defense mechanisms by interpreting as casual conversation what the manager sees as a final warning. In all instances, it will be useful if the manager follows the conference with a letter to the employee summarizing the interview, the problems discussed, and the goals set. When an interview serves a disciplinary function, it is absolutely essential that this documentation be done. While disciplining an employee is never an easy task, use of an event-focused evaluation system makes the job less difficult.

One of the best ways to maintain good communication during an evaluation interview is for the manager to avoid falling into common interview traps. These errors include:

1. Conducting a one-way conversation
2. Interrupting the employee's thoughts, explanations, questions
3. Criticizing the employee rather than the performance
4. Smoothing over real deficiencies and problems too fast
5. Failing to investigate facts before expressing opinions
6. Passing the buck by claiming that one's corrective measures originate "higher up"
7. Allowing the interview to fall into charge-countercharge cycles
8. Allowing the interview to fall into charge-denial cycles
9. Allowing the interview to fall into charge-excuse cycles
10. Allowing the interview to deteriorate into a social visit

During an interview, the manager continuously evaluates what is happening in the interaction. She must recognize what she is doing as well as what the employee is doing in order to avoid traps and to keep the interview productive. One basic rule for the manager is to keep her response options open. For every statement made by an employee, there are numerous ways to respond. Unconsidered responses tend to be limited to one of two typical patterns. The first pattern is to respond with a judgment of the employee's statement. In an interview situation, this response creates a trial-like atmosphere. The second pattern of common response is direct reaction to the content of the employee's statement. There are many times when this is an appropriate response,

but there are also many times when other responses are better. To evaluate some response options, let us examine an interview that has fallen into the charge-excuse cycle:

Head Nurse: ". . . also, you failed to give Mrs. Jones her passive exercise all last week."

Staff Nurse: "You are thinking about last Thursday, and that day she was so upset she wouldn't let anyone touch her."

Head Nurse: "I'm not thinking just of Thursday. You didn't exercise her weak side on Friday either."

Staff Nurse: "On Friday her doctor did that spinal tap and took all morning at it. No one could have gotten in there to exercise her."

Head Nurse: "But nothing went on Friday afternoon, and you still didn't exercise her."

Staff Nurse: "But I was taught that patients were to lie flat and quiet after a spinal tap to prevent a headache."

This head nurse has fallen into a deadly trap, for the staff nurse can probably find an excuse for any charge the head nurse can think up. The head nurse has in each case responded to the content of the staff nurse's statement. As long as she continues this, she will neither break the cycle nor make her point.

To break off this unproductive cycle, the head nurse needs to recognize that such a pattern takes two to keep it going. As soon as one participant refuses to play, the cycle is interrupted. One simple solution is for the head nurse to admit that this line of conversation is unproductive and break it off, going to another topic.

A better option might be to answer the last response with a question or suggestion that directs the employee out of the cycle. "Why don't you review for me your plans for Mrs. Jones last week. Maybe we can explore what happened to them.''

The head nurse also might switch from content-directed charges to feeling exploration. She could direct a question to the staff nurse concerning her feelings about Mrs. Jones.

Another choice would be for the head nurse to point out that Mrs. Jones' care is only part of a larger problem and then return to the bigger problem instead of haggling over one instance of behavior. Another useful response option is for the head nurse to call the staff nurse's attention to the excuse pattern of her responses. They might then explore why this pattern dominates her explanations of her work.

Numerous paths can be taken to restore the interview to a productive session. The critical factor is simply that the manager recognize the defective communications pattern and utilize a constructive response option.

Managers often use the evaluation interview to encourage changes in employee attitudes. It is impossible to work with attitudes that are expressed in trait language, such as ''You are hostile,'' ''You are racially prejudiced,'' ''You are headstrong and impulsive.'' The logical way to proceed to achieve desired attitude change is to identify the behavior or behaviors that give evidence of the trait. To tell an employee that he is impulsive does not tell him how to change that trait, nor does it make him wish to change. It is possible, however, to identify behaviors that demonstrate impulsiveness and impair the work process. It is quite legitimate to require that an employee change a nonfunctional work behavior.

Many authorities agree that the best way to change attitudes is to change behaviors first. Once an individual is routinely doing a particular act, he is likely to develop a positive attitude toward that act. Many nurse managers have tried to build a ''favorable attitude'' toward written nursing care plans before requiring them on the nursing units. What happens, of course, is that those favorable attitudes fail to appear, whatever steps the manager takes to induce them. On the other hand, the nurse manager who firmly and consistently requires that care plans be written by each staff nurse finds that, after a short period of time, attitudes toward writing the plans have become positive.

Managers often have difficulty knowing when and how to end an interview. While there is no absolute rule for timing, almost any interview can be easily contained within an hour. If a manager tends to hold longer conferences, she is likely to be doing one of two things: either turning the interview into a social visit, or belaboring the same essential points. Both of these patterns are to be avoided.

A good way to end the interview and give it a sense of completion is for the manager to summarize the events of the interview. She can briefly identify the problems discussed, the agreements reached, the goals set, and the proposed behavioral changes. This summary has two functions. First, it gives the employee a final chance to compare her interpretation of the interview with the manager's interpretation. Any differences in understanding can therefore be revealed and settled. Second, summarizing clearly announces to the employee that the interview is at an end. The summary includes a review of what happened in the interview, the agreements reached, and any direct orders from the manager.

There is no easy way to learn interview skills. The manager who uses postinterview evaluation, however, will improve her skills considerably. She should analyze each interview immediately after it is finished, while the dialogue still is fresh in her mind, including her responses to employee statements. Learning to recognize her weaknesses in interviewing will help the manager guard against these deficiencies in future conferences. The manager who develops skill in interviewing will be rewarded by improved employee-manager relations and by improved work performances from her staff.

REFERENCES

1. Haar, L.P. Performance Appraisal. In Rezler, A.G., and Stevens, B.J., (Eds.) *The Nurse Evaluator in Education and Service.* New York: McGraw-Hill, 1978, pp. 205–227.
2. *American Jurisprudence,* 2nd ed., vol. 48, section 606, 1970, p. 421.
3. *American Jurisprudence,* 2nd ed., vol. 48, section 624, 1970, p. 431.

BIBLIOGRAPHY

Aime, D.B. Employee evaluations—what's the difference? *Supervisor Nurse* 10(6):52.

Albrecht, S. Reappraisal of conventional performance appraisal system. *J.O.N.A.* 2(2):29, 1972.

Bernhardt, J., and Schuette, L. P.E.T.: a method of evaluating professional nurse performance. *J.O.N.A.* 5(8):18, 1975.

Bidwell, C.M., and Froebe, D.J. Development of an instrument for evaluating hospital performance. *J.O.N.A.* 1(5):10, 1971.

Cantor, M.M. Certifying competencies of personnel. *J.O.N.A.* 5(5):8, 1975.

del Bueno, D. Implementing a performance evaluation system. *Supervisor Nurse* 10(2):48, 1979.

del Bueno, D. Performance evaluation: when all is said and done, more is said than done. *J.O.N.A.* 7(10):21, 1977.

Dracup, L. Improving clinical evaluation. *Supervisor Nurse* 10(6):24, 1979.

Fitzgerald, T.H. Why motivation theory doesn't work. *Harvard Business Rev.* 49(4):37, 1971.

Fleisman, R. Disciplinary action—friend or foe? *Supervisor Nurse* 2(5):19, 1971.

Gauerke, R.D. Appraisal as a retention tool. *Supervisor Nurse* 8(6):34, 1976.

Haar, L.P., and Hicks, J.R. Performance appraisal: derivation of effective assessment tools. *J.O.N.A.* 6(7):30, 1976.

Hamric, A.B., Gresham, M.L., and Eccard, M. Staff evaluation of clinical leaders. *J.O.N.A.* 8(1):18, 1978.

Hauser, M.A. Initiation into peer review. *Am. J. Nursing* 75(12):2204, 1975.

Herzberg, F. One more time: how do you motivate employees? *Harvard Business Rev.* 46(1):53, 1968.

Huberman, J. Discipline without punishment. *Harvard Business Rev.* 42(4):62, 1964.

Johnson, K.J., and Zimmerman, M.A. Peer review in a health department. *Am. J. Nursing* 75(4):618, 1975.

Kelly, R.L. Evaluation is more than measurement. *Am. J. Nursing.* 73(1):115, 1973.

Kindall, A.F., and Garza, J. Positive program for performance appraisal. *Harvard Business Rev.* 41(6):153, 1963.

Levinson, H. Asinine attitudes toward motivation. *Harvard Business Rev.* 51(1):70, 1973.

Levinson, H. Appraisal of *what* performance? *Harvard Business Rev.* 54(4):30, 1976.

McGregor, D. An uneasy look at performance appraisal. *Harvard Business Rev.* 50(5):133, 1972.

McNamara, E.M. The caring employer helps the troubled employee. *Hospitals* 50(20):93, 1976.

Marriner, A. Evaluation of personnel. *Supervisor Nurse* 7(5):36, 1976.

Marriner, A. Discipline of personnel. *Supervisor Nurse* 7(11):15, 1976.

Oberg, W. Make performance appraisal relevant. *Harvard Business Rev.* 50(1):61, 1972.

O'Brien, M.J. Evaluation. *Supervisor Nurse* 2(4):24, 1971.

O'Donovan, T.R. Performance evaluation of subordinates. *Supervisor Nurse* 2(11):48, 1971.

Patz, A.L. Performance appraisal: useful but still resisted. *Harvard Business Rev.* 53(3):74, 1975.

Rieder, G.A. Performance review—a mixed bag. *Harvard Business Rev.* 51(4):61, 1973.

Robertson, P., and Knutson, K.E. The disciplinary conference letter. *Supervisor Nurse* 7(3):10, 1976.

South, J.C. The performance profile: a technique for using appraisals effectively. *J.O.N.A.* 8(1):27, 1978.

Waller, M., and Davids, D. Performance profiles based on nursing activity records. *J.O.N.A.* 2(5):60, 1972.

Waxman, H. Adding to the performance appraisal. *Supervisor Nurse* 2(11):44, 1971.

White, B., and Barnes, B. Power networks in the appraisal process. *Harvard Business Rev.* 49(3):101, 1971.

Chapter 24   The Inservice Education Department

In most health care institutions, nursing inservice education is a function handled by a department designated for that purpose within the nursing division. This department usually is responsible for providing education for all personnel in the nursing division, that is, for registered nurses, practical nurses, nurses' assistants, and various kinds of specialized technicians. Some inservice departments also assume responsibility for education of non-nursing personnel such as ward clerks and secretaries.

Though similar in function, nursing education departments are known by different names: nursing inservice education, staff development, continuing education, or education and training. A minority of institutions do not have a nursing service education department but instead provide nursing inservice education in one of two ways: either there is decentralized education, with tasks divided among personnel whose primary functions are in nursing service, or there may be an education division for the entire health institution, with nursing education being one part of this division. The latter arrangement indicates that the nursing division is in a weak condition regarding its own education. Since the great majority of health care institutions have a separate nursing inservice education department within the nursing division, this chapter will address the typical arrangement.

The nursing inservice education department usually is headed by a nurse administrator who has advanced preparation and experience in both nursing and education. She heads a staff of instructors who carry out the nursing education program. The number of instructors varies radically from institution to institution; an inservice administrator may have from two to 20 teachers under her direction. In this chapter the term *inservice director* refers to the administrator of the nursing inservice education department, whatever her title in a particular institution.

Program development in nursing inservice is a real challenge for the inservice director, who usually has great latitude in selection of the educational projects constituting her program. Two decision points exist in program development. The first is selection and justification of projects; the second, justification of the composite program representing the total educational services.

Program refers to the constellation of educational services offered by the inservice education department, whereas *project* refers to any one service within that program. Projects may include services planned for groups or for individuals. A course on geriatric nursing would be a project for groups; counseling on career advancement education would be a project available for individuals.

This chapter attempts to develop constructs that will enable the inservice director to produce effective education in the institutional setting. Central to the development of such constructs is the belief that objectives and plans for inservice education must consider that department's place in the nursing division. In particular, the objectives of the educational program and the projects must be planned in relation to the structure of the nursing organization, the nursing processes, and patient outcomes. These are three different perspectives from which objectives may be formulated.

That the education program must be related to nursing processes is not surprising, for inservice education is aimed at helping staff improve, maintain, or acquire specific nursing processes. The necessary relationship of the educational program to nursing organizational structure and patient outcomes can be ascertained by considering how these aspects relate to nursing processes. So-called improved nursing processes are meaningless unless they can be correlated to improved patient outcomes. Similarly, nursing management systems (structures) must be designed to achieve desired patient outcomes effectively and efficiently. For example, an alteration in the process of changing dressings for burn patients can be justified if it saves time (management) without causing increased discomfort or decreased wound healing for the patient. It also can be justified, even at decreased efficiency, if it improves wound healing (outcome). Inservice education cannot be abstracted from its environment; complex considerations of organization structure, nursing processes, and patient outcomes enter into every educational decision.

Inservice education may be viewed as a subsystem of a total nursing organization. Besides identifying its relation to the concepts of structure, process, and outcome in the nursing system, consideration must be given to inservice education as a unified program of educational resources and projects. The internal relations of selected projects to each other must be analyzed; attention is given to this aspect in the next chapter. Lastly, inservice education must be viewed from the perspective of a single educational project. Criteria for internal analysis of each project as a separate entity must be identified as is done in Chapter 26.

STRUCTURES OF THE INSERVICE DEPARTMENT

In conceiving of nursing inservice education as an organizational subsystem of the nursing division, it is useful to describe the features common to most inservice departments. The nursing organization chart usual-

ly places the inservice department on the same level with major service departments of nursing such as medical nursing, surgical nursing, and obstetric nursing. The inservice director is a peer of the other major nurse managers; her mode of relating to the other managers is coordination, and she functions in a staff, rather than line, position relative to the nursing staff. The inservice director, like the managers of major service departments, typically reports directly to the nurse executive of the institution.

Three important factors affect the inservice department and the role of the inservice director. First, the inservice director commands an education-oriented department within a larger system whose goals are not primarily educational. Second, requests for educational services usually increase faster than does the capacity of the educational staff. Last, in spite of the staff position on most organization charts, the director of inservice education tends to be a powerful person in the nursing hierarchy. These factors will each be examined in more detail.

Educational Goals Serving Patient Outcome Goals

The fact that nursing organization goals are primarily related to patient outcomes may be perceived as a constraint by the inservice director, for educational goals become means to patient-care goals rather than sufficient ends in themselves. This constraint means that the inservice educator commands only second-order goals: her goals of staff education are subsumed within primary patient outcome goals.

Second-order goals may not command the same degree of attention as do primary organizational goals. In conditions of heavy patient load, the supervisor is likely to solve immediate patient care needs by sacrificing secondary educational needs, by pulling employees from planned educational activities for immediate care services. Disruption of planned educational projects is a tactical problem to be surmounted by every inservice director. Since patient outcome goals are primary, they tend to be given higher priority than educational goals when the two functions compete for the same time.

The subservience of educational goals to patient outcome goals offers opportunities as well as constraints. If educational projects can be related directly to improved patient outcomes, the inservice director has a tangible means of evaluating the success of her projects. She can assess the effectiveness of many of her education projects by subsequent changes in the work environment; she need not rely solely on secondary measures such as paper and pencil examinations but can measure changes in patient care as instituted by those who have completed her projects.

When the inservice director can substantiate that her projects improve patient care, she can readily win the support of nursing managers. When projects are evaluated through patient outcomes, goals of both education and management are promoted.

In most hospitals, there are a few expected ongoing educational activities such as nurses' aid training or orientation of new personnel, but creation of projects is relatively open to the inservice director's discretion. The inservice director will be wise to determine her projects based on patient care deficiencies. Where good quality control systems exist, data from them will reveal deficit areas.

Multiple Requests for Services

A second factor influencing inservice education is that requests and demands for services usually exceed department resources. Continuous advances in the knowledge of disease processes and the development of new modes of nursing and medical therapy create an environment in which nurse practitioners constantly are seeking new information. Constant change also is reflected in equipment and available technologies; a rapid rate of obsolescence of knowledge and skills, necessitating their constant updating, is the result of the change tempo. In the health care institution, requests for nursing education are not admissions of inadequacy but indications of professional commitment. The health institution environment leads nursing staff members to be matter of fact about learning needs, and they tend to freely seek and use educational resources where an effective inservice department exists. In such an environment, it is almost impossible to meet all requests, even with a large and competent staff of teachers.

This excessive demand for educational services is a constraint only if the inservice director feels a compulsion to meet all requests unselectively. If she does she abdicates control of her own department to external forces. Moreover, it is likely that her productivity will be limited since what people want and what they need in educational programs frequently have little connection. It is useful for the inservice director to know the educational interests of the staff, but she is wise not to assume that these preferences automatically reflect the areas of greatest learning needs; preferences are just as likely to reflect the latest fads in nursing. If the inservice director tries to meet all requests, it also is likely departmental resources will be so diluted over multiple projects that no request will receive adequate input to produce actual change in staff behavior.

Properly viewed, a great number of requests for educational services is an opportunity for the inservice director. From a management perspective it has the psychological advantage of bringing others to her. As with any scarce service, the provider is at an advantage. In addition, these requests serve as one important source of input in the selection of projects.

Powers of the Office of Inservice Director

Perhaps the most interesting condition to analyze is the relative power of the inservice director in the overall nursing organizational structure. The typical organization chart places the inservice director equal to or higher than the major nursing managers of patient care, managers who may each be in charge of multiple functional units in the nursing division. In practice the inservice director may have even more power than organization charts would indicate, but seldom less.

Reasons for the strength of the inservice position can be found by examining both the role of the inservice director and the relation of her department to other nursing departments. It is typical that the individual filling the inservice director's role is one of the best-educated nurses in the organization. Nursing as a profession has not yet been able to meet fully the demand for well-educated nurses for high organization positions. Consequently many supervisory positions are filled by individuals whose qualifications are experiential rather than educational. The position of the inservice director, however, is seldom filled by such individuals. Usually this nurse manager is both educationally and experientially prepared for her position. In smaller hospitals, one may find that the inservice director has an education beyond that of the chief nurse officer, who may have "come up from the ranks."

The educational status of the inservice director serves two purposes. First it increases the status of the inservice position. Second, it increases the resources this individual has to offer the nursing system. It is an interesting reflection on the advancement of nursing that, less than 20 years ago, inservice positions were often used for ineffective nurses who, for humane or other reasons, could not be dismissed from the organization.

The inservice director has another advantage over other nurse managers. Because her functions are one step removed from direct patient care, she is able to avoid the trap of crisis management. Other nurse managers often are caught in situations in which immediate patient needs encourage crisis management instead of long-term planning. The inservice director, not faced with problems of such immediacy, is able to develop and implement more stable plans, and thus she

may appear to be a more capable manager than others.

The nature of inservice education also contributes to power centralization in this department. Inservice education is often the only department whose staff members interact with all other departments of the nursing division. A director of medical nursing, for example, has little interaction with a director of obstetrics in the territory of that director; their domains and staff members are not interchangeable. Staff members of inservice education, however, teach in all direct care units. This intermix provides the inservice director with a by-product of intelligence-gathering on the whole nursing division.

The inservice director is in a good position to have a disinterested but informed opinion on problems in other areas of the nursing division. Because of this position, the inservice director often is drawn into a role of troubleshooter for problems in the nursing division. Once clearly identified, the problems may or may not turn out to be problems of education. The majority of problems that are not problems of education turn out to be problems of administration; hence the tendency for the inservice director to be drawn into a triple role of consultant, educator, and administrator, thereby increasing her power base.

There are some advantages to letting this conjunctive administrative role develop. First, this role is a natural outgrowth of the problem-diagnosing activity of the inservice director; and second, there are some problems best handled by an administrator who has staff authority instead of line authority. The inservice director may be able to offer resolutions with objectivity because her position is not in the usual hierarchical structure, and her solutions may be readily acceptable to other management staff since her role is not seen as competitive with theirs. The quality of her proposed resolutions also may be enhanced by her perspective as an "outsider" to the hierarchical line.

Thus the strategic position of the inservice department and the special resources of the educator-director are likely to make the office of the inservice director particularly powerful. This power, however, arises from and promotes adoption of activities that are administrative as well as educative.

Some inservice educators feel this thrust toward administration as a constraint, as a source of additional tasks that prevent them from giving full attention to their assigned role as educators. Other inservice directors take the opposite view, that absolute division of administrative and educational functions is artificial in the organizational setting. These inservice directors see administration as complementary and related to education.

One is able to substantiate a unity between administration and education when these are viewed as complementary aspects of the same change process. Given that objectives of administration and education ultimately are improvements in patient care, both administration and education attain these goals, not primarily through effects on the patient but by producing changes in staff activities and behaviors. Where simple lack of knowledge or skill is the problem, education alone may be adequate to produce the desired change in staff behavior. In other instances simple administrative dictate may produce change. There is, however, a broad class of problems in which a conjunction of education and administrative change is most successful.

Consider, for example, an institution where nurses habitually fail to compose written care plans. Here a dual attack on the problem probably is necessary. Education in the production of appropriate plans will enhance the nurses' ability to compose quality care plans, but this education alone is not likely to make a durable change. Unless the administrative structure is altered so as to require and reward the production of care plans, the project will soon be shelved to meet more direct demands on the nurses' time.

The inservice director who sees education and administration as two conjunctive mechanisms for change may find that assuming certain administrative functions actually increases her ability to provide ef-

fective education. Therefore the press toward administrative responsibilities may be considered as an opportunity rather than as a constraint.

The inservice educator typically has greater power than her organization position would indicate, receives more demands for her services than she can supply, has more autonomy than other nursing managers, and has the peculiar necessity to make educational projects serve noneducational goals. When viewed as a subsystem in the nursing organizational structure, the inservice education department has a unique position. In contrast to other nursing departments, its objectives are different from but subservient to organizational patient-related goals. Its activities are diffused throughout the nursing organization rather than concentrated in a clearly demarcated area of nursing, and it offers unique resources, resources that will periodically be needed by all other nursing departments.

THE INSERVICE DEPARTMENT AS IT RELATES TO OTHER DEPARTMENTS

Power Relationships

While most nursing education departments have a common structure, there is less uniformity in the process by which they relate to other nursing departments. The power relations that hold between the inservice department and other nursing departments are important factors because of the constant tension between the need for immediate service from workers and the need for the workers to receive education that will enable them to improve work patterns in the future. Where inservice education is available to the employee only on his own time, this is not a problem. Most institutions, however, assume responsibility for providing employees with needed inservice education during working hours. Then a tension exists between use of employees for immediate service and investment of the employees' time toward future service abilities. This tension is exacerbated by the present stringent economy practiced in most health institutions; few institutions can now replace the worker who is attending inservice education: coworkers simply absorb that employee's share of the work.

From the perspective of the inservice director, this sacrifice of immediate service has a pay-off in the employee's future performance. Typically, other nurse managers agree with the educational pay-off in principle, but they may sell out the principle as the here and now makes demands on them. A familiar pattern develops in which the nurse manager claims a pressing need for a particular educational project, yet fails to send workers to the classes because the units are "too busy."

The scene is set for a disagreement in which the nurse manager and the inservice director haggle over custody of the worker. Educational staff hours spent in preparation for educational projects contribute to the inservice director's proprietal claim on the worker. With this problem always looming on the horizon, the mode of interaction between the education department and other nursing departments becomes critical to educational effectiveness.

There are at least four basic ways in which an inservice department can relate to the departments it serves. 1) Inservice education may have the power to compel participation of others in its projects. 2) The inservice director may operate through coordination and agreements reached together with her peer group of nurse managers. 3) The inservice department may offer projects that others attend or ignore as they choose. 4) Inservice education may be under compulsion to produce what others direct. All these forms of relationship, as well as combined forms, can be found in existing educational departments. These four power relationships will be examined in detail.

Authority to Compel Participation

If the inservice director has the authority to compel attendance at her projects by employees of other managers, this authority may be direct or mediated through the chief nurse officer. There are both advantages and disadvantages in this degree of power. First, it may produce resentment on the part of other nurse managers, who can claim interference with their authority over their own employees. One solution is to relegate control to inservice education only for projects where it can be substantiated that such power is necessary for attainment of divisional goals. In the instance of the divisional goal of economy, inservice education is given control over employees if control can be expected to save large amounts of money. It has been well established that the greatest single outlay of resources is the money spent on the nursing employee during induction into the institution[1]. Induction may include orientation for all personnel or training for aides or technical personnel. Certainly, then, the greatest financial loss occurs if an employee leaves the institution shortly after induction. Rapid turnover among new personnel usually is due to inadequate preparation (orientation and training) for responsibilities given the new employee too soon[2].

During induction periods, therefore, there are justifiable reasons for placing control with the inservice director rather than with other nursing service managers. Understandably line managers tend to solve immediate unit problems by premature assignment of new personnel. This use of the new employee works to the disadvantage of the department. Statistically a high number of new employees separate early when placed under immediately stressful work situations. Statistical probabilities, however, seldom are effective dissuasions when the nurse manager controls the new employee and has an immediate staffing need.

Some institutions, therefore, give the inservice director control over employees' schedules and activities for the orientation or training period. This control necessarily includes not only management of educational classes but also management of clinical work assignment, the latter being viewed as clinical education rather than as clinical staff-work. When an inservice education department has total responsibility for the induction period, it also is essential that the department evaluate the new employee's performance during that period. Inservice education should make the first determination of whether the new employee is to be retained or dismissed. This ancillary task of screening new employees is a logical activity for an education department since its members should be more sophisticated in evaluation techniques than are the line nurse managers.

Control of induction employees by inservice education has another advantage. While nurse managers resent inservice control over "their employees," they can view induction employees as being outside their domain. Induction employees do not "belong" to the nurse manager until they are released from the inservice department and certified as ready for practice. Nurse managers usually are quite relieved to have the original screening done by inservice education since they have less time to devote to evaluation of new employees. The inservice director's accommodation with other nurse managers also is enhanced if her trainees are not charged to the budgets of other managers. Where the cost is borne by the inservice department, new employees are not expected to "replace" other workers while they are still in orientation or training periods.

A related management function often falls to the inservice director who controls induction employees. Where large numbers of employees are oriented or trained together, the inservice director has the most reliable knowledge for matching individual employee abilities with patient unit needs. She often is drawn into the administrative function of staffing, another example of the inevitable intermixing of education and administration in the organizational setting.

Coordinative Power

The second power state by which the inservice education department may relate to other departments is through coordination and agreement between the inservice director and other nurse managers. This relationship is more in keeping with the organizational staff position typically held by the inservice director. This arrangement works well where the staff needs and inservice projects are perceived by all to correspond, and where inservice projects produce results that are evident to the line nurse managers.

Inservice education is a form of teaching-learning that must substantiate its worth if projects are derived through mutual coordination and agreement among the inservice director and other nurse managers. Nurse managers simply will not commit their limited employee resources to education if they perceive no tangible benefits.

Independent Function

In the third possible form by which inservice education may relate to other nursing departments, the inservice department presents projects that others attend or not at their own discretion and convenience. This is such a poor way of relating that it would not be mentioned were it uncommon in actual nursing organizations. The defects in the relationship are numerous. Lack of close interaction fails to assure that projects will be directed toward real learning needs. There is no way for the inservice director to calculate appropriate distribution of educational resources when the number and nature of the learners cannot be predicted. Such casual relationships encourage employees to view education as a private benefit rather than as an integral part of their work. It is difficult to hold such an audience accountable for application of its learning to the work environment. It is difficult to justify the expenditure of patients' monies on such casual education.

If the inservice director accepts this form of relationship with others, she is powerless; she can cater only to the desires (not the needs) of others. This form of relationship requires that inservice bear all the responsibility while the other departments make no commitment in return and has little to recommend it.

Dependent Function

The last form of power relationship is that in which education is subservient to the commands of others. This form occurs in organizations that decentralize education, attaching individual instructors to major service departments. In this plan there is no separate inservice department, and education is a functional part of each major nursing department.

There are both advantages and disadvantages to such decentralization. The first disadvantage is a financial one, for economies of scale are lost. Educational resources such as projectors and other audiovisual hardware tend to be duplicated in every department. In addition to increased expense in equipment, there is need for duplication of teaching facilities in each department. Where extra space is consigned for educational purposes, less space is available for patient services, which are the income-producing functions. There sometimes is an effort made to centralize educational facilities and audiovisual support services even where education, itself, is decentralized. Whether or not this works depends upon the organization and scheduling process used by the department responsible for audiovisual and space requests.

There also is increased cost in instructor salaries entailed in decentralized education, which typically requires more instructors because each instructor is limited to one area (or two) of practice. Where the instructor is eliminated totally—with the rationalization that inservice education is everyone's job—usually inservice is "decentralized" out of existence.

There also are some advantages in decentralization. The instructor whose nursing content area is delimited can develop a specialist's knowledge of that particular area with relative ease. She can keep up to date on all changes in a delimited area of nursing with minimal effort. In addition, by working with fewer personnel, the teacher can get to know the educational needs and abilities of individual employees.

The primary danger with decentralization or other arrangements in which education is subservient to service management is the loss of the healthy tension between immediate and future needs. The inservice director needs at least an equal position with other nurse managers if future needs are to receive adequate attention.

The process by which the inservice education department functions as a subsystem in the nursing division is greatly dependent on the lines of relationship established with other departments. It is important that the inservice educator be aware of, evaluate, and, when necessary, seek to alter these lines of relationship in her institution.

INSERVICE DEPARTMENT OUTCOMES

As a subsystem in the nursing organization, inservice education has the unique position of being a department whose ultimate effect is located in someone else's department—in the changed behaviors of other managers' staff and in the improved outcomes for other managers' patients. Because it may affect many parts of the nursing system, inservice education has a great potential for altering the output of the total system.

To evaluate educational outcomes, it may be necessary to control for effects of different management techniques. For example, after teaching sessions in the use of the written care plan, educational measurement may reveal that outcomes of the same educational process vary from unit to unit, depending upon management support relevant to the project. Even in evaluation there is interaction between education and management.

Because it takes time and planning to evaluate educational outcomes in staff behaviors, some educators assess their department's productivity on bases such as the expressed satisfaction of other nurse managers and staff members or quantitative head counts of numbers of teaching hours offered and numbers of staff members attending. These assessments are important input for departmental decisions, but they may be misleading if they are used as the sole estimate of educational productivity. There is no assurance that satisfaction or quantitative counts relate directly to changes in staff behaviors.

Indeed, the educational director who aims for the largest number of projects is often giving to each project too few resources to expect outcomes in terms of changed behaviors. Minimally developed projects (such as a one-hour lecture on a selected topic) usually are not adequate for effecting change. In the work setting, if education has not contributed to some lasting and worthwhile changes in the nursing division, it has been a diversion of scarce resources. Departmental outcome, therefore, is best stated as the cumulative outcome (changes in staff behavior) of all departmental projects.

A SYSTEMS VIEW OF THE INSERVICE DEPARTMENT

The inservice education department may be considered through the systems models in two different ways: as a system in itself, with its own goals and objectives, and as a control function within other systems, such as the staff behavior and patient care systems. These two views have been blended in this chapter; indeed, an effective inservice department must view itself from both of these perspectives.

As an independent system, its goals are educational. The inservice department is unique as an educational system. Unlike other educational systems, its learners (input) are diverse in background, interests, educational needs, and intellectual abilities. Further, the system must constantly revise its subject matter depending upon changes in its environment (the other nursing systems). Inservice education presents challenges never imagined in the educational setting of the neatly structured school of nursing.

With shifting goals and varying input, the thruput (program and projects) of the inservice department must be adaptable. Inservice goals aim to rectify ignorance or inabilities. They should not be expected to address management issues also. Unfortunately, many nurse managers fail to recognize managerial problems, expecting them to respond to educational treatment. Often the inservice department must educate managers as to their managerial functions and responsibilities.

As a component of other systems, inservice education is a control element; it is adjustment provided to the thruput and thus subservient to the goals of others, especially the patient care and the staff behavior systems.

Whether viewed alone or in conjunction with other systems, the major change in inservice education in today's nursing division is the resources made available to the inservice department. Many inservice budgets have been cut as a cost containment measure. Concurrently, the responsibility of many inservice education departments has been limited to job-related education. There is a well-defined trend to make nurses financially responsible for their own continuing learning if it exceeds the basic demands of the work situation.

One way that inservice departments have coped with the decrease in available resources has been to share educational projects. Indeed, the move to increase economies of scale by holding large, cooperative educational functions is evident nationwide. Further, that trend has been found to be profitable in cases where "outside" participants could be charged fees for the education offered. Ironically, then, the inservice education department often has found that it is in a position to be self-supporting if it concentrates on large educational projects that also are offered to nurses from other institutions. A problem here is the tendency to select offerings based on audience appeal rather than upon the needs of the home institution for inservice education. In other words, in an attempt to increase its resources, many an inservice department has been drawn out of inservice education into continuing education.

The opportunity is tempting, and the clientele is there, especially as laws change concerning continuing education requirements for licensure. Indeed, in taking advantage of the ready audience, nursing inservice departments are filling a need otherwise all too often filled by opportunists from outside the profession. Nevertheless, the strong move into continuing education represents a blurring of the lines between advanced education and education which is strictly work-related. Perhaps a balance is the best answer for those institutions that have elected to look to the inservice education department for profit making.

REFERENCES

1. Dane, J.H. A model for determining turnover costs. *Hospitals* 46(10):65, 1972.
2. Golub, J.C. A nurse-internship program. *Hospitals* 45(16):73, 1971.

BIBLIOGRAPHY

Cantor, M.M. Staff development: what are the qualifications? *J.O.N.A.* 5(3):7, 1975.

Cooper, S.S., and Hornback, M.S. *Continuing Nursing Education*. New York: McGraw-Hill, 1973.

Coyle, D.H. What is continuing education in nursing service? *Supervisor Nurse* 1(6):36, 1970.

Forni, P. Continuing education vs. continuing competence. *J.O.N.A.* 5(9):34, 1975.

Gatzke, H.K., and Yenney, S.L. Hospitalwide education and training. *Hospitals* 47(5):93, 1973.

Medearis, N.D., and Popiel, E.S. Guidelines for organizing inservice education. *J.O.N.A.* 1(4):30, 1971.

Rudnick, B.R., and Bolte, I.M. The case for ongoing inservice education. *J.O.N.A.* 1(2):31, 1971.

Stopera, V., and Scully, D. A workable organizational model for staff development departments. *J.O.N.A.* 3(6):14, 1972.

Tobin, H. Quality staff development—a must for change and survival: Standard IX. *J.O.N.A.* 6(4):39, 1976.

Chapter 25　　　　The Inservice Education Program

STRUCTURE OF THE INSERVICE PROGRAM

The inservice program is the totality of the activities planned and implemented by the education department; it consists of all departmental projects taken together. The inservice education department in nursing may have full or limited freedom to select its own projects. Projects undertaken by the department may differ from institution to institution. Nurses' aide training and employee orientation are typical and traditional projects. Both of these functions clearly meet the inservice criterion of improving staff performance. The training project meets the criterion by increasing skills, and the orientation project meets the criterion by making full nursing skills available faster through facilitating employee adjustment.

Whatever the set projects of the inservice department, there is usually some degree of freedom for the inservice director, particularly in the selection of continuing education for nursing staff. For most inservice managers, the chief problem is selection from the large number of potential projects. Usually there are many possible projects for any one objective desired, as well as many equally desirable and equally worthy objectives from which to choose.

In order to examine the structure of a given inservice program, it is first useful to have a taxonomy of potential projects against which to compare it. Such a taxonomy can be developed in several ways. One is to consider the purpose of the educa-

tion in relation to the job function. Table 25-1 utilizes such a perspective.

The five basic categories of educational purpose can easily be remembered as "get up," "catch up," "stay up," "move up," and "move out." Analysis of the distribution of projects over these five basic purpose categories provides a useful assessment tool for evaluating the total inservice program (Table 25-1). Clearly the proper distribution of projects among induction, remedial, maintenance, preparatory, and supplemental education depends on the departmental objectives. Nevertheless, referral to a schema is useful in identifying omissions in planning and in identifying alternative solutions to education problems.

Another useful taxonomy can be made by considering the forms of education and related services from the perspective of the recipient. In Table 25-2 common recipient needs are identified; this compilation includes direct educational needs and related administrative services.

Few inservice departments have the resources to supply all the functions listed in Table 25-2, nor are all these functions appropriate in every institution. Indeed, the greatest danger for the inservice educator is to attempt to supply a greater scope of services than can be successfully managed with her given resources. Selectivity is required in deciding what projects to attempt. A comprehensive taxonomy can give a framework from which to make such judgments.

Another taxonomy for inservice function could be topical. Appropriate topics for inservice education vary from institution to institution depending upon the kinds of patients served and the capacities of that institution's staff.

PROCESS OF PROGRAM DEVELOPMENT

Deciding the appropriate components for an inservice program necessarily involves identifying deficiencies in staff activities and in patient outcomes. When education is perceived as closely related to administration, assessment of management structures may also be perceived as essential.

Ideally, assessment of management structures, staff activities, and patient outcomes would be the function of other nurse managers, since the assessments measure goals of the whole organization. Frequently, however, other nurse managers need the assistance of the inservice educator in devising the necessary evaluation tools.

Although assessment tools are one of the primary means by which the inservice educator plans her program, they cannot be relied upon entirely unless the institution has tools to measure the total scope of services and intended outcomes. Few institutions presently can make such a claim, so that the inservice educator's experienced judgment of situational needs will supplement the evaluation tools. Evaluations made by other staff members are important too.

Table 25-1.   Taxonomy of Educational Purpose

Form	Sample Project
1. Induction Education	
a. New job	Nurses' aide training
b. New function	LPN medication course
c. Orientation	
i. New environment	New employee orientation
ii. New position	Promotion
2. Remedial Education	
a. Foundational supplement	Nurse internship
b. Reentry supplement	Refresher course
3. Maintenance Education	
a. Recurrent training	Cardiopulmonary resuscitation practice
b. Updating	Training in new technologies
4. Preparatory Education	
a. Upgrading clinical education	
i. Nurse technician programs	Coronary care course
ii. Nurse associate programs	Pediatric nurse associate
iii. Clinical nurse specialist	MA programs
b. Upgrading functional skills	
i. Educational skills	Methods-of-teaching course
ii. Management skills	Principles of team leadership
5. Supplemental Education	
a. Education applicable to direct nursing practice	Psychology, sociology, biology
b. Education facilitative to nursing practice or function	Languages, economics management theory

Subjective evaluations should not be underestimated. Simply because a judgment is not based on an objective tool does not mean that the judgment is arbitrary. Indeed one would expect that any professional staff nurse could identify weaknesses in her own performance. Since most inservice education deals with deficiencies in groups rather than in individuals, consensus about weaknesses in staff performance can be a reasonable basis for asserting that a problem exists.

The inservice director's task of identifying learning needs requires that she systematically build communications channels with all major nursing departments. The effectiveness of the inservice department is greatly dependent on the efficiency of its system for obtaining information.

Many organizations form an education committee for input into the inservice department. This provides a formal communications channel both for requests from staff members and for communications back to the staff personnel. The committee provides assurance that any educational needs overlooked by the inservice educator will be brought to her attention. Service on the education committee can also be educational for committee members, acquainting them with the problems and challenges of education in the organizational setting. Where such a committee serves to point out defi-

---

Table 25-2.   Scope of Educational Services

1. Services for
   Nursing Staff Members

   Educational projects—workshops, courses, classes

   Career education counseling— academic, certificate, and continuing education information

   Coordination and promotion of educational opportunities available outside of the home institution—conventions, seminars, workshops

   Maintenance of personnel records on educational acquisitions of all employees

   Maintenance and control of educational materials—library holdings, circulation of materials, selective distribution

   Consultation and problem solving—as needed or requested for nursing care problems

2. Services for Nursing
   Administrative Staff

   Advising and participating in formulation of policies, practices, and procedures

   Troubleshooting—analysis of problem situations in the division, proposal of solutions

   Nursing research—identification of areas of need, construction and implementation of proper research designs

   Staffing—placement of staff on the basis of individual competencies

   Serving as a catalyst in design groups or committees

   Preparation of grant proposals—initiating use of grants, helping others in preparations

   Serving as an education expert— assisting others with their own educational projects

3. Services for Patients

   Preparing programs for patient education

   Providing direct education to patients

   Teaching staff members methods of patient education

   Construction of valid patient questionnaires to identify needs for change

4. Services for Community

   Educational programs on normal health needs

   Education for special interest groups— family planning, diabetic education, emergency care education

   Nursing vocational counseling—for high school groups and others

   Managing relations with affiliating nursing, medical, or allied health students

ciencies in client outcome and general nursing problems, it is serving an appropriate function. It is important that such committees not supplant the inservice manager in making educational decisions. The inservice manager should be an expert in education, and the subsequent decisions concerning how to correct identified deficiencies should utilize that expertise.

OUTCOME OF THE INSERVICE PROGRAM

The inservice program outcome results from the totality of departmental activities examined together. The ideal program would be one that met all the learning needs of the widest scope of relevant learners and produced all the desired behaviors that could be effected by educational means. Such a program would maximize all learning potentials. Green uses the term maximization to define the greatest possible quantity of a good considered singly[1]. Thus a maximal educational program would produce the greatest quantity of every possible educational good.

The ideal of maximal outcome is unlikely to be feasible for any nursing organization for several practical reasons. First, economically, few organizations can afford an extensive teaching program. Second, resources devoted to inservice education must be balanced with resources devoted to immediate patient care provision, or education defeats its own purpose of improving patient care. Such a pattern of educational predominance exists in teaching institutions where patient needs are held secondary to teaching-learning needs of health career students. Inservice education, however, typically is subservient to patient care goals. The ideal educational situation requires a corresponding ideal care situation, and this level of care is seldom attainable in present institutions.

A third reason few organizations can claim to have an ideal teaching program is that perceived teaching-learning needs seem to expand with the available resources. The nursing department that is content to send patients home with instructions for self-care, given extra educational resources, will see the need for follow-up home visits for instructional reinforcement. The nursing department that educates staff members extensively typically expands the level of education up to the limits of its resources. Since the scope of projects contemplated tends to expand proportionate to available resources, it is virtually impossible even to define an absolute, ideal, maximal educational program.

Green offers an alternative criterion to maximization in his policy discussion[2]. He notes that policy is concerned with optimization of good and defines *optimality* as the best composition of a set of goods. In nursing inservice the set of goods is the set of projects making up the educational program. Hence, in aiming for optimality, the inservice educator aims for the best possible combination of projects. Optimality typically requires something less than maximization of each separate project. Green gives two reasons why optimality affords less total "good" than maximization. The first reason is the conflict among goods. In nursing practice, for example, there are many conflicting theories of nursing, each of which may dictate a different type of practice in any given circumstance. Even given an ideal educational situation, one is forced to select among "goods"—one nursing practice or another.

If a nursing staff is deeply involved and interested in improving team nursing, it may be counterproductive for inservice education to decide to start projects on primary nursing, even though no one would deny that knowledge about primary nursing is itself a good. Thus, given ideal and abundant resources, selection among options requires an evaluative model of optimality rather than of maximization.

Green further bases his argument for optimality on the condition of scarcity. In this condition there are more conceivably worthy projects for education than there are educational resources. Thus optimality rather than maximization of educational good can be accepted as the evaluative model for an inservice program based on the need for trade-offs among conflicting projects and the scarcity of educational resources relative to potential educational projects.

The optimality model against which the actual inservice education program is measured cannot be reduced in practice to a mathematic formula or a convenient rating scale. To build such a scale would require predictive knowledge of outcomes for all potential combinations of all conceivable projects, given in varying degrees of concentration. One is forced, therefore, to rely on the estimations of the experienced and prudent inservice educator.

The best balance among goods called for by the principle of optimality can be viewed by the inservice educator from the perspective of the department's financial resources or of the department's human resources. For example, the inservice educator must find an appropriate balance for distribution of funds between departmental teaching projects, outside workshops and seminars, and the maintenance of appropriate library holdings. The inservice educator must also find an appropriate balance for distribution of teaching resources between educational projects offered to different levels and classifications of personnel or to different nursing departments. Clearly, excessive input to one component decreases resources available to other components.

Green notes that in the extreme, an individual good reaches a point where its further increase is no longer a good but, instead, begins to have limiting consequences for realization of other goods[3]. If all educational resources are applied to maintenance of old skills, opportunity is lost to build new skills. The principle of optimality requires the calculation of opportunity costs. The calculated ''cost'' of an educational class must include not only the cost of teaching materials and salaries for both teaching personnel and attending staff members, but also the opportunities foregone by attending this class. Such foregone opportunities might be calculated to be equivalent student time given to patient care or to some other learning experience, thus involving trade-offs in light of costs expended and benefits received.

Optimality and scarcity of resources also require that priorities be set for projects and that they be based on their relative importance to client outcome. Only such projects as can fit realistically into a given time frame should be attempted. An inservice department that conducts two projects successfully (in terms of change in client outcome) has accomplished more than a department that conducts six projects without producing change.

The principle of optimality can be applied internal to and external to the inservice education program. The inservice educator will need to ask if she has an appropriate balance of projects within her department, but she also needs to determine if the education department is receiving the appropriate balance of nursing organization resources relevant to attainment of the nursing division's objectives. Both balances need to be calculated. As Green notes, the concept of optimality itself involves a balance, for it aims at a satisfactory distribution between efficiency and equity[4].

PROGRAM RECORDS

The inservice director will keep careful records of her program, its content and its participants. This is essential for two reasons. First, it is the permanent record of her performance as an educational manager. Second, such a record shows how learning opportunities have been distributed over departments and over employees. The inservice director will probably consider her yearly reports, together, every few years, in order to trace trends and to identify possible deficiencies.

Finally, such records will be important for the individual employee. There should be a system by which attendance at and completion of inservice education offerings is recorded in individual employees' files, usually kept in the personnel file. Such files may be important to the nursing division in reviewing candidates for promotions or special learning opportunities. Further, the employee himself may request that the institution sometime in the future confirm that he had such education. More and more, employees use their inservice records as an unofficial educational transcript. An employee's future career may be impeded if a given institution did not keep records of his attendance at and completion of portions of the inservice program. It is useful to devise some system whereby an employee's record is updated yearly as to educational experiences if such recordings are not made immediately upon completion of a given educational project.

REFERENCES

1. Green, T.F. What is Educational Policy? Paper presented at the University of Chicago, Department of Education, January 17, 1974, p. 10.
2. Green, T.F., 1974, pp. 8–10.
3. Green, T.F., 1974, p. 16.
4. Green, T.F., 1974, p. 11.

BIBLIOGRAPHY

Belanger, C. Staff development—a living, growing organism. *Supervisor Nurse* 9(6):16, 1978.

Calkin, J.D. Let's rethink staff development programs. *J.O.N.A.* 9(6):16, 1979.

Cantor, M.M. Education for quality care *J.O.N.A.* 3(1):49, 1973.

Cantor, M.M. Certifying competencies of personnel. *J.O.N.A.* 5(5):8, 1975.

Condon, M.B. Inservice education . . . impact on patient care. *J. Continuing Ed. Nursing* 3(3):34, 1972.

Cutler, M.J., and Siegel, F.F. Continuing education and nursing service: an example of working togetherness. *J. Continuing Ed. Nursing* 6(5):16, 1975.

del Bueno, D.J. Organizing and staffing the inservice department. *J.O.N.A.* 6(10):12, 1976.

del Bueno, D.J. What can nursing service expect from the inservice department? *J.O.N.A.* 6(7):14, 1976.

National League for Nursing, Interdivision Council on Inservice Education. Guide on inservice education. *J. Continuing Ed. Nursing* 2(3):33, 1971.

Stevenson, J.S. Developing staff research potential: Part I. *J.O.N.A.* 8(5):44, 1978.

Stevenson, J.S. Developing staff research potential: Part II. *J.O.N.A.* 8(6):8, 1978.

Tobin, H.M., and Wengerd, J.S. What makes a staff development program work? *Am. J. Nursing* 71(5):940, 1971.

Tobin, H.M., Wise, P.S., and Hull, P.K. *The Process of Staff Development: Components for Change* (2nd ed.) St. Louis: C.V. Mosby, 1979.

Chapter 26   Inservice Education Projects

STRUCTURE OF THE INSERVICE PROJECT

Selecting Subject Matter

In this chapter, as in the preceding ones, the term *project* refers to any one service within the inservice education program. Projects may include planned services for groups or individuals. Presentation of a course on care of the dying would be a project for groups; consultation on individual nursing care problems would be a project available for individuals. The term *program* refers to the total constellation of projects offered by the inservice education department.

The first problem in structuring an inservice project is that of content selection. The inservice educator will be better able to select projects if she works from the assumption that her institution funds inservice education for the sake of its clients (patients) rather than for the sake of its employees. Clearly patient-oriented goals and staff-oriented goals are not incompatible. Indeed, staff-oriented goals such as career ladder education or self-development programs usually have positive effects on patient care. Such results might be expected due to increased staff satisfaction, skills, and knowledge. For institutions with limited funds or limited educational resources, it may not be possible to run both patient-oriented and staff-oriented education. Where efficiency and economy must prevail, patient needs must take priority, with staff benefits resulting indirectly from learning or credentials acquired in client-focused projects.

Once the objective of inservice education has been placed in client outcome, a criterion for the selection of inservice projects has been established. The best inservice education will be the project that responds to identified weaknesses in client outcome. Deficient outcomes, however, are not necessarily educational problems.

The inservice educator will find that many persons tend to view all problems as amenable to correction by education. If the new aides are taking an hour instead of one-half hour for lunch, it is assumed that inservice forgot to "teach" the aides that lunch time is only one-half hour. If registered nurses are taking unsafe shortcuts in the administration of drugs, it is assumed that an educational project on drug safety will solve the problem.

The inservice educator will soon discover that half the problems she is asked to solve are not educational problems. In the drug problem, for example, a project on drug safety may produce a temporary improvement, but if the working conditions that produced the improper actions in the first place are not corrected, the problem will soon recur. Seldom is ignorance at the bottom of such a problem. Thus one of the first things an inservice educator must learn is to say "no" when she is asked to solve by educative means a problem for which education is not an appropriate solution.

Diagnosis of an identified weakness in client outcome is not accomplished merely by the classification of problems into educational and noneducational types. The weakness in client outcome is an effect and its cause, or causes, are not to be discovered simply by observing the effect. The inservice educator who takes wide latitude in considering possible causes is more likely to spot the actual problem source or sources.

The educational project selected must address the most likely agent of the deficient outcome. In some instances the connection is self-evident. The problem of patients receiving wrong medications is most likely due to poor nursing methods in the process of organization and administration of drugs. In other instances a poor effect may not immediately suggest a clear and single cause. As with any other problem solving, it is important that the inservice educator not make unwarranted cause-effect connections in determining the source of a problem.

Quite often problems are presented to the inservice educator in a diagnosed form: "This nurse can't relate to patients." "The aide doesn't know how to take accurate oral temperatures." The inservice educator must learn not to take such diagnoses at face value: in each case she needs to return to the original client outcome deficiency and make her own diagnosis of the problem. For example, it may turn out that the aide takes accurate temperatures but endeavors to remember them without committing them to writing. Thus, identifying the cause of deficient client outcome is a necessary step in selecting remedial projects. This phase is accompanied by the determination of appropriate client outcome goals.

Determining Desired Staff Behaviors

The next step in inservice planning consists in identifying staff behaviors most likely to result in the desired client outcome. The inservice educator will often have an option of several possible staff behaviors, each of which is likely to produce the desired outcome if well executed. It is important that alternative behaviors be considered so that factors of staff capabilities, organization realities, and capacities of the inservice education staff are taken into account.

Once staff behaviors have been selected, the educational experiences likely to produce those behaviors are chosen. While there is no easy way to choose those educational experiences most likely to produce the desired staff behaviors, it is important that the inservice manager weigh a wide range of alternatives. Generally the experience closest in nature to the actual desired behavior will be most effective. Supervised practice in making out actual care plans is more likely to lead to this behavior on the job than is listening to a lecture on care plans. Subsequent evaluation of changes in staff performance will soon reveal which learning experiences are effective and which are not.

Another perspective on project selection concerns how inservice education should provide for employees with different jobs and different educational levels. Many inservice educators feel the need to run multiple educational tracks—separate projects for nurses' aides, vocational nurses, registered nurses. Again, if inservice education is seen as client-related instead of as a service for employees, this problem is resolved. When the cause of a client outcome deficiency is found, it will clearly indicate which personnel need related education and which do not. It will also indicate which personnel groups can be combined for educational experiences and which cannot. For example, if an undesired outcome of patient dissatisfaction with nursing care is diagnosed as being the fault of poor interpersonal relationships between staff and patients, there is no reason why all levels of employees, from registered nurses to nurses' aides, cannot share in the program.

Mistakes in Project Planning

Four common selection mistakes must be mentioned because they dominate so much of nursing inservice education today. The first mistake is that of jumping on bandwagon topics. Trends seem to occur in nursing with regular frequency. One year every institution teaches care of the dying; the next year everyone teaches geriatric nursing. If the criterion of client outcome is used, fads will be avoided. Fad education has tended to focus on small specialty sections of nursing to the neglect of the needs of the majority of patients.

The second mistake in inservice education selection is that of letting educational efforts be directed by available audiovisual software. While it is true that many audiovisual programs are available, they should be used only when they fit the objectives of the inservice department and when they have been evaluated by the teaching staff as appropriate for a particular educational goal.

The third selection error is the one-shot project. This project gives an hour or so to a topic with no further elaboration and no follow-up for the participants. These classes have minimal effect on staff behaviors; it is surprising that they are used so frequently.

The last error to be reviewed is the reliance of nursing inservice on lectures by physicians. A lecture by a physician should be used only when it is pertinent to the educational objectives of the department and is followed by a discussion of the nursing implications. Since it is unrealistic to expect physicians to be experts in nursing, the lecture will usually need to be coordinated with input from a nursing expert in the same field.

Administrative Issues

In addition to project selection, there are several other structural issues to be considered in assuring the success of a project. The support of nursing administration is one such issue. If an inservice project is to succeed, it must have the support of nursing management, and that support must be attitudinal as well as structural. If the managers consider education as peripheral to the work, staff members will develop similar attitudes. Yet attitudinal support alone is not enough. Administration must back that support by structuring the work to facilitate and reinforce educational projects. There must be administrative follow-through on educational projects. For example, if inservice has just taught a house-wide project on use of the nursing history, the nurse managers must ascertain that completion of nursing histories becomes one of the management expectations.

Another issue in inservice education is that of planning for project attendance. It is a mistake to let staff members control their own attendance decisions. If client outcome is the criterion, it is essential that participants be matched with appropriate projects. When one considers opportunity costs, it is extravagant to let staff members attend projects that do not relate to their present or intended work. Almost all inservice projects are oversubscribed, and an attendee who will not use the knowledge in her work is likely filling a class place that could have been given to one who could use the knowledge.

Allowing an obstetric nurse to attend a two-month coronary care course costs not only the price of educating one nurse but also the opportunity cost for the nurse who could have directly benefited from that education. Employees should be selected for project attendance on a need-to-know basis, and their absence from regular duties should be anticipated in the staffing pattern. Collaboration on scheduling by inservice and nurse managers is the only way to have effective projects. When inservice is planned in this way, as an integral part of the individual's job, it is logical for the employer to hold the individual responsible for implementing the education in his job performance. Commitment to apply inservice learning should be a prerequisite for the privilege of attending any inservice project.

The foregoing arguments presume a condition of scarcity. For an institution fortunate enough to have an additional budget for staff-selected educational goals, such stringencies would not be required. Few health institutions, however, feel justified in passing on to ill clients the cost of education designed for staff interest rather than patient need.

The use of client-outcome criteria has the advantage of adaptability. Where care is poor, outcome criteria quickly identify the worst deficiencies to be remedied. In institutions where care is excellent, outcome criteria are still applicable, for it is always possible to set higher goals for patient care. A criterion of client-outcome can serve as the impetus for nursing research and improvement of professional practice. Client-outcome criteria therefore are useful sources for a variety of educational need diagnoses ranging from remedial needs to research needs.

PROCESS OF PROJECT PRESENTATION

In project presentation, the inservice educator has one advantage. The inservice educator and her learner are already immersed in the environment in which the learning will be applied. The learning is immediately applicable, and the environment provides for immediate reinforcement of learning. The inservice educator thus has an ideal situation for learning transfer. The entire institution is available to her, as it were, as a clinical laboratory for learner experience.

Ironically, many inservice educators ignore this "perfect" educational setting and mimic their school counterpart by isolating all teaching processes to a classroom removed from the practice environment. While there is no easy way to choose those educational experiences most likely to produce the desired staff behaviors, generally the experience closest in nature to the actual desired behavior will be the most effective. Supervised practice in making out actual care plans is more likely to lead to desired behavior on the job than is listening to a lecture on care plans.

One problem in a nursing division is the relation of the inservice educator's teaching processes to the teaching processes seen as inherent in every nursing role. Inservice education should not conflict with or substitute for the teaching that is a basic function of the staff nurse. When staff nurses are able to "pass the buck" to the inservice education expert for routine patient teaching, the nursing role suffers. The inservice

educator, however, can help the staff nurse to develop her talents for patient teaching. Inservice can provide the staff nurse with educational resources; it can help her to develop teaching aids and to learn to use them.

Head nurse and supervisory roles also involve both formal and informal teaching of staff. Again, inservice education must be complementary and not a substitute. Clearly there is a need for careful role definition and mutual understanding concerning the teaching processes appropriate to each nursing role.

The inservice education department can serve as a resource center for those teaching needs requiring complex educational projects. Not only should inservice education be a resource for nursing staff, but nursing staff members should serve as resource persons for inservice education. Too often inservice departments fail to utilize specialists on their own nursing staff as teachers. Inservice education should serve as a vehicle for nurses to share their expertise.

OUTCOME OF THE INSERVICE PROJECT

The last step in any inservice project is evaluation. The best way to evaluate project outcome is to look at the end product, the change in client outcome. If the results are good here, the project has justified itself and may be repeated as needed. In order to judge educational outcomes in the practice setting, the inservice educator will want to make some assessment of client outcome both before and after the educational intervention. Too often inservice assessment is done by paper and pencil testing of the participants at the end of the learning project; this is not a direct measure of client outcome. For example, staff nurses participating in a geriatric course might best be assessed by looking at the changes in the management of geriatric patients by the participants three months after completion of the course. Paper and pencil test scores are meaningless to the institution if patient care is not changed as a result of the course. Indeed, one of the rewards of creating inservice education projects is the ability to see the results of one's work in concrete form within a short period of time.

If evaluation of a project finds client outcomes unimproved, a process of reassessment should be undertaken to pinpoint the failure. The following questions should be answered:

1. Was an appropriate problem the basis of the educational project? Was the problem correctly defined and delimited? (Problem identification.)
2. Was the problem properly analyzed? Were the causes of the problem correctly identified? Was a multisource problem wrongly diagnosed as a single-source problem? Were all contributory causes considered in planning the educational project? Were administrative supports coordinated where necessary? (Problem diagnosis.)
3. Were the selected remedial staff behaviors appropriate to reach the desired client outcomes? Were the staff behaviors that were taught consistent with and realistic for the environment in which the behaviors were to be implemented? (Staff behaviors.)
4. Were the best possible learning experiences selected to teach the desired staff behaviors? Were alternate learning experiences tried? (Learning experiences.)
5. Was the desired client outcome a realistic goal? Were there noneducational factors impeding the change? (Client outcome.)
6. Were appropriate tools used to measure both change in staff behavior and change in client outcome? (Measurement tools.)

PROJECTS NOT DERIVED FROM CLIENT OUTCOME DEFICIENCY

Thus far project selection has been related primarily to identified deficiencies in client outcome, and project evaluation has been dependent on measuring change in outcome. This mode of project control is appropriate for most but not all inservice projects.

Some educational functions are so critical to life support or to recovery without irreversible damage that they cannot be handled by a criterion of response to identified deficiency. A simple example is the procedure for cardiopulmonary resuscitation. In a health care institution staff members must be ready to act immediately if a patient stops breathing and his heart stops beating. One dare not wait and accumulate evidence of deficient client outcome before initiating educational projects to teach such a vital process.

The focus of these educational needs tends to be on the nursing process rather than on client outcome. Given the particular clients served, the inservice educator needs to identify all nursing processes that are critical. For these processes the educational task is one of skill maintenance. In cardiopulmonary resuscitation, for example, the inservice educator will have to determine the frequency with which the staff requires maintenance reeducation. Reeducation cycles for each maintenance process vary from institution to institution, depending on the frequency with which the staff uses the process and the rate of turnover in staff personnel.

In determining the need for reeducation cycles, the inservice educator is likely to evaluate staff nursing process skills rather than patient outcomes. Evaluation of nursing process is preferred for two reasons. First, one does not wait for deficient patient outcomes to reinforce learning on critical processes. Second, such processes may be used with relative rarity, giving little outcome data for assessment.

The first group of projects not based on client outcome deficiencies is education in processes critical to preservation of life and body function. Ultimately these processes are identified by determining potential client need; proximally they are regulated by periodic evaluation of the staff's skill in the required nursing processes.

Another group of projects arise from examination of the nursing structure. Deficiencies in outcome here usually indicate educational needs in management, supervision, personnel administration, team leadership, or ward administration. Basic education for nursing management personnel is a major function for the inservice educator, primarily because nursing education seldom includes management concepts. While management concepts relate to efficiency of client outcome, they are not likely to be derived from examination of client outcome deficiencies.

The major inservice education projects may be derived from client outcome (needs-oriented projects), nursing process (critical life and function preserving projects), and organization structure (management-related projects).

Not all inservice educators accept the primarily deficiency-based criterion formulated here. Some prefer to act from a basis of "building on strengths"; others combine both principles in planning inservice programs. Certainly the two principles (deficiency-based and strength-based) are not incompatible. For an institution to take pride in maintaining and improving its areas of excellence does not conflict with its efforts to improve areas of care that are less exemplary.

INSERVICE VERSUS SCHOOL SETTING

Inservice education as a teaching process differs from education in the school setting in the nature of its interaction with its environment (structure) and its interdependence on evaluation procedures (outcome) for feedback and direction. The fact that the educational process is directed toward immediate change in the present environment enforces on the inservice educator a high degree of accountability. Her successes or failures are there to be seen and measured. As with most human enterprises, failures are readily evident to others, whereas successes are often taken for granted. It is up to the inservice educator, constructing and utilizing evaluation tools, to make her successes as evident as are her failures.

Some nurse administrators fail to recognize the talents required for successful inservice management. An inservice educator must combine the talents of an educator and a manager, for her projects require the conceptualization of nursing ideas, the application of effective teaching techniques, and the consequent change in staff behavior in everyday work situations. Teaching in inservice departments also requires great expertise. Inservice education places greater demands on the instructor than does the teaching role in a school of nursing, for example. An obvious reason is that it requires more nursing knowledge to teach graduate nurses than it does to teach nursing students. An even more important reason is that the inservice educator must be adept at teaching many different kinds of people, with different levels and kinds of education, different career goals, different life-styles, and different atttudes toward education. Compared with this population, student nurse groups are still fairly homogeneous.

Successful change implementation is the ultimate justification for nursing inservice. It matters little how well the inservice department is organized or how thoughtfully the program is derived if the individual projects are not effective in producing change. Assessment of project effectiveness requires careful measurement of changes in client outcome and changes in staff behaviors. The inservice educator must be guided constantly by the interaction between the educational project and the environment in which that education is to be applied.

BIBLIOGRAPHY

del Bueno, D.J. Need to know versus nice to know. *J.O.N.A.* 6(8):6, 1976.

Dyche, J. Accountability in inservice education. *J. Continuing Ed. Nursing* 3(1):27, 1972.

Guinee, K.K. *Teaching and Learning in Nursing.* New York: Macmillan, 1978.

Hospital Research and Education Trust. *Training and Continuing Education—A Handbook for Health Care Institutions.* Chicago: HRET, 1970.

Knowles, M.S. *The Modern Practice of Adult Education: Androgyny Versus Pedagogy.* New York: Association Press, 1970.

McMahon, J., and Neuman, M.M. Tool for evaluating the impact of an inservice program on nursing care. *J. Continuing Ed. Nursing* 3(2):5, 1972.

Taylor, M.L. Mobilizing nursing department resources for educational programming. *J.O.N.A.* 8(12):39, 1978.

Chapter 27

The Nursing Administration Control System

The major system by which the nurse executive regulates all activities in her division is the nursing administration control system. It is in this system that nursing care and nursing management are synthesized, and the input to the system includes all the nursing division's activities and organizing frameworks. The goals of the system are reflected in the major operating documents of the division, which state its objectives, functions, and subordinate objectives and functions. The thruput for this system consists in the managerial moves and structures that regulate overall activities of the division. Major components of that thruput system include the logistic systems that move people and supplies, the communication systems that regulate and influence behavior, and the responsibility or accountability system as reflected in the organization patterns and charts.

This chapter will focus upon the cybernetic, or control, function of the administrative system. How, then, does the nurse executive establish control over these multiple and diverse components for her division? The control function may be divided into internal and external control subsystems. External controls are those that originate outside of the nursing division itself; internal controls are originated as part of self-regulation within the division.

An extensive and excellent review of external regulation and control is given by Westwick[1]. External controls are federal, state, local, and professional controls for the health care institution (including its nursing division). Federal control rests primarily with the Social Security Administration, which sets institutional qualifications for receipt of Medicare and Medicaid payments.

While such control is accepted "voluntarily" by an institution, few health care agencies can afford the luxury of rejecting participation in federal reimbursement plans. Other federal regulations and controls are imposed by the Fair Labor Standards Act and the Occupational Safety and Health Act. National and state constitutional and contractual law also acts to regulate the institution and the nursing division.

State regulations affect the health care organization; professional standards review organizations top the list, with rate-setting and health care building regulations following. Since the state is the organ of government that licenses health care organizations, each state has developed various codes and requirements. State board of health regulations represent one application of such codes. Local units of government may add additional constraints and regulations to institutions within their borders.

As is the case with federal regulation, an institution does not have to accept accreditation by the Joint Commission on Accreditation of Hospitals, but the benefits associated with such accreditation usually make it more than advantageous to accede to this control mechanism.

At present the nursing professional organization does not have an accreditation program for nursing divisions. But it does have published standards, and the effective nurse executive administrator will feel a professional obligation to conform to these basic standards[2]. In addition to publishing standards for nursing service, the American Nurses' Association also publishes standards for individual nursing practice[3] and standards for practice in specialized areas of nursing[4]. Further, the ANA has certification programs for individuals who wish to testify to their advanced practice. The first certification examinations for nursing service administrators were offered late in 1979. These exams allow for two levels of nursing service certification[5].

Within the institution, yet external to the nursing division, the nurse executive will be subjected to control systems devised by her boss. Frequently the institutional administrator is not a professional nurse and will allow the nurse executive great leeway in the administration of her own division. Even so, the nurse executive will be expected to report her activities and administrative decisions through a yearly or twice-yearly report. The formulation of such a report is an important activity for the executive. Not only does it report her activities for the period, but it serves as a history of her accomplishments. The nurse executive should prepare for the writing of this report by systematically accumulating data. If she merely tries to remember at one sitting what she has accomplished during the last year, she is likely to miss some of the most important accomplishments. She should keep an ongoing record to refresh her mind for the annual report. This report serves several secondary functions as well as the formal one. First, all or part of the report may be communicated to nursing managers and staff. When staff are constantly involved in the change process, it is easy for them to forget the achievements of the past. The yearly report serves as a pleasant reminder of these achievements. Moreover, copies of their yearly reports have been known to help more than one nurse executive obtain a desired job. Keeping detailed yearly records of her achievements proved particularly important to one director, who was fired by a reactionary boss. Her yearly reports assured a potential new employer that her goals were not "radical and unrealistic" as had been asserted to him by her former employer. The ability to put together a clear, organized, coherent annual report is an important skill, and this task should not be given less than serious attention by the executive.

INTERNAL CONTROLS

Interdivisional feedback for the administration control system comes from diverse sources: results from quality control of patient care, summaries of performance appraisals, feedback concerning inservice education offerings and attendance, incident/accident reports, personnel files, reports of patient census and classification, staffing and scheduling data, budget reports, and weekly (or less frequent) reports from subordinate managers.

All of these sources provide information and either directly provide control or become the initiating source for other control activities. It is important for each of these feedback systems that the nurse executive determine what information should be communicated. And the nature of that information will direct activities within the division. Nurses and managers spend time on what is seen as important by their superiors, not on what they judge to be insignificant. By requiring data on a given subject, the nurse executive is asserting its importance to her.

THE NURSING INFORMATION SYSTEM

The nursing information system may be divided into two discrete though related systems. The first is the participation of the nursing division in the hospital information system (HIS), sometimes called the management information system (MIS). These labels usually refer to the data that are managed on the institution's computerized systems. The second nursing system component is the official, written and verbal communication among division members. Routine reports and records will be discussed here.

Computerized Nursing Information

Often nursing is one of the last divisions to participate in a computerized system. Initially, such systems were small, with limited capabilities and were devoted to patient admission data, charges for service and supplies, payroll and budgetary functions, and logistic system information—such as who is on what diet or receiving what treatment when. Most institutions now have more extensive computer capabilities and offer computerized handling of certain aspects of care, such as computerized laboratory studies and computerized handling of physician orders. When a system is this advanced, it is advisable for the nursing division to request that data of significance to it be placed on computer. Computerized nursing data typically deal with staffing and scheduling and with patient classification, which is often correlated with patient census and nursing staffing data. Many nursing divisions already have their quality control systems included in the nursing information package. Some nursing divisions are now exploring adding nursing diagnoses and nursing regimens to the data bank. Certainly, the nurse executive will see that data needed routinely for any purpose, such as reports to the board of health or CASH reports or other data reported to the local hospital association are computerized.

The nurse executive will need expert help in learning what can and what cannot be done by computerized information systems. Essentially, they can handle and correlate easily quantifiable variables of the nurse executive's choosing. Not all computer systems have similar capabilities, so the executive will have to have generalized knowledge about computer systems and also information concerning the specific capabilities of the system in her institution.

If installation of a computer system is being planned, it is imperative that the nursing division be part of the planning. Otherwise, it is unlikely that anyone will consider the nursing needs that can be served by the system. A computer system is a good example of a sunk cost; once a given system is installed, it is often too late to get services which were not considered when the system was selected. Nursing must plan for its needs and make its requests long before computer purchases or leases are finalized.

When a computer system is new to a nursing staff, the nurse executive must include orientation to the system in her planning. Such system may be intimidating to the supervisor (or staff nurse) who has never interacted with such a system before.

The Noncomputerized Information System

Official communications channels that are noncomputerized still dominate the work of the nursing division. These channels include supervisors' reports, head nurses' reports, change-of-shift reports, managers' verbal reports, and whatever other lines of communication are devised in a given nursing system to manage its ongoing work. The importance of these channels for control by nursing management often is overlooked. Even the verbal exchange can direct activities of subordinates. Let us consider both informal and formal communications channels as they relate to control issues.

The superior controls the perceptions of subordinates by controlling the flow of input to others and by controlling the form of response from others. March and Simon note that the organization's vocabulary screens out some parts of reality while magnifying others[6]. This mode of control also applies to the selection of vocabulary and subject matter addressed by the nurse executive. Her vocabulary is attention-directing and cue-establishing since it predisposes the employee to a certain mind-set by supplying the accepted categories and classifications of thought. Attention-directing and cue-establishing communications are unobtrusive but effective means for control.

The manager does not have to change the individual to change his behavior. The manager need change only the premises for the decisions of others. If promotions and other rewards go to those who have the "right perspective," for example, the ambitious members will soon adopt the desired perspective.

One way to establish the desired mind-set is the directive use of the questioning technique. Staff members take on the purposes of their manager, not through the philosophy of nursing she espouses, but through those requirements that are impressed upon them in the everyday work situation. The informal use of the question is one of the best devices for establishing desired work and thought patterns.

The nurse executive who asks a supervisor, "How are things going?" misses a valuable training opportunity. She has lost the chance to convey to the supervisor the kinds of things to be thinking about and acting on in her supervisory role. A question such as, "What are you doing about the teaching needs of your Spanish-speaking patients?" is directive.

Supervisors and head nurses can be taught which issues are important to the nurse executive and which are not by using the directive question. If the conversation of the nurse executive with her supervisors is primarily about scheduling, the supervisors will think primarily about scheduling. If, however, the nurse executive's questions to the supervisors are primarily patient-oriented, the supervisors soon take on this same pattern in dealing with their head nurses. (They have to, in order to get the answers that they need for the nurse executive's questions.) Thus the real philosophy of nursing and nursing management in operation soon filters down through the whole organization. Conscious monitoring of the kinds of questions she uses will give the nurse executive a good informal mechanism for directing staff behavior.

The nurse executive can also utilize communication channels for promulgating her philosophy of management, of nursing, or of nursing education. Routine report forms provide an excellent set for thinking patterns. For example, the nurse executive who wishes to promote problem solving among her supervisors, might structure her weekly supervisory report form as shown in Figure 27-1. On the other hand, the nurse executive who is trying to encourage management by objectives might use a weekly report form to encourage that mind-set. (See Figure 27-2.)

Even before the nurse executive has said a word, her required report systems have directed staff managers into the desired thought patterns. When structured reports are used only at the highest administrative level, one soon finds supervisors using

SUPERVISOR'S WEEKLY REPORT OF ACTIVITIES		
Problem Situation	Solutions Considered	Present Status of Problem Solving

Figure 27-1. Problem-Oriented Supervisory Report

SUPERVISOR'S WEEKLY REPORT OF ACTIVITIES			
Objective	Planned Activities	Present Status	Evaluation

Figure 27-2. MBO-Oriented Supervisory Report

similar forms for input from lower level staff. It may be useful periodically to alter the nature of routine communication forms and reports so that different objectives can be accomplished.

Precise orientation to such forms is essential so that they are not misinterpreted. One director in a new position requested that her supervisors inform her daily about "important" patients. She soon discovered that the feedback information was meaningless, because her supervisors' interpretations of "important" and her interpretation were quite different. The supervisors, relying upon past practices, filled in the form with the names of patients who were newly admitted, recently discharged, on the critical list, had recently expired, or were VIPs. The director soon discovered she had to publish criteria for "important" patients. Her criteria included patients with complex nursing needs, patients whose medical and nursing regimes might conflict, patients who presented potential legal or administrative problems. Once the criteria were published, she got the information that she wanted.

Thus both the directive question and the carefully constructed communications form can be used to control the work that gets done. Both can be used to establish the mind-set that will reinforce the decisions of the nurse executive.

Establishing appropriate ways of thinking in subordinates is only part of the task toward implementing decisions. The implications of each decision for the routine work patterns of staff members must be analyzed, for these routinized work patterns are the systems by which most decisions will be implemented. If a decision conflicts with a well-established system, that decision is likely to be ignored unless the system is made compatible with the decision.

Suppose a nurse executive decides that qualified LPNs should have the opportunity to maintain their skills in the administration of medications. If such a directive is sent to units where the ingrained assignment "system" is that RNs administer medications and LPNs give bedside care, it is unlikely that many head nurses will carry out the directive in any manner other than tokenism. To regularize the assigning of medications to LPNs, the nurse executive will have to interfere with the assignment system. One way would be to require supervisors to sample assignment sheets on their units monthly to check LPN assignments relative to medications, thereby providing the nurse executive with feedback and control in the affected system.

In establishing controls for implementing any given decision, it is necessary to assess what systems are affected by the decision. These systems then must be systematically controlled by reporting devices or managerial acts of other types in order that the managerial decision actually is implemented in the work of the nursing division.

SUMMARY

This chapter has focused on the nursing administration control system—on the data that are routinely collected, interpreted, and communicated within the nursing division. Collection of data structures the nursing division in that it points out which elements of the environment are considered significant, and that the data, once interpreted, initiate changes in the nursing systems. Major sources of administrative control data include patient information, personnel data, reports and records of logistic movements of materiel, managerial status reports, and routine interdivisional communication systems.

In determining what data to collect, the nurse executive may apply the following criteria:

1. Data are relatively easy to collect.
2. Data are meaningful and necessary to the nursing operations.
3. Data actually are used in making improvements in the nursing system.

What are the purposes of the nursing administration control system? All of the following are included:

1. To improve patient care.
2. To evaluate the effectiveness of the division as a managerial unit.
3. To meet demands of licensure, accreditation, and review by other legal or quasilegal bodies.
4. To protect employees and employer.
5. To implement nursing research by identifying deficiencies meriting serious inquiry.
6. To facilitate the work process.

REFERENCES

1. Westwick, C.R. Evaluation of nursing organization and structure. In Rezler, A.G., and Stevens, B.J. (Eds.) *The Nurse Evaluator in Education and Service.* New York: McGraw-Hill. 1978, pp. 249–263.
2. American Nurses' Association. *Standards for Nursing Services.* Kansas City, Mo.: ANA, 1973.
3. American Nurses' Association. *Standards for Nursing Practice.* Kansas City, Mo.: ANA, 1973.
4. ANA publishes standards for such groups as emergency room nursing, orthopedic nursing, cardiovascular nursing, rehabilitation nursing, and many other specialized groups of practice.
5. American Nurses' Association. *Nursing Administration/Nursing Administration, Advanced.* (Certification bulletin and application) Kansas City, Mo.: ANA, 1979.
6. March, J.G., and Simon, H.A. *Organizations.* New York: Wiley, 1958, pp. 161–169.

BIBLIOGRAPHY

Alexander, E.L. *Nursing Administration in the Hospital Health Care System.* (2nd ed.) St. Louis: C.V. Mosby, 1978.

Arndt, C., and Huckabay, L.M.D. *Nursing Administration—Theory for Practice with a Systems Approach.* St. Louis: C.V. Mosby, 1975.

Bigham, G.D. Developing staff and records where traditional roles are changing. *J.O.N.A.* 3(1):36, 1973.

Birckhead, L.M. The need for nurse support systems in affecting computer systems. *J.O.N.A.* 8(3):51, 1978.

Cantor, M.M. (Ed.) *The JCAH Standards for Nursing Service.* Wakefield, Mass. Nursing Resources, 1975.

Clark, C.C., and Shea, C.A. *Management in Nursing: A Vital Link in the Health Care System.* New York: McGraw-Hill, 1979.

DiVincenti, M. *Administering Nursing Service.* (2nd ed.) Boston: Little, Brown, 1977.

Donovan, H.M. *Nursing Service Administration: Managing the Enterprise.* St. Louis: C.V. Mosby, 1975.

Ganong, J.M., and Ganong, W.L. *Nursing Management.* Germantown, Md.: Aspen Systems, 1976.

Harman, R.J. Nursing services information system. *J.O.N.A.* 7(3):14, 1977.

Heskett, J.L. Logistics—essential to strategy. *Harvard Business Rev.* 55(6):85, 1977.

Schmitz, H.H., Ellerbrake, R.P., and Williams, T.M. Study evaluates effects of new communication system. *Hospitals* 50(21):129, 1976.

Shanks, M.D., and Kennedy, D.A. *Administration in Nursing.* (2nd ed.) New York: McGraw-Hill, 1970.

Somers, J.B. Information systems: the process of development. *J.O.N.A.* 9(1):53, 1979.

Veninga, R. Interpersonal feedback: a cost-benefit analysis. *J.O.N.A.* 5(2):40, 1975.

Zielstorff, R.D. The planning and evaluation of automated systems: a nurse's point of view. *J.O.N.A.* 5(6):22, 1975.

Zielstorff, R.D. Orienting personnel to automated systems. *J.O.N.A.* 6(3):14, 1976.

Zielstorff, R.D. Designing automated information systems *J.O.N.A.* 7(4):14, 1977.

Zielstorff, R.D. Nursing CAN affect computer systems. *J.O.N.A.* 8(3):49, 1978.

Index

357